External Disease and Cornea

Section 8

2011–2012

(Last major revision 2010–2011)

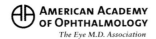

**AMERICAN ACADEMY
OF OPHTHALMOLOGY**
The Eye M.D. Association

LEO

LIFELONG
EDUCATION FOR THE
OPHTHALMOLOGIST

The Basic and Clinical Science Course is one component of the Lifelong Education for the Ophthalmologist (LEO) framework, which assists members in planning their continuing medical education. LEO includes an array of clinical education products that members may select to form individualized, self-directed learning plans for updating their clinical knowledge. Active members or fellows who use LEO components may accumulate sufficient CME credits to earn the LEO Award. Contact the Academy's Clinical Education Division for further information on LEO.

The American Academy of Ophthalmology is accredited by the Accreditation Council for Continuing Medical Education to provide continuing medical education for physicians.

The American Academy of Ophthalmology designates this enduring material for a maximum of 15 *AMA PRA Category 1 Credits*™. Physicians should claim only credit commensurate with the extent of their participation in the activity.

The Academy provides this material for educational purposes only. It is not intended to represent the only or best method or procedure in every case, nor to replace a physician's own judgment or give specific advice for case management. Including all indications, contraindications, side effects, and alternative agents for each drug or treatment is beyond the scope of this material. All information and recommendations should be verified, prior to use, with current information included in the manufacturers' package inserts or other independent sources, and considered in light of the patient's condition and history. Reference to certain drugs, instruments, and other products in this course is made for illustrative purposes only and is not intended to constitute an endorsement of such. Some material may include information on applications that are not considered community standard, that reflect indications not included in approved FDA labeling, or that are approved for use only in restricted research settings. **The FDA has stated that it is the responsibility of the physician to determine the FDA status of each drug or device he or she wishes to use, and to use them with appropriate, informed patient consent in compliance with applicable law.** The Academy specifically disclaims any and all liability for injury or other damages of any kind, from negligence or otherwise, for any and all claims that may arise from the use of any recommendations or other information contained herein.

Cover image courtesy of Vincent P. deLuise, MD.

Basic and Clinical Science Course

Gregory L. Skuta, MD, Oklahoma City, Oklahoma, *Senior Secretary for Clinical Education*

Louis B. Cantor, MD, Indianapolis, Indiana, *Secretary for Ophthalmic Knowledge*

Jayne S. Weiss, MD, Detroit, Michigan, *BCSC Course Chair*

Section 8

Faculty Responsible for This Edition

James J. Reidy, MD, *Chair,* Buffalo, New York

Charles S. Bouchard, MD, Maywood, Illinois

George J. Florakis, MD, New York, New York

Kenneth M. Goins, MD, Iowa City, Iowa

Kristin Hammersmith, MD, Philadelphia, Pennsylvania

David S. Rootman, MD, Toronto, Canada

Robert W. Weisenthal, MD, De Witt, New York

Minas T. Coroneo, MD, MS, *Consultant,* Randwick, Australia

Carolyn M. Parrish, MD, Nashville, Tennessee
Practicing Ophthalmologists Advisory Committee for Education

The Academy wishes to acknowledge Holly Hindman, MD, *Committee on Aging,* and William Crane, MD, *Vision Rehabilitation Committee,* for their reviews of this edition.

The Academy also wishes to acknowledge The Cornea Society for recommending faculty members to the BCSC Section 8 committee.

Financial Disclosures

The authors state the following financial relationships:

Dr Coroneo: Allergan, consultant, lecturer/honoraria recipient; DORC International, lecturer/honoraria recipient, patent and/or royalty holder; Eagle Vision, patent and/or royalty holder; Sydney Biotech, equity ownership, patent and/or royalty holder; Transcend Medical, employee, equity ownership, patent and/or royalty holder.

Dr Reidy: Alcon Laboratories, lecturer/honoraria recipient; Allergan, consultant

The other authors state that they have no significant financial interest or other relationship with the manufacturer of any commercial product discussed in the chapters that they contributed to this course or with the manufacturer of any competing commercial product.

Recent Past Faculty

M. Reza Dana, MD, MPH

John E. Sutphin, Jr, MD

In addition, the Academy gratefully acknowledges the contributions of numerous past faculty and advisory committee members who have played an important role in the development of previous editions of the Basic and Clinical Science Course.

American Academy of Ophthalmology Staff

Richard A. Zorab, *Vice President, Ophthalmic Knowledge*

Hal Straus, *Director, Publications Department*

Christine Arturo, *Acquisitions Manager*

Stephanie Tanaka, *Publications Manager*

D. Jean Ray, *Production Manager*

Brian Veen, *Medical Editor*

Steven Huebner, *Administrative Coordinator*

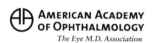

**AMERICAN ACADEMY
OF OPHTHALMOLOGY**
The Eye M.D. Association

655 Beach Street
Box 7424
San Francisco, CA 94120-7424

Contents

12   Clinical Approach to Depositions and Degenerations of the Conjunctiva, Cornea, and Sclera **331**

13   Clinical Aspects of Toxic and Traumatic Injuries of the Anterior Segment **351**

General Introduction

The Basic and Clinical Science Course (BCSC) is designed to meet the needs of residents and practitioners for a comprehensive yet concise curriculum of the field of ophthalmology. The BCSC has developed from its original brief outline format, which relied heavily on outside readings, to a more convenient and educationally useful self-contained text. The Academy updates and revises the course annually, with the goals of integrating the basic science and clinical practice of ophthalmology and of keeping ophthalmologists current with new developments in the various subspecialties.

The BCSC incorporates the effort and expertise of more than 80 ophthalmologists, organized into 13 Section faculties, working with Academy editorial staff. In addition, the course continues to benefit from many lasting contributions made by the faculties of previous editions. Members of the Academy's Practicing Ophthalmologists Advisory Committee for Education serve on each faculty and, as a group, review every volume before and after major revisions.

Organization of the Course

The Basic and Clinical Science Course comprises 13 volumes, incorporating fundamental ophthalmic knowledge, subspecialty areas, and special topics:

1 Update on General Medicine
2 Fundamentals and Principles of Ophthalmology
3 Clinical Optics
4 Ophthalmic Pathology and Intraocular Tumors
5 Neuro-Ophthalmology
6 Pediatric Ophthalmology and Strabismus
7 Orbit, Eyelids, and Lacrimal System
8 External Disease and Cornea
9 Intraocular Inflammation and Uveitis
10 Glaucoma
11 Lens and Cataract
12 Retina and Vitreous
13 Refractive Surgery

In addition, a comprehensive Master Index allows the reader to easily locate subjects throughout the entire series.

References

Readers who wish to explore specific topics in greater detail may consult the references cited within each chapter and listed in the Basic Texts section at the back of the book.

These references are intended to be selective rather than exhaustive, chosen by the BCSC faculty as being important, current, and readily available to residents and practitioners.

Related Academy educational materials are also listed in the appropriate sections. They include books, online and audiovisual materials, self-assessment programs, clinical modules, and interactive programs.

Study Questions and CME Credit

Each volume of the BCSC is designed as an independent study activity for ophthalmology residents and practitioners. The learning objectives for this volume are given on page 1. The text, illustrations, and references provide the information necessary to achieve the objectives; the study questions allow readers to test their understanding of the material and their mastery of the objectives. Physicians who wish to claim CME credit for this educational activity may do so by mail, by fax, or online. The necessary forms and instructions are given at the end of the book.

Conclusion

The Basic and Clinical Science Course has expanded greatly over the years, with the addition of much new text and numerous illustrations. Recent editions have sought to place a greater emphasis on clinical applicability while maintaining a solid foundation in basic science. As with any educational program, it reflects the experience of its authors. As its faculties change and as medicine progresses, new viewpoints are always emerging on controversial subjects and techniques. Not all alternate approaches can be included in this series; as with any educational endeavor, the learner should seek additional sources, including such carefully balanced opinions as the Academy's Preferred Practice Patterns.

The BCSC faculty and staff are continuously striving to improve the educational usefulness of the course; you, the reader, can contribute to this ongoing process. If you have any suggestions or questions about the series, please do not hesitate to contact the faculty or the editors.

The authors, editors, and reviewers hope that your study of the BCSC will be of lasting value and that each Section will serve as a practical resource for quality patient care.

Objectives

Upon completion of BCSC Section 8, *External Disease and Cornea*, the reader should be able to

- describe the anatomy and molecular biology of the cornea

- explain the pathogenesis of common disorders affecting the eyelid margin, conjunctiva, cornea, and sclera

- recognize the distinctive signs of specific diseases of the ocular surface and cornea

- describe how the environment can affect the structure and function of the ocular surface

- outline the steps in an ocular examination for corneal or external eye disease and choose the appropriate laboratory and other diagnostic tests

- summarize the developmental and metabolic alterations that lead to structural changes of the cornea

- identify topographic changes of the cornea and describe the risks and benefits of corrective measures

- assess the indications and techniques of surgical procedures for managing corneal disease, trauma, and refractive error

- apply the results of recent clinical research to the management of selected disorders of the conjunctiva and cornea

- integrate the discipline of corneal and external eye disease into the practice of ophthalmology

CHAPTER 1

Structure and Function of the External Eye and Cornea

The Outer Eye and Cornea in Health and Disease

The external eye is the most crucial part of the body exposed to the outside world. The normal structure and function of the healthy eye rely on homeostasis of the entire body for protection against an adverse environment. Genetics and nutrition determine the embryogenesis and growth of the eye. Intact vascular and nervous systems ensure stable metabolism, and the immune system maintains surveillance.

The cushioning effect of the periocular tissues and local barriers such as the orbital rim are needed to safeguard the globe. The eyebrows and eyelashes catch small particles, and the cilia also work as sensors to stimulate reflex eyelid closure. Blinking augments the lacrimal pump to rinse tears over the eye and flush off foreign material. The tear film also dilutes toxins and allergens and contains proteins that control the normal flora. Mucin stabilizes the tear film and demarcates the living cells of the ocular surface from the surrounding environment.

The epidermis and epithelium of healthy eyelids, conjunctiva, and cornea adhere tightly to their basement membranes. Regulation of cellular growth and metabolism is critical to the maintenance of an intact ocular surface and a transparent cornea. The underlying extracellular matrix of the eye's mucous membrane is rich in blood vessels and conjunctiva-associated lymphoid tissue (CALT). The anterior segment of the eye provides a clear, protected entrance for light that is to be processed by the visual pathways through the central nervous system.

Understanding the eye's innate defenses requires study of ocular histology and biochemistry and the observation of many people, both healthy and ill. Ophthalmologists who specialize in corneal and external eye disease build on this understanding, which extends from clinical examination to clinicopathologic problem solving, molecular medicine, and microsurgery. Readers should become familiar with ocular embryology, anatomy, physiology, and biochemistry (in BCSC Section 2, *Fundamentals and Principles of Ophthalmology*); ocular immunology (in BCSC Section 9, *Intraocular Inflammation and Uveitis*); and ophthalmic pathology (in BCSC Section 4, *Ophthalmic Pathology and Intraocular Tumors*).

Development of the Anterior Segment

The eye begins to develop during week 4 of gestation as an evagination from the *neuroectoderm*. Invagination of the optic vesicle forms the double-layered optic cup of neuroectoderm at week 5. At this time, the surface ectoderm forms the lens placode and gives rise to the corneal and conjunctival epithelium and the eyelid epidermis. Also at week 5 to 6, the first wave of *mesenchymal cells* from the *neural crest* of the surface ectoderm extends under the epithelium from the limbus to begin forming the corneal endothelium. A subsequent wave of mesenchymal cells of neural crest origin at week 7 begins forming the corneal stroma and sclera. Greater detail is available in BCSC Section 2, *Fundamentals and Principles of Ophthalmology.*

At 2 months' gestation, the eyelids fuse and the conjunctiva begins to develop within the eyelid folds. The ocular surface epithelium differentiates shortly afterward. At 3 months, all corneal components are present except the Bowman layer, which appears in the fourth month as the scleral spur is also forming. The eyelids begin to open between the fifth and seventh months. At birth, the infant's globe is 80% of its adult size. The postnatal sclera and cornea are somewhat distensible, gradually becoming more rigid during the first 2 years of life.

Anatomy

Eyelids

The eyelid skin blends into the surrounding periorbital skin, varying from 0.5 mm thick at the eyelid margin to 1 mm thick at the orbital rim. Except for fine vellus hairs, the only hairs of the eyelids are the eyelashes, or *cilia,* which are twice as numerous along the upper eyelid margin as along the lower. Cilia are replaced every 3–5 months; they usually regrow in 2 weeks when cut and within 2 months if pulled out.

The epidermis of the eyelids abruptly changes to nonkeratinized stratified squamous epithelium at the mucocutaneous junction of the eyelid margin, along the row of *meibomian gland* orifices. Holocrine sebaceous glands and eccrine sweat glands are present in the eyelid skin. Near the eyelid margin are the apocrine sweat glands (the *glands of Moll*) and numerous sebaceous glands (the *glands of Zeis*) (Fig 1-1).

Wolfley DE. Eyelids. In: Krachmer JH, Mannis MJ, Holland EJ, eds. *Cornea.* 2nd ed. Vol 1. Philadelphia: Elsevier/Mosby; 2005:53–58.

Conjunctiva

The conjunctival sac includes the *bulbar conjunctiva,* a *fornix* on 3 sides and a medial *semilunar fold,* and the *palpebral conjunctiva.* Smooth-muscle fibers from the levator muscle maintain the superior fornix, and fibrous slips extend from the horizontal rectus tendons into the temporal conjunctiva and plica to form cul-de-sacs during horizontal gaze. The *caruncle* is a fleshy tissue mass containing hairs and sebaceous glands. The *tarsal conjunctiva* is tightly adherent to the underlying tarsus, and the bulbar conjunctiva is loosely

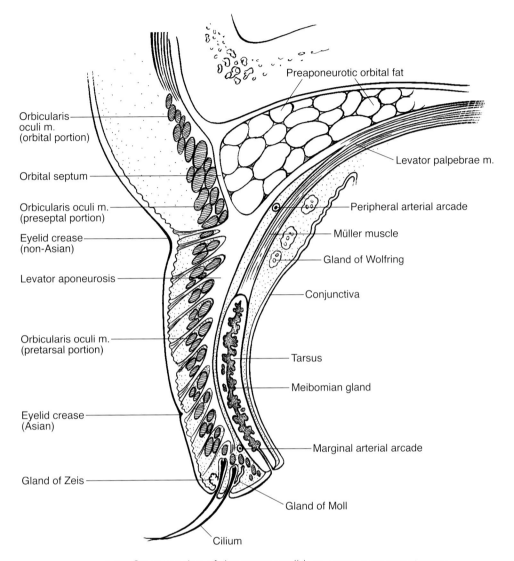

Orbicularis
oculi m.
(orbital portion)

Orbital septum

Orbicularis oculi m.
(preseptal portion)

Eyelid crease
(non-Asian)

Levator aponeurosis

Orbicularis oculi m.
(pretarsal portion)

Eyelid crease
(Asian)

Gland of Zeis

Preaponeurotic orbital fat

Levator palpebrae m.

Peripheral arterial arcade

Müller muscle

Gland of Wolfring

Conjunctiva

Tarsus

Meibomian gland

Marginal arterial arcade

Gland of Moll

Cilium

Figure 1-1 Cross section of the upper eyelid. *(Illustration by Christine Gralapp.)*

adherent to Tenon capsule. These tissues blend at the limbus, where a series of radiating ridges called the *palisades of Vogt* appear. This area contains corneal stem cells.

The cell morphology of the conjunctival epithelium varies from stratified cuboidal over the tarsus to columnar in the fornices to squamous on the globe. Multiple surface folds are present. Goblet cells account for up to 10% of basal cells of the conjunctival epithelium; they are most numerous in the tarsal conjunctiva and the inferonasal bulbar conjunctiva.

The *substantia propria* of the conjunctiva consists of loose connective tissue. CALT, which consists of lymphocytes and other leukocytes, is present, especially in the fornices.

Lymphocytes interact with mucosal epithelial cells through reciprocal regulatory signals mediated by growth factors, cytokines, and neuropeptides.

The palpebral conjunctiva shares its blood supply with the eyelids. The bulbar conjunctiva is supplied by the anterior ciliary arteries branching off the ophthalmic artery. These capillaries are fenestrated and leak fluorescein just like the choriocapillaris. Sensory innervation is controlled by the lacrimal, supraorbital, supratrochlear, and infraorbital branches of the ophthalmic division of cranial nerve V.

> Nelson JD, Cameron JD. The conjunctiva: anatomy and physiology. In: Krachmer JH, Mannis MJ, Holland EJ, eds. *Cornea*. 2nd ed. Vol 1. Philadelphia: Elsevier/Mosby; 2005:37–43.

Cornea

The cornea is a transparent, avascular tissue that measures 11–12 mm horizontally and 10–11 mm vertically. Its refractive index is 1.376, although, in calibrating a keratometer, a refractive index of 1.3375 is used to account for the combined optical power of the anterior and posterior curvatures of the cornea. The cornea is aspheric, although its radius of curvature is often recorded as a spherocylindrical convex mirror representing the central anterior corneal surface, also called the *corneal cap.*

The average radius of curvature of the central cornea is 7.8 mm. The cornea thus contributes 74%, or 43.25 diopters (D), of the total 58.60 dioptric power of a normal human eye. The cornea is also the major source of astigmatism in the optical system. See Measurement of Corneal Topography in Chapter 2 for more information on corneal optics.

For its nutrition, the cornea depends on glucose diffusing from the aqueous humor and oxygen diffusing through the tear film. In addition, the peripheral cornea is supplied with oxygen from the limbal circulation.

The cornea has one of the body's highest densities of nerve endings, and the sensitivity of the cornea is 100 times that of the conjunctiva. Sensory nerve fibers extend from the long ciliary nerves and form a subepithelial plexus. Neurotransmitters in the cornea include acetylcholine, catecholamines, substance P, calcitonin gene–related peptide, neuropeptide Y, intestinal peptide, galanin, and methionine-enkephalin.

Epithelium

The corneal epithelium is composed of stratified squamous epithelial cells and makes up about 5% (0.05 mm) of the total corneal thickness (Fig 1-2; see also Chapter 2, Fig 2-1). The epithelium and tear film form an optically smooth surface. Tight junctions between superficial epithelial cells prevent penetration of tear fluid into the stroma. Continuous proliferation of perilimbal basal epithelial cells (limbal stem cells; see Chapter 3) gives rise to the other layers that subsequently differentiate into superficial cells. With maturation, these cells become coated with microvilli on their outermost surface (which causes them to appear dark by scanning electron microscopy and bright by specular microscopy) and then desquamate into the tears. This process of differentiation takes about 7–14 days. Basal epithelial cells secrete a continuous, 50-nm-thick basement membrane, composed of type IV collagen, laminin, and other proteins.

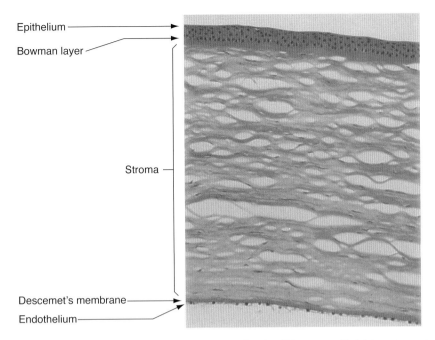

Epithelium
Bowman layer
Stroma
Descemet's membrane
Endothelium

Figure 1-2 Normal cornea. The epithelium, normally 5 cell layers, will thicken to maintain a smooth surface (H&E ×32).

Stroma

Optimal corneal optics requires a smooth surface with a healthy tear film and epithelium. Clarity of the cornea depends on the tight packing of epithelial cells to produce a layer with a nearly uniform refractive index and minimal light scattering. The regular arrangement of stromal cells and macromolecules is also necessary for a clear cornea. Keratocytes vary in density and size throughout the stroma and form a spiraling 3-dimensional network throughout the cornea. They are found as flattened fibroblasts between the collagen lamellae (Fig 1-3). These corneal fibroblasts continually digest and manufacture stromal molecules. The density of keratocytes declines in the normal population but to a lesser degree than does that of endothelial cells. The density also declines with corneal surgery and may not recover completely.

Beneath the acellular *Bowman layer,* the corneal stroma is composed of an extracellular matrix formed of collagens and proteoglycans. Type I and type V fibrillar collagens are intertwined with filaments of type VI collagen. The major corneal proteoglycans are decorin (associated with dermatan sulfate) and lumican (associated with keratan sulfate). The concentrations and ratio of proteoglycans vary from anterior to posterior. Similarly, the posterior stroma is "wetter" than the anterior (3.85 mg H_2O/mg dry weight vs 3.04). Other water-soluble proteins, analogous to lens crystallins, may be secreted by keratocytes or contained in the epithelial cells to control the optical properties of the cornea. The lamellae of the anterior stroma are short, narrow sheets with extensive interweaving between layers, whereas the posterior stroma has long, wide, thick lamellae extending from

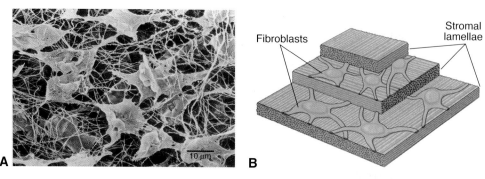

Figure 1-3 Keratocytes **(A)** are flattened fibroblasts **(B)** situated between the corneal lamellae. *(Reproduced with permission from Oyster CW.* The Human Eye: Structure and Function. *Sunderland, MA: Sinauer Associates; 1999:331.)*

limbus to limbus with minimal interlamellar connections. The human cornea has little elasticity and stretches only 0.25% at normal IOP.

The lattice arrangement of collagen fibrils embedded in the extracellular matrix is partly responsible for corneal transparency. This pattern acts as a diffraction grating to reduce light scattering by means of destructive interference. Scattering is greater anteriorly, resulting in a higher refractive index that decreases from 1.401 at the epithelium to 1.380 in the stroma and 1.373 posteriorly. The cornea is transparent because the size of the lattice elements is smaller than the wavelength of visible light.

Transparency also depends on keeping the water content of the corneal stroma at 78%. Corneal hydration is largely controlled by intact epithelial and endothelial barriers and the functioning of the endothelial pump, which is linked to an ion-transport system controlled by temperature-dependent enzymes such as Na^+,K^+-ATPase. In addition, negatively charged stromal glycosaminoglycans tend to repel each other, producing a *swelling pressure (SP)*. Because the IOP tends to compress the cornea, the overall imbibition pressure of the corneal stroma is given as IOP – SP. The total transendothelial osmotic force is calculated by adding the imbibition pressure and the various electrolyte gradients produced by the endothelial transport channels. Corneal hydration varies from anterior to posterior, with increasing wetness closer to the endothelium and resistance of the movement of water laterally within the stroma. See also BCSC Section 2, *Fundamentals and Principles of Ophthalmology.*

Hollingsworth J, Perez-Gomez I, Mutalib HA, Efron N. A population study of the normal cornea using an in vivo, slit-scanning confocal microscope. *Optom Vis Sci.* 2001;78(10):706–711.

Jester JV, Moller-Pedersen T, Huang J, et al. The cellular basis of corneal transparency: evidence for "corneal crystallins." *J Cell Sci.* 1999;112(Pt 5):613–622.

Piatigorsky J. Review: a case for corneal crystallins. *J Ocul Pharmacol Ther.* 2000;16(2): 173–180.

Endothelium

The endothelium is made up of closely interdigitated cells arranged in a mosaic pattern of mostly hexagonal shapes. Human endothelial cells do not proliferate in vivo, but they can divide in cell culture. Although some recent evidence cites the possibility of peripheral corneal endothelial stem cells, cell density declines throughout life. Cell loss results in enlargement and spread of neighboring cells to cover any defective area, especially as a result of trauma or surgery. Cell density varies over the endothelial surface; normally, the concentration is highest in the periphery.

Descemet's membrane is the basement membrane of the corneal endothelium. It increases in thickness from 3 µm at birth to 10–12 µm in adults, as the endothelium gradually lays down a posterior amorphous nonbanded zone.

Bourne WM, Nelson LR, Hodge DO. Central corneal endothelial cell changes over a ten-year period. *Invest Ophthalmol Vis Sci.* 1997;38(3):779–782.

Foster CS, Azar DT, Dohlman CH, eds. *Smolin and Thoft's The Cornea: Scientific Foundations and Clinical Practice.* 4th ed. Philadelphia: Lippincott Williams & Wilkins; 2004.

Nishido T. Cornea. In: Krachmer JH, Mannis MJ, Holland EJ, eds. *Cornea.* 2nd ed. Vol 1. Philadelphia: Elsevier/Mosby; 2005:3–26.

Whikehart DR, Parikh CH, Vaughn AV, Mishler K, Edelhauser HF. Evidence suggesting the existence of stem cells for the human corneal endothelium. *Mol Vis.* 2005;11:816–824.

Biomechanics of the cornea

The cornea is a composite material consisting of collagen fibrils that stretch from limbus to limbus packaged in lamellae that are arranged in parallel fashion and embedded in an extracellular matrix of glycosaminoglycans. The layers slide easily over each other, indicating a very low shear resistance, but the stroma itself is an inelastic, anisotropic structure that distributes tensile stress unequally throughout its thickness, depending on corneal hydration.

When the cornea is in a dehydrated state, stress is distributed either principally to the posterior layers or uniformly over the entire structure. When the cornea is healthy or edematous, the anterior lamellae take up the strain.

Corneal rigidity affects the results of IOP measurements and procedures. In vivo measurements using a forced air jet generate force or pressure on the cornea that can measure its rigidity *(corneal hysteresis).* Such measurements infer that corneal biomechanics consists of more than central pachometry alone but also includes viscosity, bioelasticity, hydration, regional pachometry, and probably other factors that have yet to be elucidated.

Sclera

The sclera is composed primarily of type I collagen and proteoglycans (decorin, biglycan, and aggrecan). Other components include elastin and glycoproteins such as fibronectin. Fibroblasts lie along collagen bundles. The long posterior ciliary nerves supply the anterior sclera. An intrascleral loop *(Axenfeld loop)* from a branch of one of these nerves sometimes forms a visible nodule over the ciliary body.

Normally a densely white tissue, sclera becomes more translucent when thinning occurs or the water content changes, falling below 40% or rising above 80%. For example, senile scleral plaques are areas of calcium phosphate deposits just anterior to the insertions of the medial and lateral rectus muscles that become dehydrated and reveal the blue color of the underlying uvea.

Rada JA, Johnson JM. Sclera. In: Krachmer JH, Mannis MJ, Holland EJ, eds. *Cornea.* 2nd ed. Vol 1. Philadelphia: Elsevier/Mosby; 2005:27–35.

CHAPTER 2

Examination Techniques for the External Eye and Cornea

Examination of the patient begins the moment the examiner enters the room. Because readers should already be familiar with the basic techniques of the complete ocular examination, this chapter describes how to recognize abnormalities produced by disorders of the external eye and cornea. *Practical Ophthalmology: A Manual for Beginning Residents* (5th ed, American Academy of Ophthalmology; 2005) offers a concise review of examination techniques.

Vision

Visual acuity testing is an essential part of an examination, and the refraction of a patient with an abnormal cornea requires special attention. If visual acuity is reduced because of corneal irregularity, it may be necessary to use a rigid gas-permeable (RGP) contact lens with overrefraction. One method for obtaining a patient's best visual acuity is to take keratometry readings and select a large-diameter RGP contact lens with a base curve halfway between the 2 powers and with a power near the patient's spherical equivalent. Topical anesthesia helps reduce tearing as the spherical overrefraction is performed.

BCSC Section 3, *Clinical Optics*, discusses various methods of evaluating visual function.

External Examination

Physical examination of the eye begins with inspection and palpation. The examiner observes the patient's appearance and notes the condition of the skin, the position and action of the eyelids, the presence of preauricular lymph nodes, and the placement of the globes. Eversion of the eyelids permits examination of the palpebral conjunctiva. Infants and frightened patients may need to have their eyelids gently pried open with the thumbs or a retractor.

Common measurements include palpebral fissure height and levator function. The examiner should also measure any visible or palpable mass by its height and longest dimension. Tear production may be measured with sterile filter-paper strips.

External examination of the outer eye and adnexa begins with the examiner looking at the patient, preferably in daylight or bright room light, and then proceeding to magnification with focal illumination. The simplest magnifying instruments are loupes and condensing lenses like those used for indirect ophthalmoscopy. Many handheld penlights and transilluminators are also available; these tools are helpful at the bedside and for external surgical procedures.

Slit-Lamp Biomicroscopy

The slit-lamp biomicroscope has 2 rotating arms—1 for the slit illuminator and the other for the biomicroscope—mounted on a common axis. The illumination unit is essentially a projector with a light beam that is adjustable in width, height, direction, intensity, and color. The biomicroscope is a binocular Galilean telescope with multiple magnifications. A headrest immobilizes the patient, and a joystick lever and adjustable eyepieces allow the examiner to focus the stereoscopic image.

The illumination and microscope arms are parfocal, arranged so that both focus on the same spot, with the slit beam centered in the field of view. This setup provides direct illumination, and purposeful shifting of alignment allows for indirect illumination. Variations of these illumination techniques, using both dark-field and bright-field contrast, are used to examine the anterior segment of the eye.

> Leibowitz HM, Waring GO III, eds. *Corneal Disorders: Clinical Diagnosis and Management.* 2nd ed. Philadelphia: Saunders; 1998:34–81.

Direct Illumination Methods

Diffuse illumination
With diffuse illumination, the light beam is broadened, reduced in intensity, and directed at the eye from an oblique angle. Diffuse illumination is usually used at low magnification to give an overview of the eyelids, conjunctiva, sclera, and cornea. Swinging the illuminator arm to produce highlights and shadows can enhance the visibility of surface changes.

Slit illumination
With slit illumination, the light and the microscope are focused on the same spot, and the slit aperture is adjusted from wide to narrow. Broad-beam illumination, using a slit width of around 3 mm, can help the examiner visualize opaque lesions. Slit-beam illumination, using a beam width of about 1 mm or less, gives an optical section of the cornea (Fig 2-1). A very narrow slit beam helps identify refractive index differences in transparent structures as light rays pass through the cornea, anterior chamber, and lens. The examiner can reduce the height of a narrow beam to determine the presence and amount of cell and flare in the anterior chamber.

Specular reflection
Specular reflections are normal light reflexes bouncing off a surface. An example is the bright round or oval spot seen reflected from the ocular surface in a typical flash

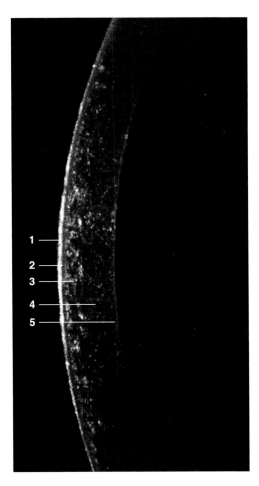

Figure 2-1 Slit section of normal cornea. *1,* Tear film. *2,* Epithelium. *3,* Anterior stroma with high density of keratocytes. *4,* Posterior stroma with lower density of keratocytes. *5,* Descemet's membrane and endothelium. *(Reproduced with permission from Krachmer JH, Mannis MJ, Holland EJ, eds. Cornea. 2nd ed. Vol 1. Philadelphia: Elsevier/Mosby; 2005:201. © CL Mártonyi, WK Kellogg Eye Center, University of Michigan.)*

photograph of an eye. These mirror images of the light source can be annoying, and it is tempting to ignore them during slit-lamp examination. However, the clarity and sharpness of these reflections from the tear film give clues to the condition of the underlying tissue.

A faint reflection also comes from the posterior corneal surface. The examiner can enhance this specular reflection by using a light beam at an appropriate angle, revealing the corneal endothelium (Fig 2-2). Following are the steps for examining the corneal endothelium with specular reflection:

1. Begin by setting the slit-beam arm at an angle of 60° from the viewing arm and using a short slit or 0.2-mm spot.
2. Identify the very bright mirror image of the lightbulb's filament and the paired epithelial and endothelial Purkinje light reflexes.
3. Superimpose the corneal endothelial light reflex onto the filament's mirror image, giving a bright glare.
4. Use the joystick to move the biomicroscope slightly forward in order to focus the endothelial reflex.

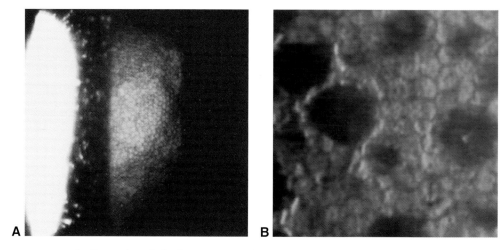

Figure 2-2 **A,** Corneal endothelium seen with specular reflection using the slit-lamp biomi-croscope at ×40 magnification. **B,** Fuchs endothelial dystrophy seen in specular microscopy showing guttae. *(Part A reproduced with permission from Krachmer JH, Mannis MJ, Holland EJ, eds. Cornea. 2nd ed. Vol 1. Philadelphia: Elsevier/Mosby; 2005:208. © CL Mártonyi, WK Kellogg Eye Center, University of Michigan; part B photograph courtesy of John E. Sutphin, MD.)*

Specular microscopy is monocular, and 1 eyepiece may require focusing. A setting of ×25 to ×40 is usually needed to obtain a clear view of the endothelial mosaic. Cell density and morphology are noted; guttae and keratic precipitates appear as nonreflective dark areas.

Indirect Illumination Methods

Proximal illumination
Turning a knob on the illumination arm slightly decenters the light beam from its isocen-tric position, causing the light beam and the microscope to be focused at different but ad-jacent spots. This technique, proximal illumination, highlights an opacity against deeper tissue layers and allows the examiner to see small irregularities that have a refractive index similar to that of their surroundings. Moving the light beam back and forth in small oscil-lations can help the examiner detect small 3-dimensional lesions.

Sclerotic scatter
Total internal reflection in the cornea makes possible another form of indirect illumina-tion, sclerotic scatter. Decentering the isocentric light beam so that an intense beam shines on the limbus and scatters off the sclera causes a very faint glow of the cornea. Reflective opacities stand out against the dark field, whereas areas of reduced light transmission in the cornea are seen as shades of gray. This technique is effective in demonstrating epithe-lial edema and nebulae (Fig 2-3).

Retroillumination
Retroillumination can be used to examine more than one area. Retroillumination from the iris is performed by displacing the beam tangentially while examining the cornea. The

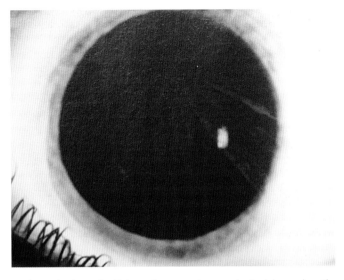

Figure 2-3 Corneal verticillata in Fabry disease demonstrated by sclerotic scatter against the dark background of a well-dilated pupil. *(Reproduced with permission from Krachmer JH, Mannis MJ, Holland EJ, eds.* Cornea. *2nd ed. Vol 1. Philadelphia: Elsevier/Mosby; 2005:212. © CL Mártonyi, WK Kellogg Eye Center, University of Michigan.)*

examiner observing the zone between the light and dark backgrounds can detect subtle corneal abnormalities. Retroillumination from the fundus is performed by aligning the light beam nearly parallel with the examiner's visual axis and rotating the light so it shines through the edge of the pupil. Opacities in the cornea or lens are highlighted against the red reflex, and iris defects are transilluminated (Fig 2-4).

Farrell TA, Alward WLM, Verdick RE. Fundamentals of slit-lamp biomicroscopy. In: *The Eye Exam and Basic Ophthalmic Instruments* [DVD]. San Francisco: American Academy of Ophthalmology; 1993. (Reviewed for currency 2007.)

Mártonyi CL. Slit lamp examination and photography. In: Krachmer JH, Mannis MJ, Holland EJ, eds. *Cornea.* 2nd ed. Vol 1. Philadelphia: Elsevier/Mosby; 2005:191–223.

Clinical Use

Slit-lamp examination is performed in a logical sequence:

1. eyelids
2. eyelid margins
3. tear film
4. conjunctiva
5. cornea
6. aqueous humor
7. iris
8. lens
9. vitreous

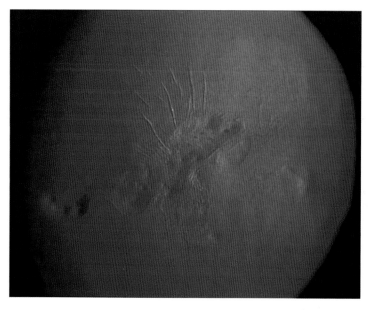

Figure 2-4 Epithelial fingerprint dystrophy is best visualized in retroillumination from the fundus. *(Reproduced with permission from Krachmer JH, Mannis MJ, Holland EJ, eds. Cornea. 2nd ed. Vol 1. Philadelphia: Elsevier/Mosby; 2005:217. © CL Mártonyi, WK Kellogg Eye Center, University of Michigan.)*

After adjusting the focus of the eyepieces, the clinician usually begins the examination with direct illumination of the eyelids, conjunctiva, and sclera. A broad beam illuminates the cornea and overlying tear film in the optical section. Details are examined with a narrow beam. The clinician estimates the height of the tear meniscus and looks for mucin cells and other debris in the tear film. Discrete lesions are measured with a slit-beam micrometer or an eyepiece reticule. Retroillumination and indirect illumination accentuate fine changes. The examiner then uses specular reflection to inspect the endothelium and has the patient shift gaze in different directions so that each corneal quadrant can be surveyed. A slit beam is used to judge the corneal thickness and the depth of the anterior chamber. A short beam or spot will show flare or cells in the aqueous humor. Direct, slit, and retroillumination techniques are used to identify abnormalities of the iris and lens.

The experienced examiner actively controls the light beam with multiple illumination methods to sweep across the eye, using shadows and reflections to bring out details. Having the patient blink can also help the examiner distinguish changes of the ocular surface from tiny opacities floating in the tear film. After initial low-power screening, much of the slit-lamp examination is performed using higher magnifications.

Except for the anterior vitreous humor, deeper and peripheral intraocular structures require special lenses. A contact lens allows examination of the intermediate and posterior portions of the eye and is often combined with angled mirrors and prisms for gonioscopy and peripheral fundus examination.

Stains

Hydroxyxanthene dyes such as fluorescein have been in clinical use for more than a century. They are commonly used to detect corneal epithelial lesions, to aid in applanation tonometry, and to evaluate lacrimal drainage and deficient tear flow. In clinical practice, fluorescein is used to detect disruption of intercellular junctions, and rose bengal and lissamine green are used to evaluate abnormal epithelial cells and ocular surface changes associated with insufficient tear-film protection.

Fluorescein

Topical fluorescein is a nontoxic, water-soluble dye that is available in several forms: as a 0.25% solution with an anesthetic (benoxinate or proparacaine), an antiseptic (povidone-iodine), and a preservative; as a 2% nonpreserved unit-dose eyedrop; and in impregnated paper strips. Fluorexon is a related macromolecular compound available as a 0.35% nonpreserved solution that will not stain most contact lenses. Staining is easily detected with a cobalt blue filter.

Fluorescein is most commonly used for applanation tonometry and evaluation of the tear film. *Tear breakup time (TBUT)* is measured by instilling fluorescein, asking the patient to hold the eyelids open after 1 or 2 blinks, and counting the seconds until a dry spot appears. The appearance of dry spots in less than 10 seconds is considered abnormal. TBUT is further discussed in Chapter 3. Fluorescein will stain punctate and macroulcerative epithelial defects *(positive staining),* and it can highlight nonstaining lesions that project through the tear film *(negative staining).* Different disease states can produce various punctate staining patterns (Fig 2-5). Fluorescein that collects in an epithelial defect will diffuse into the corneal stroma and cause a green flare in the anterior chamber. In the *dye disappearance test,* the tear meniscus is observed for the disappearance of fluorescein. Prolonged presence of the dye suggests a blockage of the drainage system.

The *Seidel test* is used to detect seepage of aqueous humor through a corneal perforation. The examiner applies fluorescein using a moistened strip or concentrated drop to the site of suspected leakage and looks for a flow of clear fluid streaming through the orange dye under cobalt blue light (Fig 2-6).

Rose Bengal and Lissamine Green

Rose bengal and lissamine green (both available as a 1% solution or on impregnated strips) are other water-soluble dyes; they stain the cornea and conjunctiva when a disruption occurs in the protective mucin coating. These dyes are routinely used for evaluating tear deficiency states and detecting various epithelial lesions. Lissamine green is better tolerated and has fewer toxic effects on cultured human corneal epithelial cells. See also Chapters 3 and 4.

Bron AJ, Evans VE, Smith JA. Grading of corneal and conjunctival staining in the context of other dry eye tests. *Cornea.* 2003;22(7):640–650.

Faulkner WJ, Varley GA. Corneal diagnostic techniques. In: Krachmer JH, Mannis MJ, Holland EJ, eds. *Cornea.* 2nd ed. Vol 1. Philadelphia: Elsevier/Mosby; 2005:229–235.

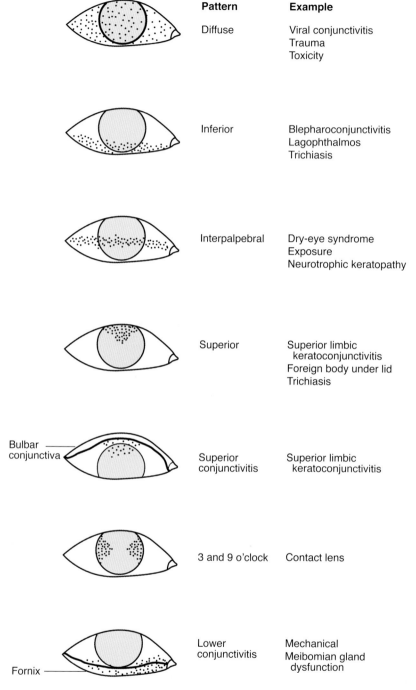

Pattern	Example
Diffuse	Viral conjunctivitis Trauma Toxicity
Inferior	Blepharoconjunctivitis Lagophthalmos Trichiasis
Interpalpebral	Dry-eye syndrome Exposure Neurotrophic keratopathy
Superior	Superior limbic keratoconjunctivitis Foreign body under lid Trichiasis
Superior conjunctivitis	Superior limbic keratoconjunctivitis
3 and 9 o'clock	Contact lens
Lower conjunctivitis	Mechanical Meibomian gland dysfunction

Bulbar conjunctiva

Fornix

Figure 2-5 Punctate staining patterns of the ocular surface. *(Illustration by Joyce Zavarro.)*

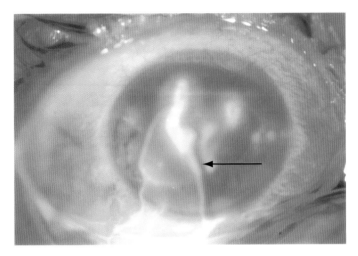

Figure 2-6 Leakage of aqueous from the anterior chamber *(arrow)* following a corneal laceration. Concentrated fluorescein on the edge of the aqueous rivulet (Seidel test) indicates an active flow of fluid from a leaking anterior chamber.

Clinical Evaluation of Ocular Inflammation

In clinical practice, it is helpful to use key distinctive features to categorize a patient's problem. The major disease mechanisms of the outer eye that the clinician should recognize by the history and examination are the following:

- infection
- immune alteration
- neoplasia
- maldevelopment
- degeneration
- trauma

These pathogenic categories are discussed in greater detail in individual chapters later in this volume. Because redness is often a feature of infection, allergy, neoplasia, injury, and other conditions, the following sections introduce the most common signs of ocular inflammation. (Table 2-1 is a summary of changes seen in the external eye and cornea.)

Leibowitz HM, Waring GO III, eds. *Corneal Disorders: Clinical Diagnosis and Management.* 2nd ed. Philadelphia: Saunders; 1998:502–542.

Eyelid Signs of Inflammation

Individual skin changes should be described by their size, shape, and borders. Multiple lesions or a generalized skin eruption should be characterized by arrangement and distribution, using such terms as *disseminated, grouped,* or *confluent.* Several commonly encountered cutaneous lesions and their accompanying characteristics are described in Table 2-1.

Table 2-1 Common Clinical Changes of the External Eye and Cornea

Tissue	Finding	Description
Eyelid	Macule	Spot of skin color change
	Papule	Solid, raised spot
	Vesicle	Blister filled with serous fluid
	Bulla	Large blister
	Pustule	Pus-filled blister
	Keratosis	Scaling from accumulated keratinizing cells
	Eczema	Scaly crust on a red base
	Erosion	Excoriated epidermal defect
	Ulcer	Epidermal erosion with deeper tissue loss
Conjunctiva	Hyperemia	Focal or diffuse dilation of the subepithelial plexus of conjunctival blood vessels, usually with increased blood flow; other changes include fusiform vascular dilations, saccular aneurysms, petechiae, and intra-conjunctival hemorrhage
	Chalasis	Laxity of conjunctiva, sometimes with prolapse over the eyelid
	Chemosis	Conjunctival edema caused by a transudate leaking through fenestrated conjunctival capillaries as a result of altered vascular integrity (eg, inflammation and vasomotor changes) or hemodynamic changes (eg, impaired venous drainage or intravascular hyposmolarity)
	Tearing	Excess tears from increased lacrimation or impaired lacrimal outflow
	Mucus excess	Increased amount of mucin relative to aqueous component of tears
	Discharge	Exudate on the conjunctival surface, varying from proteinaceous (serous) to cellular (purulent)
	Papilla	Dilated, telangiectatic conjunctival blood vessels, varying from dotlike changes to enlarged tufts surrounded by edema and inflammatory cells
	Follicle	Focal lymphoid nodule with accessory vascularization
	Pseudomembrane	Inflammatory coagulum on the conjunctival surface that does not bleed during removal
	Membrane	Inflammatory coagulum suffusing the conjunctival epithelium that bleeds when stripped
	Granuloma	Nodule of chronic inflammatory cells with fibrovascular proliferation
	Phlyctenule	Nodule of chronic inflammatory cells, often at or near the limbus
	Punctate epithelial erosion	Loss of individual epithelial cells in a stippled pattern
	Epithelial defect	Focal area of epithelial loss
Cornea	Punctate epithelial erosion	Fine, slightly depressed stippling caused by altered or desquamated superficial epithelium
	Punctate epithelial keratitis	Swollen, slightly raised epithelial cells that can be finely scattered, coarsely grouped, or arranged in an arborescent pattern
	Epithelial edema	Swollen epithelial cells (intraepithelial edema) or intercellular vacuoles (microcystic edema)

(Continued)

Table 2-1 *(continued)*

Tissue	Finding	Description
	Bulla	Fluid pocket within or under the epithelium
	Epithelial defect	Focal area of epithelial loss, caused by trauma (abrasion) or other condition
	Dendrite	Branching linear epithelial ridge with swollen cells, terminal end bulbs, and possible central ulceration
	Ulcer	Epithelial defect, stromal loss, stromal inflammation, or any combination of these changes
	Filament	Strand (filament) or clump (mucous plaque) of mucus and degenerating epithelial cells attached to an altered ocular surface
	Subepithelial infiltrate	Coin-shaped inflammatory opacity in the anterior portion of Bowman layer
	Suppurative stromal keratitis	Focal yellow-white infiltrate composed of neutrophils
	Nonsuppurative stromal keratitis	Focal gray-white infiltrate of lymphocytes and other mononuclear cells; also called interstitial keratitis, especially when accompanied by stromal neovascularization
Sclera	Episcleritis	Focal or diffuse dilation of radial superficial episcleral vessels
	Nonnecrotizing scleritis	Dilated deep episcleral vessels with scleral edema
	Necrotizing scleritis	Area of avascular sclera

Cellular infiltration and edema of the upper eyelid can cause eyelid drooping, called *mechanical blepharoptosis.* Protective ptosis is a result of ocular surface discomfort and photophobia.

Conjunctival Signs of Inflammation

Most forms of conjunctivitis heal without complications, but permanent changes may occur with more severe or chronic inflammation. Keratinization of the ocular surface epithelium may occur over a chronically inflamed, indurated lesion. Chemosis may occur acutely or develop into conjunctivochalasis over time, with redundant folds that may even protrude over the lower eyelid. Conjunctival scarring can range from subepithelial reticular or lacy fibrosis to extensive symblepharon formation, with eyelid distortion and secondary dry-eye changes. Identifying the principal clinical feature of ocular inflammation can help in the differential diagnosis of common causes of conjunctivitis (Table 2-2). Two common changes are papillae and follicles.

Papillae

Papillae are vascular changes seen most easily in the palpebral conjunctiva where fibrous septae anchor the conjunctiva to the tarsus. With progression, these dilated vessels sprout spokelike capillaries that become surrounded by edema and a mixed inflammatory cell infiltrate, producing raised elevations under the conjunctival epithelium (Fig 2-7).

Table 2-2 Common Causes of Conjunctival Inflammation

Finding	Examples
Papillary conjunctivitis	Allergic conjunctivitis
	Bacterial conjunctivitis
Follicular conjunctivitis	Adenovirus conjunctivitis
	Herpes simplex virus conjunctivitis
	Molluscum contagiosum blepharoconjunctivitis
	Chlamydial conjunctivitis
	Drug-induced (eg, dipivefrin) conjunctivitis
Conjunctival pseudomembrane or membrane	Severe viral or bacterial conjunctivitis
	Stevens-Johnson syndrome
	Chemical burn
Conjunctival granuloma	Cat-scratch disease
	Sarcoidosis
	Foreign-body reaction
Conjunctival erosion or ulceration	Stevens-Johnson syndrome
	Ocular cicatricial pemphigoid
	Graft-vs-host disease
	Factitious conjunctivitis
	Mechanical or chemical trauma

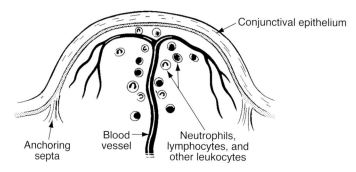

Figure 2-7 Cross-sectional diagram of conjunctival papilla with a central vascular tuft surrounded by acute and chronic leukocytes.

A mild papillary reaction produces a smooth, velvety appearance (Fig 2-8A). Chronic or progressive changes result in enlarged vascular tufts that obscure the underlying blood vessels (Fig 2-8B). Connective tissue septae restrict inflammatory changes to the fibrovascular core, producing the appearance of elevated, polygonal, hyperemic mounds. Each papilla has a central red dot that represents a dilated capillary viewed end-on. The palpebral and forniceal conjunctiva beyond the tarsus is less helpful in revealing the nature of an inflammatory reaction because the anchoring septae become sparser toward the fornix and permit undulation of less adherent tissue. With prolonged, recurrent, or severe conjunctival inflammation, the anchoring fibers of the tarsal conjunctiva stretch and weaken, leading to confluent papillary hypertrophy (Fig 2-8C). The furrows between these enlarged fibrovascular structures collect mucus and pus.

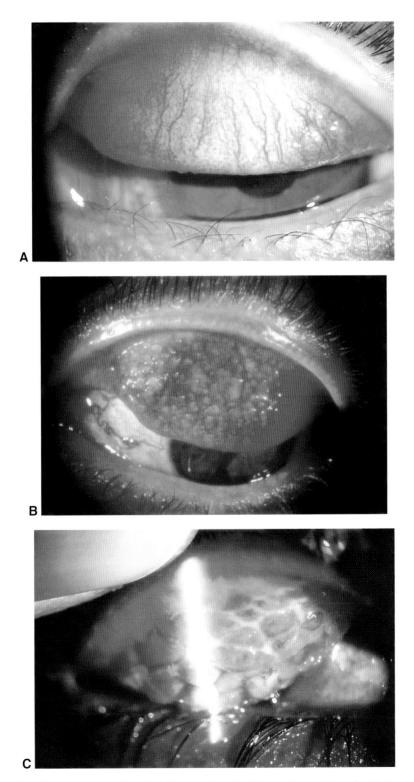

Figure 2-8 Papillary conjunctivitis. **A,** Mild papillae. **B,** Moderate papillae. **C,** Marked (giant) papillae.

Follicles

Conjunctival lymphoid tissue is normally present within the substantia propria except in neonates, who do not have visible follicles. Conjunctival follicles are round or oval clusters of lymphocytes (Fig 2-9). Small follicles are often visible in the normal lower fornix. Clusters of enlarged, noninflamed follicles are occasionally seen in the inferotemporal palpebral and forniceal conjunctiva of children and adolescents, a condition known as *benign lymphoid folliculosis* (Fig 2-10).

    Follicular conjunctivitis involves redness and new or enlarged follicles (Fig 2-11). Vessels surround and encroach on the raised surface of follicles but are not prominently visible within the follicle. Follicles can be seen in the inferior and superior tarsal conjunctiva and, less often, on the bulbar or limbal conjunctiva. They must be differentiated from cysts produced by tubular epithelial infoldings during chronic inflammation.

Corneal Signs of Inflammation

Inflammation can affect any layer of the cornea. The pattern of corneal inflammation, or *keratitis,* can be described according to the following:

- *distribution:* diffuse, focal, or multifocal
- *depth:* epithelial, subepithelial, stromal, or endothelial

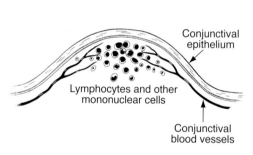

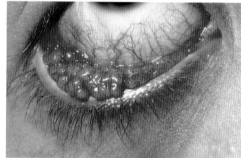

Figure 2-9 Cross-sectional diagram of conjunctival follicle with mononuclear cells obscuring conjunctival blood vessels.

Figure 2-10 Benign folliculosis. *(Courtesy of Kirk R. Wilhelmus, MD.)*

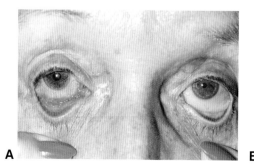

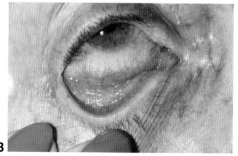

A

B

Figure 2-11 Follicular conjunctivitis. **A,** Inflammation of the right eye from glaucoma medication. **B,** Right eye showing follicular conjunctivitis in the inferior fornix. *(Courtesy of John E. Sutphin, MD.)*

- *location:* central or peripheral
- *shape:* dendritic, disciform, and so on

The clinician should also note any structural or physiologic changes associated with keratitis, such as ulceration or endothelial dysfunction.

Punctate epithelial keratopathy is a nonspecific term that includes a spectrum of biomicroscopic changes from punctate epithelial granularity to erosive and inflammatory changes (Fig 2-12).

Stromal inflammation may be manifested by the presence of new blood vessels. Active corneal blood vessels most commonly come from the limbal vascular arcades and migrate into the peripheral cornea. Cells can also enter the stroma from the tear film through an epithelial defect or, less often, from direct interlamellar infiltration of leukocytes at the limbus. Inflammatory cells enter from aqueous humor in the presence of endothelial injury. In a vascularized cornea, inflammatory cells can emanate directly from infiltrating blood and lymphatic vessels.

Stromal inflammation is characterized as *suppurative* or *nonsuppurative* (Fig 2-13). It is further described by distribution (*focal* or *multifocal* infiltrates) and by location *(central, paracentral,* or *peripheral). Necrotizing* stromal keratitis is a severe form of infiltrate without the liquefaction associated with suppuration. The various morphologic changes of corneal inflammation, categorized by the principal clinical features, aid in differential diagnosis (Table 2-3).

Endothelial dysfunction often accompanies corneal stromal inflammation and contributes to epithelial and stromal edema. Swollen endothelial cells called *inflammatory pseudoguttae* are visible by specular reflection as dark areas of the normal mosaic pattern. *Keratic precipitates (KP)* are clumps of inflammatory cells on the back of the cornea that come from the anterior uvea during the course of keratitis or uveitis. The clinical appearance of KP depends on the composition:

- Fibrin and other proteins coagulate into small dots and strands.
- Neutrophils and lymphocytes aggregate into punctate opacities.
- Macrophages form larger "mutton-fat" clumps.

Inflammation can lead to corneal opacification. Altered stromal keratocytes fail to produce some water-soluble factors and, consequently, make new collagen fibers that are disorganized, scatter light, and form a nontransparent scar. Scarring can also incorporate calcium complexes, lipids, and proteinaceous material. Dark pigmentation of a residual corneal opacity is often a result of incorporated melanin or iron salts.

Corneal inflammation can also lead to neovascularization. Superficial stromal blood vessels originate as capillary buds of limbal vascular arcades in the palisades of Vogt. New lymphatic vessels may also form but cannot be seen clinically. Subepithelial fibrous ingrowth into the peripheral cornea is called a *pannus* or vascularized pannus (Fig 2-14). Neovascularization may invade the cornea at deeper levels depending on the nature and location of the inflammatory stimulus. Any vessel tends to remain at a single lamellar plane as it grows unless stromal disorganization has occurred.

Leibowitz HM, Waring GO III, eds. *Corneal Disorders: Clinical Diagnosis and Management.* 2nd ed. Philadelphia: Saunders; 1998:432–479.

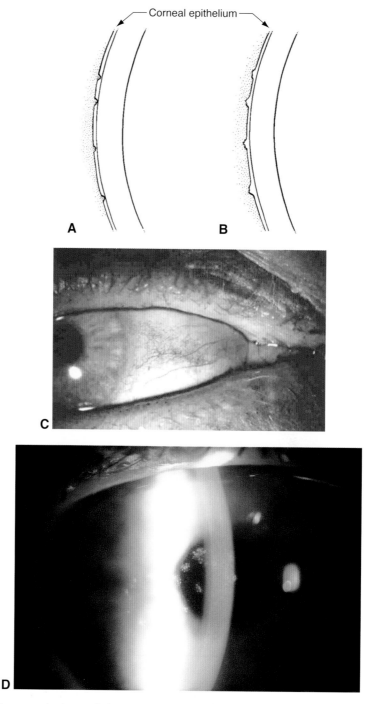

Figure 2-12 Punctate lesions of the corneal epithelium. **A,** Punctate epithelial erosions. **B,** Punctate epithelial keratitis. **C,** Punctate epithelial erosions in dry eye with lissamine green staining most apparent in the nasal and temporal conjunctiva. **D,** Punctate epithelial keratitis. *(Part C courtesy of Minas Coroneo, MD.)*

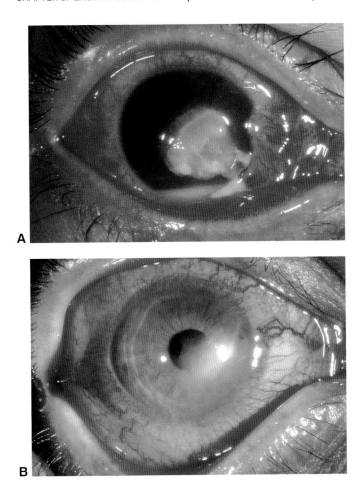

Figure 2-13 Inflammation of the corneal stroma. **A,** Suppurative keratitis. **B,** Nonsuppurative, nonnecrotizing (disciform) stromal keratitis.

Table 2-3 Common Causes of Corneal Inflammation

Finding	Examples
Punctate epithelial erosions	Dry-eye syndrome
	Toxicity
	Atopic keratoconjunctivitis
Punctate epithelial keratitis	Adenovirus keratoconjunctivitis
	Herpes simplex virus epithelial keratitis
	Thygeson superficial punctate keratitis
Stromal keratitis, suppurative	Bacterial keratitis
	Fungal keratitis
Stromal keratitis, nonsuppurative	Herpes simplex virus stromal keratitis
	Varicella-zoster virus stromal keratitis
	Syphilitic interstitial keratitis
Peripheral keratitis	Blepharitis-associated marginal infiltrates
	Peripheral ulcerative keratitis caused by connective tissue diseases
	Mooren ulcer

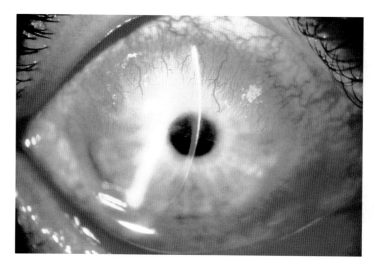

Figure 2-14 Corneal pannus. *(Courtesy of Kirk R. Wilhelmus, MD.)*

Scleral Signs of Inflammation

Episcleritis and scleritis may be *nodular* or *diffuse,* and anterior scleritis may be *necrotizing* or *nonnecrotizing.* The red-free light filter can help identify which layer of blood vessels is dilated. Areas of increased translucency *(scleromalacia)* are detected by direct observation and by transillumination.

Corneal Pachometry

A corneal pachometer measures corneal thickness, a sensitive indicator of endothelial physiology that correlates well with functional measurements such as aqueous fluorophotometry. The normal cornea has an average central thickness of about 540 μm. Note that in the Ocular Hypertension Treatment Study, the average corneal thickness was higher, at 573 ± 39 μm, but it was acknowledged that these numbers were probably higher than those of the general population. The cornea becomes thicker in the paracentral zone and peripheral zone. The thinnest zone is about 1.5 mm temporal to the geographic center.

Brandt JD, Beiser JA, Kass MA, Gordon MO. Central corneal thickness in the Ocular Hypertension Treatment Study (OHTS). *Ophthalmology.* 2001;108:1779–1788.

Optical pachometry can be performed using a device that attaches to the slit-lamp biomicroscope, but the device is somewhat imprecise. Ultrasonic pachometry is both easier and more accurate. Instrumentation is based on the speed of sound in the normal cornea (1640 m/sec). The applanating tip must be perpendicular to the surface because errors are induced by tilting. Improved signal processing and other methods, such as laser interferometry, allow the examiner to map the corneal thickness very precisely. Scanning slit and Scheimpflug anterior segment imaging can produce maps of the entire corneal thickness (Fig 2-15).

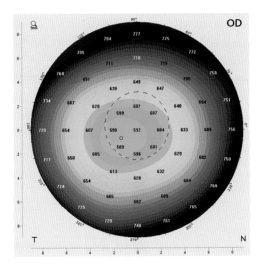

Figure 2-15 Scheimpflug image map depicting multiple points of corneal thickness measurement (in micrometers). *(Courtesy of George J. Florakis, MD.)*

Corneal pachometry can help in diagnosing corneal thinning disorders and can also be used to assess the function of the corneal endothelium. Folds in Descemet's membrane are first seen when corneal thickness increases by 10% or more; epithelial edema occurs when corneal thickness exceeds 700 μm. A central corneal thickness greater than 650 μm suggests a higher risk for symptomatic corneal edema after intraocular surgery.

Optical coherence tomography (OCT) and *high-resolution ultrasonography* are newer techniques that can be used to image the cornea, including curvature and thickness, as well as the anterior segment.

Corneal Edema

The corneal endothelium maintains corneal clarity through 2 functions: by acting as a barrier to the aqueous humor and by providing a metabolic pump. Alteration of either function by damage or maldevelopment leads to corneal edema, a condition of abnormal homeostasis resulting in excess fluid within the corneal stroma and/or epithelium. Increased permeability and insufficient pump sites occur with decreased endothelial cell density lower than 500 cells/mm², although the critical number for clinically evident edema is not an absolute.

Acute corneal edema is often the result of an altered barrier effect of the endothelium or epithelium. *Chronic corneal edema* is usually caused by an inadequate endothelial pump. When functioning normally, the endothelial pump balances the leak rate to maintain the corneal stromal water content at 78% and the central corneal thickness at about 540 μm. *Stromal edema* alters corneal transparency, but visual loss is most severe when epithelial microcysts or bullae occur. A *posterior collagenous layer,* or *retrocorneal membrane,* can arise after endothelial cell damage. The physiology of the endothelium is discussed in BCSC Section 2, *Fundamentals and Principles of Ophthalmology.*

Various traumatic, inflammatory, and dystrophic mechanisms can produce corneal edema (Table 2-4). The examiner should consider duration, laterality, and the presence

Table 2-4 Causes of Corneal Edema

Type	Cause
Acute	Trauma (eg, epithelial defect, intraocular surgery)
	Inflammation (eg, infectious or immune-mediated keratitis, corneal graft rejection)
	Hypoxia (eg, contact lens overwear)
	Hydrops from ruptured Descemet's membrane (eg, keratoconus)
	Increased intraocular pressure
Chronic	Trauma or toxins (eg, intraocular surgery)
	Fuchs dystrophy
	Posterior polymorphous dystrophy
	Iridocorneal endothelial syndrome
	Retained lens fragment

of associated ocular disease in identifying the underlying etiology. Clinical examination should use the various illumination techniques of slit-lamp biomicroscopy. Early signs include patchy or diffuse haze of the epithelium, mild stromal thickening, faint deep stromal wrinkles *(Waite-Beetham lines)*, Descemet's membrane folds, and a patchy or diffuse posterior collagenous layer. Endothelial alterations include reversible changes such as pseudoguttata and permanent alterations such as corneal guttae *(cornea guttata)*.

Corneal thickness and intraocular pressure

Corneal thickness affects the measurement of IOP. Thicker corneas cause falsely higher IOP readings and thinner corneas cause falsely lower pressure readings. Thicker corneas resist the indentation inherent to nearly all methods of IOP measurement, including applanation, air-puff, Tonopen, and pneumotonometry. Therefore, patients with normal (nonedematous) but thick corneas may have artifactually elevated IOP because of increased corneal rigidity and resistance to deformation. Conversely, edematous corneas with a corresponding decrease in rigidity and resistance to deformation may have an artifactually lower IOP. Thin corneas (which may have an artifactually lower IOP reading) may be an independent risk factor for glaucomatous damage to the optic nerve by a mechanism not yet determined. Correction of IOP for pachometry does not fully explain the lower risk for thicker corneas. See BCSC Section 10, *Glaucoma*.

Brandt JD. Corneal thickness in glaucoma screening, diagnosis, and management. *Curr Opin Ophthalmol.* 2004;15(2):85–89.

Doughty MJ, Zaman ML. Human corneal thickness and its impact on intraocular pressure measures: a review and meta-analysis approach. *Surv Ophthalmol.* 2000;44(5):367–408.

Esthesiometry

Esthesiometry is the measurement of corneal sensation, which is a function of the ophthalmic branch of cranial nerve V. Its primary use is in the evaluation of neurotrophic keratopathy. In most clinical circumstances, reduced corneal sensitivity can be diagnosed qualitatively without special instruments, but quantitative esthesiometry is useful in unusual cases and for research. The examiner does not apply topical anesthesia (or any other topical agent, preferably) to the eye if corneal sensation is to be evaluated. The patient, too, should be advised not to apply topical medications before the examination.

Corneal sensation is most easily tested in comparison to a normal fellow eye. A rolled wisp of cotton from a cotton-tipped applicator is touched lightly to corresponding quadrants of each cornea. The patient is asked to report the degree of sensation in the first eye relative to that of the fellow eye, and sensation is recorded as normal, reduced, or absent for each quadrant. This method can be used to detect most clinically relevant cases of reduced corneal sensation.

The handheld esthesiometer (Coche-Bonnet) is a contact device that gives quantitative information about corneal sensation. This device contains a thin, flexible, retractable nylon filament. The patient's cornea is touched with the filament, which is extended to the full length of 6 cm. The filament is then retracted incrementally in 0.5-cm steps until it becomes rigid enough to allow the patient to feel its contact. This length is then recorded. Esthesiometry readings may vary with user technique, but in general a lower number, or shorter filament, indicates reduced corneal sensation. After the central cornea's sensitivity is measured, a map is produced of the cornea (and sometimes of the bulbar conjunctiva) by testing the superior, temporal, inferior, and nasal quadrants sequentially.

Two noncontact esthesiometry methods have also been described, one using air, the other using air mixed with carbon dioxide. Noncontact corneal esthesiometry stimulates the corneal nerves by releasing a controlled pulse of air at a predetermined pressure (in millibars). The subject indicates verbally whether the stimulus is felt, and a stimulus threshold can be determined.

Faulkner WJ, Varley GA. Corneal diagnostic techniques. In: Krachmer JH, Mannis MJ, Holland EJ, eds. *Cornea.* 2nd ed. Vol 1. Philadelphia: Elsevier/Mosby; 2005:229–235.

Goins KM. New insights into the diagnosis and treatment of neurotrophic keratopathy. *Ocul Surf.* 2005;3(2):96–110.

Anterior Segment Photography

External and Slit-Lamp Photography

External eye photography is usually performed with a single-lens reflex camera. Magnification up to 1:1 (life-size) can be obtained with a bellows, extension ring, or close-focusing lens. Digital or 35-mm cameras may also be attached with an adapter to a slit lamp and will produce excellent-quality images, particularly if used with external illumination.

Slit-lamp photography and videophotography allow a permanent record of most anterior segment conditions.

Mártonyi CL. Slit lamp examination and photography. In: Krachmer JH, Mannis MJ, Holland EJ, eds. *Cornea.* 2nd ed. Vol 1. Philadelphia: Elsevier/Mosby; 2005:191–221.

Specular Photomicroscopy

Because slit-lamp illumination techniques are only semiquantitative and slit-lamp photography is difficult, clinicians may want to use specular photomicroscopes to photograph the endothelium for closer evaluation. Specular reflection allows visualization of the corneal endothelial mosaic. Wide-field specular microscopy can be performed throughout the entire cornea, thus allowing the study of regional variability. Specular microscopy can be an important diagnostic tool, especially for differentiating between difficult or overlapping diagnostic entities, such as between the iridocorneal endothelial (ICE) syndrome and posterior polymorphous corneal dystrophy.

Contact specular microscopy techniques involve the use of a photomicroscope attached to an applanating cone and a coupling fluid. They are best performed following the application of a topical anesthetic (although noncontact techniques also exist). A relatively clear cornea is generally required to obtain a good specular image. As fine focus is obtained, the endothelial mosaic comes into view (Fig 2-16). The stroma and epithelium can also be examined and photographed. Most instruments have a pachometer attached to the focusing apparatus so that corneal thickness can be measured. Both contact and noncontact specular microscopes may include a computer for analyzing the images. The following parameters can be calculated from a specular or confocal image. (Note that these parameters have implications for the cornea's response to surgical manipulation.)

- *Density.* The normal endothelial cell density decreases with age. Endothelial cell density normally exceeds 3500 cells/mm² in children and gradually declines with age to about 2000 cells/mm² in older people. An average value for adults is 2400 cells/mm² (1500–3500), with a mean cell size of 150–350 μm². Corneas with low cell density (eg, fewer than 1000 cells/mm²) might not tolerate intraocular surgery.
- *Coefficient of variation.* The standard deviation of the mean cell area divided by the mean cell area gives the coefficient of *variation,* a unitless number normally less than 0.30. *Polymegathism* is increased variation in individual cell areas; it typically increases with contact lens wear. Corneas with significant polymegathism (>0.40) might not tolerate intraocular surgery.
- *Percentage of hexagonal cells.* The percentage of cells with 6 apices should ideally approach 100%. Lower percentages indicate a diminishing state of health of the endothelium. *Pleomorphism* is increased variability in cell shape. Corneas with

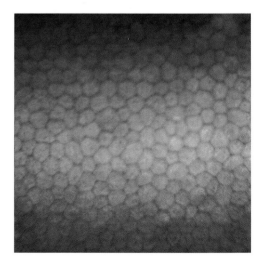

Figure 2-16 Confocal videomicrograph of normal corneal endothelium, with cell density of 2470 cells/mm².

high pleomorphism (more than 50% nonhexagonal) might not tolerate intraocular surgery.

American Academy of Ophthalmology. *Corneal Endothelial Photography*. Ophthalmic Technology Assessment. San Francisco: American Academy of Ophthalmology; 1996. (Reviewed for currency 2003.)

Phillips C, Laing R, Yee R. Specular microscopy. In: Krachmer JH, Mannis MJ, Holland EJ, eds. *Cornea*. 2nd ed. Vol 1. Philadelphia: Elsevier/Mosby; 2005:261–281.

Anterior Segment Fluorescein Angiography

Anterior segment fluorescein angiography has occasionally been used to study the circulatory dynamics of normal and pathologic bulbar conjunctival, episcleral, scleral, and iris blood vessels. This technique is particularly applicable to patients who might have areas of vascular nonperfusion, as in necrotizing scleritis and some forms of iritis.

Anterior Segment Imaging

Imaging of the anterior segment has significantly improved over the past decade, allowing the diagnosis and treatment of various conditions in a more precise and rapid manner. Techniques include the use of high-frequency ultrasound, Scheimpflug analysis, and scanning slit and OCT. The superficial location of the cornea and anterior chamber allows images that can detect foreign bodies, assess iris and ciliary body tumors, evaluate the extent of trauma, assess the anterior chamber angle, and determine the position of the crystalline lens or IOL.

Anterior segment echography, or ultrasound biomicroscopy—specifically high-frequency ultrasonography—uses a water-bath immersion technique. With this technique, the depth of tissue penetration is approximately 5 mm and structures can be viewed through opaque media. Figure 2-17 is an example of ultrahigh frequency biomicroscopy of the normal limbus.

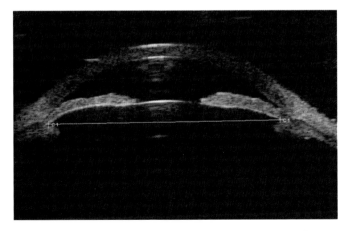

Figure 2-17 Ultrasound biomicroscopic visualization of the entire anterior segment, including structures behind the iris pigment epithelium, thereby permitting precise determination of the sulcus-to-sulcus measurements prior to phakic refractive implant. *(Reproduced with permission from Goins KM, Wagoner MD. Imaging the anterior segment. Focal Points: Clinical Modules for Ophthalmologists. San Francisco: American Academy of Ophthalmology; 2009, module 11.)*

Techniques involving the Scheimpflug camera, scanning-slit topography devices, and OCT are noncontact, which offers some practical advantages, including less training for image acquisition. The Scheimpflug-based imaging system uses a rotating Scheimpflug camera that is perpendicular to the slit beam and takes 50 slit images of the anterior segment in less than 2 seconds. A 3-dimensional image is constructed assessing the anterior and posterior corneal curvature, corneal thickness, anterior chamber depth, lens opacification and lens thickness. Pachometry and topography of the entire anterior and posterior surface of the cornea can be displayed (Fig 2-18).

The scanning-slit topography devices (eg, Orbscan; Bausch & Lomb, Rochester, NY) assess the curvature of the anterior and posterior surfaces along with the anterior surface of the lens and iris. The posterior elevation map created with this instrument is derived mathematically and may overestimate the posterior curvature, especially after LASIK procedures (Fig 2-19).

The anterior segment OCT devices are analogous to ultrasonographic devices but emit and reflect light rather than sound. The images are obtained in a noncontact, noninvasive fashion, and high-resolution corneal and angle scans measuring the depth, width, and angle of the anterior chamber can be obtained (Fig 2-20).

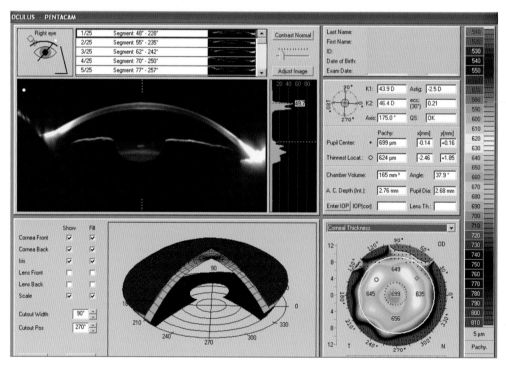

Figure 2-18 Scheimpflug image of a 65-year-old patient with Fuchs endothelial dystrophy and cataract. The general display clearly depicts epithelial and endothelial opactiy of the cornea with a densitometry measurement of 49.7 (normal 22–30) and the lenticular opacity with a densitometry reading of 37.0. In addition, keratometry, axis of astigmatism, corneal thickness, and anterior chamber depth are provided. *(Reproduced with permission from Goins KM, Wagoner MD. Imaging the anterior segment. Focal Points: Clinical Modules for Ophthalmologists. San Francisco: American Academy of Ophthalmology; 2009, module 11.)*

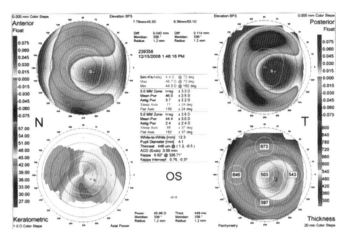

Figure 2-19 Orbscan scanning-slit topography of a keratoconus patient. *(Courtesy of James J. Reidy, MD.)*

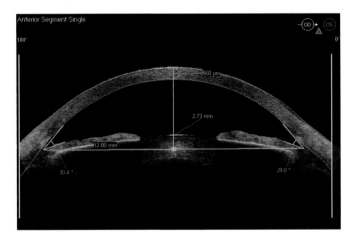

Figure 2-20 Anterior segment OCT image in a phakic eye. The central anterior chamber depth is 2.73 mm, and there is moderate narrowing of the anterior chamber angle. *(Reproduced with permission from Goins KM, Wagoner MD. Imaging the anterior segment. Focal Points: Clinical Modules for Ophthalmologists. San Francisco: American Academy of Ophthalmology; 2009, module 11.)*

Goins KM, Wagoner MD. Imaging the anterior segment. *Focal Points: Clinical Modules for Ophthalmologists.* San Francisco: American Academy of Ophthalmology; 2009, module 11.

Konstantopoulos A, Hossain P, Anderson DF. Recent advances in ophthalmic anterior segment imaging: a new era for ophthalmic diagnosis? *Br J Ophthalmol.* 2007;91(4):551–557.

Confocal Microscopy

The scanning confocal microscope can be used to study cell layers of the cornea even in cases with edema and scarring. Compared with ultrasonography or OCT, confocal

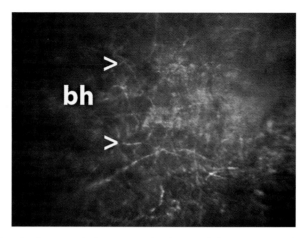

Figure 2-21 Confocal microscopic image at the level of deep stroma demonstrates fungal hyphae. Carets denote branching hyphae *(bh)*. *(Reproduced with permission from Goins KM, Wagoner MD. Imaging the anterior segment. Focal Points: Clinical Modules for Ophthalmologists. San Francisco: American Academy of Ophthalmology; 2009, module 11.)*

microscopy provides more spatial resolution and magnification, particularly in the z-axis. This allows in vivo optical sections of the cornea with a resolution at cellular and subcellular levels. Confocal microscopy can detect infectious crystalline keratopathy, fungal keratitis, and amebic keratitis. It has also been used to follow refractive surgery patients to analyze haze formation and the complications of LASIK flaps, such as epithelial ingrowth.

Four types of confocal microscopes have been described for clinical use: (1) the tandem-scanning (TSCM), (2) the scanning-slit (SSCM), (3) the laser scanning (LSCM), and (4) a single-sided disk design that is not commercially available. The first 3 are approved by the FDA in the United States. They differ in several ways, but, in general, the TSCM provides a shallower depth of field and better anterior-posterior localization and reconstruction. The SSCM is more user-friendly and, as a result, is the most used technique. The LSCM provides the highest resolution: to approximately 1–2 µm (Fig 2-21).

Cavanagh HD, Petroll WM, Jester JV. Confocal microscopy. In: Krachmer JH, Mannis MJ, Holland EJ, eds. *Cornea.* 2nd ed. Vol 1. Philadelphia: Elsevier/Mosby; 2005:283–297.

Chiou AG, Kaufman SC, Kaufman HE, Beuerman RW. Clinical corneal confocal microscopy. *Surv Ophthalmol.* 2006;51(5):482–500.

Goins KM, Wagoner MD. Imaging the anterior segment. *Focal Points: Clinical Modules for Ophthalmologists.* San Francisco: American Academy of Ophthalmology; 2009, module 11.

Measurement of Corneal Topography

Zones of the Cornea

For more than 100 years, the corneal shape has been known to be aspheric. Typically, the central cornea is about 3 D steeper than the periphery, a positive shape factor. Clinically, the cornea is divided into zones that surround fixation and blend into one another.

The *central zone* of 1–2 mm closely fits a spherical surface. Adjacent to the central zone is a 3–4-mm doughnut with an outer diameter of 7–8 mm. Called the *paracentral zone,* this doughnut represents an area of progressive flattening from the center. Together, the paracentral and central zones constitute the *apical zone,* as used in contact lens fitting. The central and paracentral zones are primarily responsible for the refractive power of the cornea (Fig 2-22). Adjacent to the paracentral zone is the *peripheral zone,* with an outer diameter of approximately 11 mm, and adjoining this is the limbus, with an outer diameter that averages 12 mm.

The peripheral zone is also known as the *transitional zone,* as it is the area of greatest flattening and asphericity of the normal cornea. The *limbus* is adjacent to the sclera and is the area where the cornea steepens prior to joining the sclera at the limbal sulcus.

The *optical zone* is the portion of the cornea that overlies the entrance pupil of the iris; it is physiologically limited to approximately 5.4 mm because of the Stiles-Crawford effect. The *corneal apex* is the point of maximum curvature, typically temporal to the center of the pupil. The *corneal vertex* is the point located at the intersection of the patient's line of fixation and the corneal surface. It is represented by the corneal light reflex when the cornea is illuminated coaxially with fixation. The corneal vertex is the center of the keratoscopic image and does not necessarily correspond to the point of maximum curvature at the corneal apex (Fig 2-23).

Shape, Curvature, and Power

Three topographic properties of the cornea are important to its optical function: the underlying *shape,* which determines its *curvature* and hence its refractive *power.* Shape and curvature are *geometric* properties of the cornea, whereas power is a *functional* property. Historically, power was the first parameter of the cornea to be described, and a unit representing the refractive power of the central cornea, the *diopter,* was accepted as the basic unit of measurement. However, with the advent of contact lenses and refractive surgery,

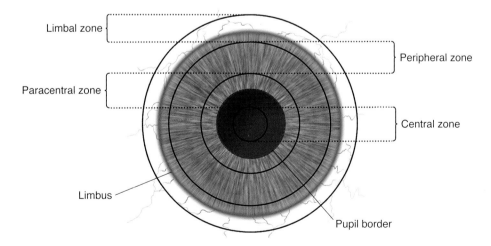

Figure 2-22 Topographic zones of the cornea. *(Illustration by Christine Gralapp.)*

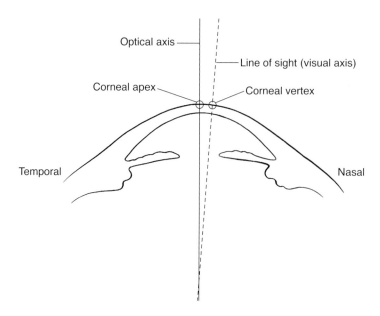

Figure 2-23 Corneal vertex and apex. *(Illustration by Christine Gralapp.)*

knowing the overall shape and the related property of curvature has become increasingly important.

The refractive power of the cornea is determined by *Snell's law,* the *law of refraction.* Snell's law is based on the difference between 2 refractive indices (in this case, of the cornea and of air), divided by the radius of curvature. The anterior corneal power using air and corneal stromal refractive indices is higher than clinically useful because it does not take into account the negative contribution of the posterior cornea. Thus, for most clinical purposes, a derived corneal refractive index of 1.3375 is used in calculating central corneal power. This value was chosen to allow 45 D to equate to a 7.5-mm radius of curvature. Average refractive power of the central cornea is about +43 D, which is the sum of the refractive power at the air–stroma interface of +49 D minus the endothelium–aqueous power of 6 D. The refractive index of air is 1.000; aqueous and tears, 1.336; and corneal stroma, 1.376. Although the air–tear interface of the cornea is responsible for most of the eye's refraction, the difference between total corneal power based on stroma alone and with tears is only –0.06 D.

BCSC Section 3, *Clinical Optics,* covers these topics in greater depth.

Keratometry

The ophthalmometer (keratometer) empirically estimates corneal power by reading 4 points of the central 2.8- to 4.0-mm zone. These points do not represent the corneal apex or vertex but are a clinically useful estimation of central corneal power. The radius of curvature is calculated from the simple vergence formula using the known circular object size and measuring the distance with doubling prisms to stabilize the image. The longer axis of the elliptical image is produced by the flattest portion of the cornea (ie, that part of the central cornea that has the longest radius of curvature and the lowest dioptric power). The axial radius of curvature is then used in computing the corneal power in this region. Results are reported as *radius of curvature* in millimeters or *refracting power* in diopters.

For most normal corneas, keratometry is sufficiently accurate for contact lens fitting or IOL power calculation. Keratometry is also useful in detecting irregular astigmatism, in which keratometric images cannot be superimposed or are not regular ovals. However, in some circumstances, such as with keratoconus or after radial keratotomy, the optical properties of the cornea are affected by zones other than those measured by keratometry. Topographic keratometry can be performed with a special attachment to the keratometer. See also BCSC Section 3, *Clinical Optics.*

Keratoscopy

Information about corneal curvature can be obtained with a variety of instruments that reflect the images of multiple concentric circles from the corneal surface. These devices allow analysis of corneal curvature in zones both central and peripheral to those measured by keratometry. In general, on steeper parts of the cornea, the reflected mires appear closer together and thinner, and the axis of the central mire is shorter (Fig 2-24). Conversely, along the flat axis, the mires are farther apart and thicker, and the central mire is longer. The handheld *Placido disk* is a keratoscope with a flat target. *Collimating keratoscopes* use rings inside a column or a curve to maximize the area of the ocular surface that can reflect the target mires. Photokeratoscopy preserves the virtual image of concentric circles on film, and videokeratoscopy stores the images on video.

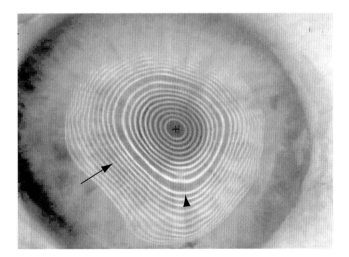

Figure 2-24 Videokeratoscopic mires are closer together in the axis of steep curvature *(arrow),* and farther apart in the flat axis *(arrowhead)* in this post–penetrating keratoplasty patient. Major axes are not orthogonal. *(Courtesy of John E. Sutphin, MD.)*

Computerized Corneal Topography

See BCSC Section 13, *Refractive Surgery,* for a more detailed discussion of computerized corneal topography.

Keratoscopy images can be digitally captured and analyzed by computers. Placido disk–based computerized topographers have been the type most commonly available. These units assume the angle of incidence to be nearly perpendicular and the radius of curvature to be the distance from the surface to the intersection with the line of sight or visual axis of the patient *(axial distance)* (Fig 2-25). However, the assumption that the visual axis is coincident to the corneal apex may lead to some misinterpretations, such as the overdiagnosis of keratoconus. *Axial curvature* closely approximates the power of the central 1–2 mm of the cornea but fails to describe the true shape and power of the peripheral cornea.

Another method of describing the corneal curvature uses the *instantaneous radius of curvature* (also called *tangential power*) at a certain point. This radius is determined by taking a perpendicular path through the point in question from a plane that intersects the point and the visual axis but allowing the radius to be the length necessary to correspond to a sphere with the same curvature at that point. The instantaneous radius of curvature, with curvature given in diopters, is estimated by the difference between the corneal index of refraction and 1.000 divided by this tangentially determined radius. The tangential map typically shows better sensitivity to peripheral changes with less "smoothing" of the curvature than the axial maps (Fig 2-26). (In these maps, diopters are relative units of curvature and not the equivalent of diopters of corneal power.)

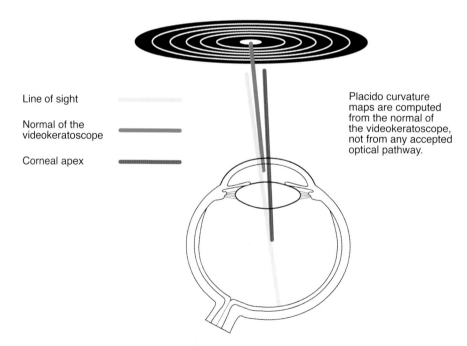

Line of sight

Normal of the
videokeratoscope

Corneal apex

Placido curvature
maps are computed
from the normal of
the videokeratoscope,
not from any accepted
optical pathway.

Figure 2-25 Placido imagery for calculating the corneal curvature. The assumption that the perpendicular to the videokeratograph, the patient's line of sight, and the corneal apex are coincident is rarely correct. *(Courtesy of Michael W. Belin, MD; rendered by C. H. Wooley.)*

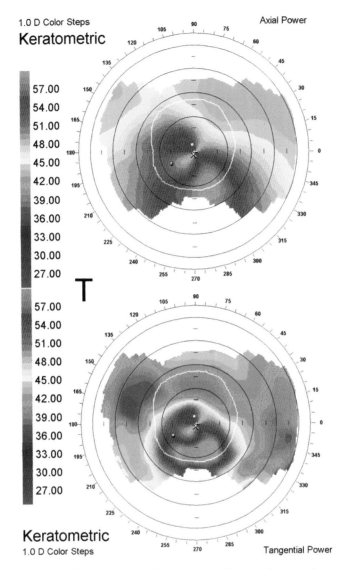

Figure 2-26 Topography of a patient with keratoconus. The top image shows axial curvature, the bottom, tangential curvature. Note that the steeper curve on the bottom is more closely aligned to the cone. *(Courtesy of John E. Sutphin, MD.)*

A third map, the *mean curvature map*, does not require the perpendicular ray to cross the visual axis. It uses an infinite number of spheres to fit the curvature at that point. The algorithm determines a minimum and maximum size best-fit sphere and, from their radii, determines an average curvature (arithmetic mean of principal curvatures) known as the *mean curvature* for that point. These powers are then mapped using standard colors to represent diopter changes, allowing for more sensitivity to peripheral changes of curvature (Fig 2-27).

In addition to power maps, computerized topographic systems may display other data: pupil size and location, indexes estimating regular and irregular astigmatism, estimates of the probability of having keratoconus, simulated keratometry, and more.

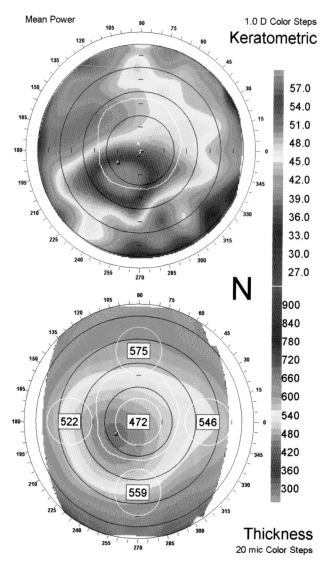

Figure 2-27 The top image shows mean curvature in keratoconus for the same patient as in Figure 2-26. The local curvature outlines the cone, as shown by the thinnest point in the pachometry map in the bottom figure. *(Courtesy of John E. Sutphin, MD.)*

All of these maps attempt to depict the underlying shape of the cornea by scaling curvature through the familiar dioptric notation instead of the less familiar millimeters of radius. A more accurate way to describe curvature would be to use the true shape of the cornea; some systems directly derive corneal shape by means of scanning slits or rectangular grids and then determine power from that shape.

To represent shape directly, maps may display a *z-height* from an arbitrary plane (iris plane, limbal plane, or frontal plane) using color maps. Just as viewing the curvature of the earth in an appropriate scale fails to show the details of mountains and basins, these

z maps do not show clinically important variations. Geographic maps show land elevation relative to sea level. Similarly, corneal surface maps are plotted to show differences from best-fit spheres or other objects that closely mimic the normal corneal shape.

The American National Standards Institute (ANSI) in the United States is currently developing standards for the corneal topography industry that will make the comparison of maps more uniform and clarify the confusion of terminology.

Indications

About two thirds of patients with normal corneas have a symmetric pattern that is round, oval, or bowtie-shaped, as in Figure 2-28. The others are classified as having an asymmetric pattern: inferior steepening, superior steepening, asymmetric bowtie patterns, or nonspecific irregularity. However, many corneas are found to have a complex shape that is oversimplified by the use of such qualitative pattern descriptions.

Corneal topography detects irregular astigmatism from contact lens warpage, keratoconus and other thinning disorders, corneal surgery, trauma, and postinflammatory and degenerative conditions. Different values obtained at subsequent examinations can signal a change in corneal contour if the alignment of the eye and the instrument is the same. Computer-assisted topographic modeling systems allow the clinician to detect subtle and minor variations in power distribution of the anterior corneal surface.

Corneal topography is important in the preoperative evaluation of cataract and refractive surgery patients. Patients with corneal warpage (irregular astigmatism and/or peripheral steepening, distorted keratoscopic mires) should discontinue contact lens wear and allow the corneal map and refraction to stabilize prior to undergoing surgery. Patients with keratoconus are not routinely considered for LASIK surgery, as the thin cornea has an unpredictable response and reducing its thickness may lead to progression of the condition. The forme fruste, or subclinical, keratoconus recognized by Placido disk–based topography

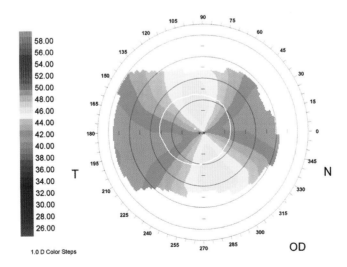

Figure 2-28 Keratography of a normal cornea with regular astigmatism. The white circle indicates the pupil. Simulated keratometry is 41.3, 46.2@102. *(Courtesy of John E. Sutphin, MD.)*

requires caution on the part of the ophthalmologist and is now considered to be a contraindication to LASIK and possibly surface ablation. Forme fruste keratoconus or early pellucid marginal degeneration may show a peripheral steepening or "crab claw" configuration (Fig 2-29). Furthermore, topographic corneal abnormalities may preclude the use of advanced IOL technologies such as toric, multifocal, or pseudoaccommodative IOLs.

Corneal topography can also be used to show the effects of keratorefractive procedures. Pre- and postoperative maps may be algebraically subtracted to determine whether the desired effect was achieved. Corneal mapping may help to explain unexpected results, including undercorrections, aberrations, induced astigmatism, or glare and halos, by detecting decentered surgery or inadequate surgery, such as shallow incisions in radial keratotomy. Corneal topography also confirms the expected physiologic effects of refractive surgery. For example, in LASIK for myopia, the ablation profile leads to flattening of the central cornea and a relative peripheral steepening.

Corneal topography is useful in managing congenital and postoperative astigmatism, particularly following penetrating keratoplasty. Complex peripheral patterns may result in a refractive axis of astigmatism that is not aligned with topographic axes. Failure to correct the underlying shape by removing appropriate sutures or operating on the appropriate axis may lead to unexpected results. The appropriate axis depends on the type of surgery (incisional surgery is done on the steep axis, compression sutures on the flat axis, and minus cylinder ablation on the flat axis).

Finally, detection of irregular astigmatism by means of corneal topography can be used in managing ocular surface disorders such as map-dot-fingerprint dystrophy.

Limitations

Besides the limitations of the algorithms and variation in terminology by manufacturer, the accuracy of corneal topography may be affected by various other potential problems:

- misalignment
- stability (test-to-test variation)

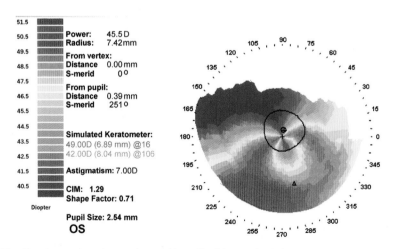

Figure 2-29 Keratography of a patient with pellucid marginal degeneration. The "crab claw" appearance is fully developed, with central flattening and inferior steepening; forme fruste keratoconus may have a similar but less definite appearance. *(Courtesy of John E. Sutphin, MD.)*

- sensitivity to focus errors
- tear-film effects
- distortions
- area of coverage (central and limbal)
- nonstandardized data maps
- colors that may be absolute or varied (normalized)

Corbett MC, O'Brart DPS, Rosen E, et al. *Corneal Topography: Principles and Applications.* London: BMJ Books; 1999.

Courville CB, Klyce SD. Corneal topography. In: Foster CS, Azar DT, Dohlman CH, eds. *Smolin and Thoft's The Cornea: Scientific Foundations and Clinical Practice.* 4th ed. Philadelphia: Lippincott Williams & Wilkins; 2004:175–185.

Maguire LJ. Keratometry, photokeratoscopy, and computer-assisted topographic analysis. In: Krachmer JH, Mannis MJ, Holland EJ, eds. *Cornea.* 2nd ed. Vol 1. Philadelphia: Elsevier/Mosby; 2005:171–184.

Roberts C. Principles of corneal topography. In: Elander RE, Rich LF, Robin JB, eds. *Principles and Practice of Refractive Surgery.* Philadelphia: Saunders; 1997:475–497.

Retinoscopy

Retinoscopy can detect irregular astigmatism by showing nonlinear or multiple reflexes that cannot be completely neutralized with a spherocylindrical lens. With a multifocal cornea, retinoscopy reveals multiple regular reflexes that move in different directions. Irregular astigmatism and multifocal cornea can occur in keratoconus and after keratorefractive surgery. Abnormalities found with retinoscopy can help explain why a patient with a clear cornea cannot see well. In addition, retinoscopy can disclose disrupted light reflexes caused by disturbances of the corneal surface. In cases where retinoscopic findings exceed the corresponding slit-lamp findings, retinoscopy can help gauge the relative effect of corneal surface changes on vision. See also BCSC Section 3, *Clinical Optics.*

Krachmer JH, Mannis MJ. Refraction of the abnormal cornea. In: Krachmer JH, Mannis MJ, Holland EJ, eds. *Cornea.* 2nd ed. Vol 1. Philadelphia: Elsevier/Mosby; 2005:167–170.

Prevention Practices in Ophthalmology

Some corneal and external eye diseases can be prevented. Strategies for prevention include adequate hygiene and nutrition, aseptic surgical techniques, protective spectacles to minimize ocular trauma, and prophylactic antibiotics. Prevention begins with immunization. Practicing ophthalmologists should provide their office staff with an opportunity for hepatitis B vaccination and follow other regulations of the Occupational Safety and Health Administration. Universal precautions that safeguard the health of patients' eyes, as well as the health of the ophthalmologist's and staff's eyes, should be a part of daily practice.

Universal Precautions

Optimal infection control is based on the assumption that all specified human body fluids are potentially infectious. Many transmissible diseases of the external eye, such as adenoviral conjunctivitis, cause redness that immediately indicates infection. Other infectious agents, however, can be present on the ocular surface without causing inflammation. Human immunodeficiency virus (HIV), hepatitis B virus, hepatitis C virus, rabies virus, and the agent of Creutzfeldt-Jakob disease are not immediately obvious without systemic clues or laboratory testing. Every patient must be approached as potentially contagious. Guidelines for routine ophthalmic examinations include the following:

- Wash hands between patient examinations. Use disposable gloves if an open sore, blood, or blood-contaminated fluid is present. Using cotton-tipped applicators to manipulate the eyelids can also minimize direct contact.
- Avoid unnecessary contact. Eyedropper bottles used in the office should not directly touch the eyelids, eyelashes, or ocular surface of any patient. Individual sterile strips impregnated with dye are preferred where available.
- Disinfect all contact instruments after each use. Tonometer tips and pachometer tips should be soaked in diluted bleach or hydrogen peroxide after every use. Trial contact lenses must be disinfected between patients. BCSC Section 10, *Glaucoma*, discusses infection control in clinical tonometry in greater detail.
- Handle sharp devices carefully. Needles must always be discarded into puncture-resistant (sharps) containers.

Universal precautions are also discussed in BCSC Section 9, *Intraocular Inflammation and Uveitis*.

Minimizing transmission of bloodborne pathogens and surface infectious agents in ophthalmic offices and operating rooms. Information Statement. San Francisco: American Academy of Ophthalmology; 2002.

Segal WA, Pirnazar JR, Arens M, Pepose JS. Disinfection of Goldmann tonometers after contamination with hepatitis C virus. *Am J Ophthalmol.* 2001;131(2):184–187.

Smith CA, Pepose JS. Disinfection of tonometers and contact lenses in the office setting: are current techniques adequate? *Am J Ophthalmol.* 1999;127(1):77–84.

CHAPTER 3

Ocular Surface Disease: Diagnostic Approach

Ocular Cytology

An important step in the diagnosis of many infectious and inflammatory conditions of the ocular surface is the examination of conjunctival or corneal specimens by light microscopy. Standard staining procedures are widely used to facilitate the detection of microbial and human cells. This section discusses the procedures used in these investigations and the implications that can be drawn from their results. See also BCSC Section 4, *Ophthalmic Pathology and Intraocular Tumors*.

Specimen Collection

Scraping or swabbing

Conjunctival scraping is generally preferred to swabbing because it yields more epithelial cells and causes less contamination due to inflammatory debris from the ocular surface. To obtain a conjunctival specimen for cytologic examination, the clinician applies a topical anesthetic and everts the upper eyelid. The tarsal conjunctiva is lightly scraped with a sterile spatula. When epithelial cells are removed during scraping, the conjunctival surface should blanch slightly, but not bleed excessively. An alternative method of gathering conjunctival cells involves the use of a cytobrush. After the conjunctiva is rubbed, the brush is dipped into buffer solution, and the cells that float to the surface are concentrated on a Millipore filter. Rapid immersion into fixative avoids excessive air drying of material on a glass slide or filter paper.

Conjunctival swabbing for culture should be done before a topical anesthetic is instilled. Calcium alginate or Dacron swabs, slightly moistened with liquid broth, are preferable for collecting specimens of epithelial cells and microflora; cotton swabs may inhibit bacterial and viral growth. Specimens can also be obtained from the contralateral conjunctiva for comparison.

Procedures for obtaining and culturing specimens for suspected infectious conditions are discussed further in Chapter 4.

Impression cytology

Impression cytology is primarily a research tool, but it allows for precise assessment of the ocular surface epithelium. A piece of filter paper is pressed against a specific area of the conjunctival (or, in rare cases, the corneal) surface to lift off epithelial cells. This procedure can be considered a noninvasive superficial biopsy that provides a means for mapping specific cell changes topographically and quantifying surface abnormalities. Cells thus harvested can be examined directly as attached epithelial sheets for morphologic and histologic studies or may be processed as free cells for flow cytometry; the latter technique allows quantification of the expression of specific proteins (eg, cytokines, receptors, and so on) by the epithelial cells. The technique is both powerful and quantitative, and it precludes the need for a biopsy, which is not always convenient in a clinic setting.

Baudouin C, Hamard P, Liang H, Creuzot-Garcher C, Bensoussan L, Brignole F. Conjunctival epithelial cell expression of interleukins and inflammatory markers in glaucoma patients treated over the long term. *Ophthalmology.* 2004;111(12):2186–2192.

Koh S, Maeda N, Hirohara Y, et al. Serial measurements of higher-order aberrations after blinking in patients with dry eye. *Invest Ophthalmol Vis Sci.* 2008;49(1):133–138.

Preferred Practice Patterns Committee, Cornea/External Disease Panel. *Conjunctivitis.* San Francisco: American Academy of Ophthalmology; 2008.

Tseng SC. Staging of conjunctival squamous metaplasia by impression cytology. *Ophthalmology.* 1985;92(6):728–733.

Interpretation of Ocular Cytology

Microscopic examination of material collected from the ocular surface can reveal cells, cellular elements, and microorganisms that can be helpful in diagnostic evaluation; such examination is perhaps best carried out in conjunction with a laboratory experienced in these evaluations.

Dry-Eye Syndrome

The term *dry-eye syndrome* has been defined as "a multifactorial disease of the tears and ocular surface that results in symptoms of discomfort, visual disturbance, and tear-film instability with potential damage to the ocular surface. It is accompanied by increased osmolarity of the tear film and inflammation of the ocular surface" (DEWS, 2007).

Dry eye represents a disturbance of the *lacrimal functional unit (LFU)*, an integrated system comprising the lacrimal glands, ocular surface (cornea, conjunctiva, and meibomian glands), and eyelids, as well as the sensory and motor nerves that connect them (Fig 3-1). The LFU regulates the major components of the tear film and responds to environmental, endocrinologic, and cortical influences. Its overall functions are to preserve

- tear-film integrity: lubricating, antimicrobial, and nutritional roles
- ocular surface health: maintaining corneal transparency and surface stem cell population
- quality of image projected onto the retina

Tear-film stability is threatened when the interactions among stabilizing tear-film constituents are compromised by decreased tear secretion, delayed clearance, and altered tear composition. A consequence of such compromise is ocular surface inflammation. Although the initial reaction to ocular irritation may be reflex tear secretion, eventually

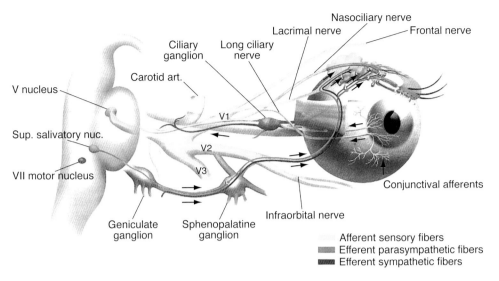

Figure 3-1 The lacrimal functional unit. *(Reproduced with permission from Pflugfelder SC, Beuerman RW, Stern ME, eds.* Dry Eye and Ocular Surface Disorders. *New York: Marcel Dekker; 2004.)*

inflammation, accompanying chronic secretory dysfunction and a decrease in corneal sensation, compromises the reflex response and results in even greater tear-film instability. Perturbation of the LFU is considered to play an important role in the evolution of different forms of dry eye.

> The definition and classification of dry eye disease: report of the Definition and Classification Subcommittee of the International Dry Eye WorkShop (2007). *Ocul Surf.* 2007;5(2):75–92.

Mechanisms of Dry Eye

The core mechanisms of dry eye are believed to be driven by tear hyperosmolarity and tear-film instability. The cycle of events is shown in Figure 3-2. Tear hyperosmolarity causes damage to the surface epithelium by activating a cascade of inflammatory events at the ocular surface and a release of inflammatory mediators into the tears. Epithelial damage involves cell death by apoptosis, a loss of goblet cells, and disturbance of mucin expression leading to tear-film instability. This instability exacerbates ocular surface hyperosmolarity and completes the vicious cycle. Tear-film instability can also be initiated by several etiologies, including xerosing medication, xerophthalmia, ocular allergy, topical preservative use, and contact lens wear.

Epithelial injury caused by dry eye stimulates corneal nerve endings, leading to symptoms of discomfort, increased blinking, and, potentially, compensatory reflex lacrimal tear secretion. Loss of normal mucins at the ocular surface contributes to symptoms by increasing frictional resistance between the lids and globe. During this period, the high reflex input may cause neurogenic inflammation within the lacrimal gland.

The major causes of tear hyperosmolarity are reduced aqueous tear flow, resulting from lacrimal failure, and/or increased evaporation from the tear film (see the arrow at the top

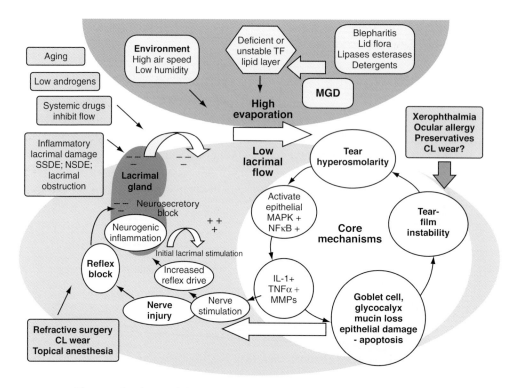

Figure 3-2 The mechanisms of dry eye. *(Reproduced with permission from The definition and classification of dry eye disease: report of the Definition and Classification Subcommittee of the International Dry Eye WorkShop (2007). Ocul Surf. 2007;5(2):75–92.)*

center of Fig 3-2). Low humidity and high air flow help increase evaporative loss, which may be caused clinically, in particular, by meibomian gland dysfunction (MGD), which leads to an unstable tear-film lipid layer. The quality of eyelid oil is modified by the action of esterases and lipases released by normal eyelid commensals, whose numbers are increased in blepharitis. Reduced aqueous tear flow is due to impaired delivery of lacrimal fluid into the conjunctival sac. It is unclear whether this is a feature of normal aging, but it may be induced by some systemic drugs, such as certain antihypertensive agents, antihistamines, and antimuscarinic agents. The most common cause is inflammatory lacrimal damage, which is seen in autoimmune disorders such as Sjögren syndrome and also in non–Sjögren syndrome dry eye (NSSDE). Inflammation causes both tissue destruction and a potentially reversible neurosecretory block. A receptor block may also be caused by circulating antibodies to the M3 receptor. Inflammation is favored by low tissue androgen levels.

Tear delivery may be obstructed by cicatricial conjunctival scarring or reduced by a loss of sensory reflex drive to the lacrimal gland from the ocular surface. Eventually, the chronic surface damage of dry eye leads to a reduction in corneal sensitivity and reflex tear secretion. Various etiologies, acting, at least in part, by the mechanism of reflex secretory block, may cause dry eye, including refractive surgery (LASIK dry eye), contact lens wear, and the chronic abuse of topical anesthetics. Individual etiologies often cause dry eye by several interacting mechanisms.

Classification: Major Etiologic Causes of Dry Eye

Interpreting studies that investigate the risk factors, pathogenesis, and therapy of dry-eye conditions has been complicated in the past by a lack of accepted diagnostic criteria and standardized, specific diagnostic tests. However, a diagnostic classification scheme for dry-eye disorders has now been established, along with uniform guidelines for evaluating both the disorder and its response to therapy. The major subclassification in this scheme, shown in Figure 3-3, separates dry-eye patients into those with ATD and those with evaporative tear dysfunction (ETD). The term *environment* is used broadly to include bodily states habitually experienced by an individual both internally and externally.

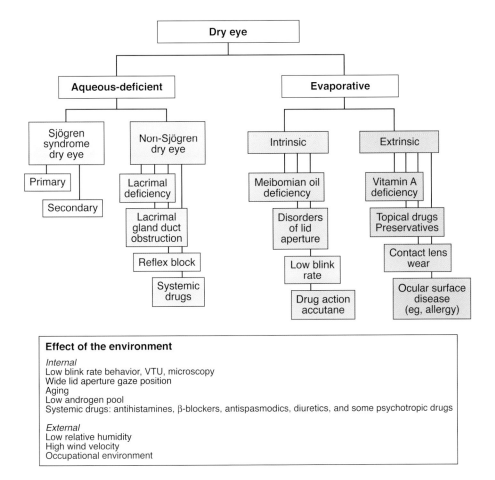

Effect of the environment

Internal
Low blink rate behavior, VTU, microscopy
Wide lid aperture gaze position
Aging
Low androgen pool
Systemic drugs: antihistamines, β-blockers, antispasmodics, diuretics, and some psychotropic drugs

External
Low relative humidity
High wind velocity
Occupational environment

Figure 3-3   Diagnostic classification scheme for dry-eye disorders. *(Courtesy of Minas T. Coroneo, MD.)*

This background may influence the onset and type of dry-eye disease in an individual, which may be aqueous-deficient or evaporative in nature.

Aqueous-deficient dry eye has 2 major groupings: Sjögren syndrome dry eye and non–Sjögren syndrome dry eye. *Evaporative dry eye* may be intrinsic, where the regulation of evaporative loss from the tear film is directly affected (eg, by meibomian lipid deficiency; poor lid congruity and lid dynamics; low blink rate; and the effects of drug action, such as that of systemic retinoids). Extrinsic evaporative dry eye is caused by conditions that are associated with evaporation through pathologic effects on the ocular surface. These include vitamin A deficiency; the action of toxic topical agents such as preservatives; contact lens wear; and a range of ocular surface diseases, including allergic eye disease.

Dry-eye syndrome is one of the commonest reasons for ophthalmic consultation and becomes increasingly prevalent with age, affecting approximately 10% of those aged 30–60 and increasing to 15% of adults over the age of 65. Most epidemiologic studies have demonstrated a higher prevalence among women, and it seems to occur with equal prevalence in all racial and ethnic groups.

There has been renewed interest in dry eye with the growth and development of refractive procedures, which demand high ocular surface quality on the one hand, yet interfere with ocular surface innervation and shape on the other. Related technologies (such as double-pass retinal image–based scatter indices) may allow more sensitive measures of tear-film failure.

Tear-Film Evaluation

Tests for dry eye lend some degree of objectivity to what is essentially a clinical diagnosis, although no one test is sufficiently specific to permit an absolute diagnosis. The best approach is to combine information from the history and examination with the results of one or more of the following diagnostic tests. The tests described may be performed in the following sequence to minimize the potential for alteration of subsequent test results by preceding procedures. However, any of the tests may affect the outcome of subsequent ones. An ongoing issue in assessing patients with dry eye is the frequent lack of correlation between symptoms and signs.

Inspection

A "foot-of-the-bed" inspection may reveal signs of associated systemic disease (such as rheumatoid arthritis), indications of personal habits (eg, smoking), or signs of associated ocular disease (pseudoptosis, blepharospasm), as well as eyelid malposition. External examination may also reveal the characteristic facial telangiectasia and eyelid margin hyperemia associated with ocular rosacea.

Inspection of the tear meniscus between the globe and the lower eyelid (normally 1.0 mm in height and convex) is essential. A tear meniscus 0.3 mm or less is considered abnormal. Tear breakup is a functional measure of tear stability; if stability is perturbed (as in lipid or mucin deficiency), the *tear breakup time (TBUT)* can become more rapid (lower). TBUT is determined by instilling fluorescein and then evaluating the stability of the tear film. The examiner moistens a fluorescein strip with sterile saline and applies it to the tarsal conjunctiva (fluorescein-anesthetic combination drops are not suitable for this purpose). After several blinks, the tear film is examined using a broad beam of the slit lamp with a blue filter. The time lapse between the last blink and the appearance of the first randomly distributed dry spot on the cornea is the tear breakup time. Dry spots appearing in less than 10 seconds are considered abnormal.

Noninvasive assessment of the TBUT (without applying any fluorescein to the ocular surface) can also be made by using optical (eg, videokeratoscopic) imaging devices that can similarly detect a break in the tear film. TBUT should be measured before any eyedrops are instilled and before the eyelids are manipulated in any way. It is best to wait at least 1 minute after fluorescein instillation to evaluate the corneal surface for fluorescein staining. Afterward, an additional dye, such as lissamine green or rose bengal, can be used to evaluate bulbar conjunctival staining.

Evidence of tear-film debris should be sought. The eye should be carefully inspected for conjunctivochalasis, especially in patients with poor-quality tear film who complain of epiphora (Fig 3-4). Also, besides an assessment of staining, a complete inspection of the ocular surface, including eversion of the eyelids, must be performed. Evaluation of eyelid laxity in floppy eyelid syndrome can be done at this time. Some of the symptomatology of dry eye can occur in patients with multiple concretions, often seen in patients with chronic blepharitis (Fig 3-5; see also Chapter 5).

Tests of Tear Production

Aqueous tear production can be assessed in a variety of ways (Table 3-1). *Schirmer testing* is performed by placing a thin strip of filter paper in the inferior cul-de-sac (Fig 3-6). The amount of wetting can be measured to quantify aqueous tear production. There are several variations of the Schirmer test. The *basic secretion test* is performed following the instillation of a topical anesthetic, followed by lightly blotting residual fluid out of the

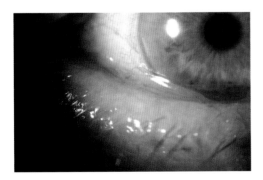

Figure 3-4 Conjunctivochalasis is frequently seen in dry-eye patients and may require repair. *(Courtesy of Robert W. Weisenthal, MD.)*

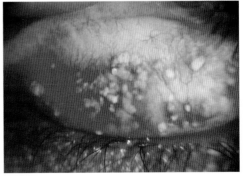

Figure 3-5 Multiple concretions in a patient with dry eye and chronic blepharitis. Symptoms were more easily controlled after the concretions were removed. *(Courtesy of Minas T. Coroneo, MD.)*

Table 3-1 Assessment of Aqueous Tear Production

Test	Topical Anesthesia	Time	Nasal Stimulation	Normal Value
Basic tear secretion	+	5 min	–	≥10 mm
Schirmer I	–	5 min	–	≥10 mm
Schirmer II	–	5 min	+	≥15 mm

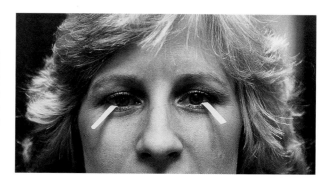

Figure 3-6 The Schirmer test uses the amount of wetting of the paper strips as a measure of tear flow. *(Reproduced with permission from Carr T, ed.* Ophthalmic Medical Assisting. *3rd ed, rev. San Francisco: American Academy of Ophthalmology; 2003:93.)*

inferior fornix. A thin filter-paper strip (5 mm wide, 35 mm long) is placed at the junction of the middle and lateral thirds of the lower eyelids to minimize irritation to the cornea during the test. The test can be performed with open or closed eyes, although some recommend the eyes be closed to limit the effect of blinking. Although normal measurements are quite variable, repeated measurements of less than 5 mm of wetting, with anesthetic, are highly suggestive of aqueous tear deficiency (ATD), whereas 5–10 mm is equivocal. The *Schirmer I test,* which is similar to the basic secretion test but *without* topical anesthetic, measures both basic and reflex tearing combined. Less than 10 mm of wetting after 5 minutes is diagnostic of ATD. Although this test is relatively specific, the level of sensitivity is poor. Using lower cutoff measurements increases the specificity of these tests but decreases their sensitivity. The *Schirmer II test,* which measures reflex secretion, is performed in a similar manner without topical anesthetic. However, after the filter-paper strips have been inserted into the inferior fornices, a cotton-tipped applicator is used to irritate the nasal mucosa. Wetting of less than 15 mm after 5 minutes is consistent with a defect in reflex secretion. Although an isolated abnormal result for any of these tests can be misleading, serially consistent results are highly suggestive. Schirmer testing is also useful in demonstrating to patients the presence of an ATD. An alternative to classic Schirmer strips is the phenol red–impregnated cotton thread test, which allows for quicker assessment of tear secretion but has not been fully validated.

Tear Composition Assays

Other procedures may be useful in helping diagnose ATD. Cultures of the eyelid margins are rarely helpful, but they may provide useful information in selected cases. Additional tests include tear-film osmolarity (virtually all forms of dry eye are associated with increased osmolarity; benchtop osmometers are becoming more available), tear lysozyme, and tear lactoferrin. In lacrimal gland dysfunction states, the normal production of proteins by the lacrimal gland is diminished, so a decreased tear lysozyme or lactoferrin level is highly suggestive of dry eye. A commercial assay is available for measuring lactoferrin in tears. Many of these tests have been used in clinical trials assessing the efficacy of novel treatments for dry eye. At the present time, no consensus has been reached as to which of these tests is most sensitive and/or specific for the diagnosis of ATD, and some are not readily available.

Newer Imaging Technologies and Dry Eye

An important symptom of dry eye is reduced quality of vision, and many new technologies brought about by refractive surgery may prove useful in functional assessments of dry eye. Wavefront sensing, for example, appears to be a useful objective method for evaluating sequential changes in visual performance related to tear-film dynamics. Serial measurement of higher-order aberrations, increased in some forms of dry eye, may show a relationship between tear dynamics and quality of vision. More recently, retinal image double-pass–based scattering indices have been developed as an objective means of assessing the tear film.

Confocal microscopy has been used to image the tear film and assess dry-eye–associated corneal neuropathy. It has also been used to assess meibomian gland morphology; mean acinar unit diameter is significantly larger in patients with meibomian gland disease. Both the density and diameter of acinar units has been shown to be associated with the severity of meibomian gland dropout.

Aqueous Tear Deficiency

Findings that are particularly indicative of ATD include, by definition, decreased aqueous tear production, as measured by Schirmer testing. In addition, the characteristic exposure pattern of conjunctival and/or corneal staining with either lissamine green or rose bengal, corneal staining by fluorescein, and filamentary keratopathy support a diagnosis of ATD. Patients who display signs and symptoms of ATD can be subdivided into those who have Sjögren syndrome and those who do not (non–Sjögren syndrome).

CLINICAL PRESENTATION   The spectrum of ATD ranges from mild irritation with minimal ocular surface disease to severe and disabling irritation, occasionally associated with sight-threatening corneal complications. Advanced stages can include the development of corneal calcification, particularly in association with certain topical medications (especially antiglaucoma medications); band keratopathy; and keratinization of the cornea and conjunctiva.

Symptoms tend to be worse toward the end of the day, with prolonged use of the eyes, or with exposure to environmental extremes. Patients who live in temperate climates and are exposed to the lower levels of humidity associated with indoor heating systems during the winter months tend to become particularly symptomatic. Foreign-body sensation is a symptom frequently associated with punctate epithelial keratopathy. Associated complaints include burning, a dry sensation, photophobia, and blurred vision. Rapid assessment of dry eye can be achieved by the "stare test": after a few blinks, a patient is asked to look at a visual acuity chart; the time until the image blurs should be more than 8 seconds.

Signs of a dry eye include bulbar conjunctival hyperemia, conjunctivochalasis (redundancy of the bulbar conjunctiva), a decreased tear meniscus, irregular corneal surface, and debris in the tear film. Epithelial keratopathy, which can be fine and granular, coarse, or confluent, is best demonstrated following the instillation of lissamine green, rose bengal, or fluorescein. Fluorescein stains epithelial erosions and exposed basement membrane and may produce fine or coarse granular staining of the inferior or central cornea. Rose bengal and lissamine green stain not only dead and devitalized cells and mucus but also epithelial cells that are inadequately protected by ocular surface mucins. Rose bengal and lissamine green staining can be more sensitive than fluorescein in revealing early or mild cases of keratoconjunctivitis sicca (KCS); the staining may be seen at the nasal and temporal limbus and/or inferior paracentral cornea *(exposure staining)* (Fig 3-7; see also Fig 2-12C, in Chapter 2). Alternatively, it can be most prominent along the inferior cornea and inferior conjunctiva *(linear staining)*, as seen in MGD. Lissamine green has some advantages over rose bengal: it does not stain healthy conjunctival epithelium, it is far less irritating, and it does not inhibit viral growth.

In more severe dry-eye states, filaments and mucous plaques may be seen. *Filaments* represent strands of epithelial cells attached to the surface of the cornea over a core of mucus. Filamentary keratopathy can be quite painful, as these strands are firmly attached to the richly innervated surface epithelium (Fig 3-8). Marginal or paracentral thinning and even perforation can occur in more severe disease. Incomplete blinking is frequently noted. Associated local eye disease, such as blepharitis, MGD, and eyelid abnormalities, can contribute significantly to the patient's level of discomfort. Clinicians may find useful a classification based on disease severity (Table 3-2).

A reliable means of assessing clinical disease severity by questionnaire is the Ocular Surface Disease Index (OSDI). The questionnaire is useful in evaluating the effects of various treatment regimes, and the scoring system allows patients to follow their progress. In some patients, although ocular surface health improves, discomfort does not (this is thought to be due to corneal neuropathy).

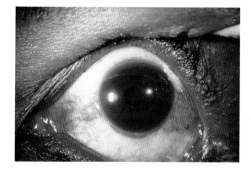

Figure 3-7 Keratoconjunctivitis sicca with punctate epithelial erosions, shown by rose bengal stain. *(Courtesy of Vincent P. deLuise, MD.)*

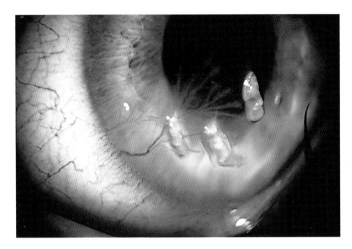

Figure 3-8 Filamentary keratopathy in a vascularized cornea. *(Courtesy of Minas T. Coroneo, MD.)*

LABORATORY EVALUATION Although lacrimal gland biopsy is rarely performed to help diagnose Sjögren syndrome, minor (labial) salivary gland biopsy is easily carried out (Fig 3-9). After local anesthetic gel is applied, followed by local infiltration, a chalazion clamp is applied to the buccal mucosa inside the lower lip. A 1- to 2-mm incision is made with a 30° blade, and tissue deep to this is grasped, teased through the incision, and excised. Clumps of glands usually emerge, 2–3 clumps per incision site. Patients are warned of the possibility of localized labial numbness, although with this small incision technique, it is rare.

Conjunctival impression cytology can be used to monitor the progression of ocular surface changes, beginning with decreased goblet cell density, followed by squamous metaplasia and, in later stages, keratinization.

Patients with ATD may have circulating autoantibodies, including antinuclear antibody (ANA), rheumatoid factor (RF), or SS antibodies (SS-A and SS-B). The presence of these antibodies has been correlated with the severity of symptoms and ocular surface changes, including a higher incidence of sterile and bacterial keratitis, suggesting that a disturbance in immune regulation may play a role in pathogenesis. As previously noted, many systemic diseases have been associated with ATD (Table 3-3).

MEDICAL MANAGEMENT The selection of treatment modalities for patients with dry eye depends largely on the severity of their disease (Table 3-4). Mild cases of dry eye may require no more than the use of artificial tear solutions. Preservative-free lubricants can be useful, even at early stages of the disease. Changing or discontinuing any topical or systemic medications that contribute to the condition should be considered, although it is not always practical. Smoking is a risk factor, and advice regarding cessation should be sought. Warm compresses with eyelid massage can also help by bolstering the lipid layer. If the condition is not sufficiently managed with artificial tears, the use of sustained-release ocular lubricants may be considered. It may also be appropriate to modify the patient's environment in an effort to reduce evaporation of the tear film; a humidifier and/or moisture shields on glasses can be helpful. Therapy for patients with severe dry-eye syndrome

Table 3-2 Dry-Eye Severity Grading Scheme

Dry-Eye Severity Level	1	2	3	4*
Discomfort, severity & frequency	Mild and/or episodic; occurs under environmental stress	Moderate episodic or chronic, stress or no stress	Severe frequent or constant without stress	Severe and/or disabling and constant
Visual symptoms	None or episodic mild fatigue	Annoying and/ or activity-limiting episodic	Annoying, chronic and/or constant, limiting activity	Constant and/ or possibly disabling
Conjunctival injection	None to mild	None to mild	+/–	+/++
Conjunctival staining	None to mild	Variable	Moderate to marked	Marked
Corneal staining (severity/ location)	None to mild	Variable	Marked central	Severe punctate erosions
Corneal/tear signs	None to mild	Mild debris, ↓ meniscus	Filamentary keratitis, mucus clumping, ↑ tear debris	Filamentary keratitis, mucus clumping, ↑ tear debris, ulceration
Lid/meibomian glands	MGD variably present	MGD variably present	Frequent	Trichiasis, keratinization, symblepharon
TBUT (sec)	Variable	≤10	≤5	Immediate
Schirmer score (mm/5 min)	Variable	≤10	≤5	≤2

*Must have signs AND symptoms.
TBUT = fluorescein tear break-up time, MGD = meibomian gland disease.

Reprinted with permission from The definition and classification of dry eye disease: report of the Definition and Classification Subcommittee of the International Dry Eye Workshop (2007). *Ocul Surf.* 2007;5(2):75–92.

includes all of the previously noted measures as well as punctal occlusion and occasionally lateral tarsorrhaphy.

The mainstay of treatment for dry-eye syndrome is the use of topical tear substitutes (eyedrops, gels, and ointments). Preservative-free tear substitutes are recommended to avoid toxicity in patients who use these agents frequently. Demulcents are polymers added to artificial tear solutions to improve their lubricant properties. Demulcent solutions are mucomimetic agents that can briefly substitute for glycoproteins lost late in the disease process. Demulcents alone, however, cannot restore lost glycoproteins or conjunctival goblet cells, reduce corneal cell desquamation, or decrease osmolarity. Until relatively recently, all demulcent solutions contained preservatives. Preservative-free demulcent solutions were introduced after it was recognized that preservatives increased corneal desquamation. The elimination of preservatives from traditional demulcent solutions has

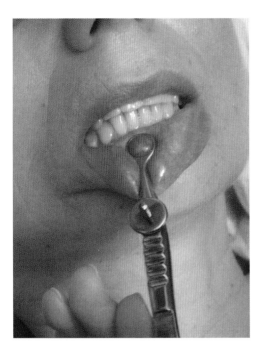

Figure 3-9 Labial gland biopsy. *(Courtesy of Minas T. Coroneo, MD.)*

Table 3-3 Systemic Diseases Associated With Dry Eye

Autoimmune disorders
  Primary Sjögren syndrome
  Secondary Sjögren syndrome associated with
    Rheumatoid arthritis
    Systemic lupus erythematosus
    Progressive systemic sclerosis (scleroderma)
    Polymyositis and dermatomyositis
    Primary biliary cirrhosis
  Graft-vs-host disease
  Immune reactions after radiation to head and neck
Infiltrative processes
  Lymphoma
  Amyloidosis
  Hemochromatosis
  Sarcoidosis
Infectious processes
  HIV-diffuse infiltrative lymphadenopathy syndrome
  Trachoma
Neuropathic dysfunction
  Multiple sclerosis
  Cranial neuropathies (Bell palsy, vasculitis)
  Parkinson disease
  Alzheimer disease
Endocrine dysfunction
  Androgen deficiency

Table 3-4 **Recommended Treatment for Dry Eye**

Severity	Therapeutic Options
Mild	Artificial tears with preservatives up to 4× daily Lubricating ointment at bedtime Hot compresses and eyelid massage
Moderate	Artificial tears without preservatives 4× daily to hourly Lubricating ointment at bedtime Topical anti-inflammatory treatment (cyclosporine A 0.05% 2× daily) Reversible occlusion, lower puncta (plugs)
Severe	All of the above Punctal occlusion (lower and upper) Topical serum drops (20%) 4–6× daily Topical corticosteroids (nonpreserved if available) Moist environment (humidifier, moisture shields) Tarsorrhaphy (lateral and medial) Bandage lenses (rarely)

led to improved corneal barrier function, and subsequent attempts have been made to improve function even further by adding various ions to the solutions.

Topical cyclosporine A 0.05% has been approved by the FDA as a treatment for the inflammatory component of dry eye and is considered to be a major advance. Modulation of the ocular surface inflammatory response might reduce destruction of lacrimal acini and increase neural responsiveness, thereby improving lacrimal secretion. Topical cyclosporine is thus being used earlier in the course of this disease; a small percentage of patients may even gain long-term benefit after an initial course of cyclosporine is stopped. Approximately 70% of patients with moderate to severe dry eye seem to benefit from the use of topical cyclosporine, which to date has shown minimal side effects.

Also, short courses of topical corticosteroids have been used off-label to interrupt the inflammatory cycle in dry-eye patients. Other treatments that have been successfully used in the treatment of severe dry eye are dilute solutions of hyaluronic acid and autologous serum drops (requiring special formulation). The composition of diluted autologous serum is somewhat similar to that of normal tears, particularly in relation to growth factors, and therefore some of the benefit may relate to the trophic function of these substances. Pharmacologic stimulation of tear secretion has been attempted with many compounds, with varying degrees of success. The cholinergic agonists pilocarpine and cevimeline stimulate muscarinic receptors present in salivary and lacrimal glands, thereby increasing secretion. Although studies have shown both to be effective in treating both xerostomia and dry eye in patients with Sjögren syndrome, they are approved only for the treatment of xerostomia. It is uncertain as to whether these agents show long-term benefits.

Treatment of filamentary keratopathy, which sometimes accompanies severe dry-eye conditions, is best directed at controlling the underlying condition, particularly if ATD is responsible. Acetylcysteine 10%, dispensed in an eyedrop container, can be used as a mucolytic agent and is helpful in alleviating these symptoms. Topical anti-inflammatory agents may also be helpful. Wearing goggles, shields, or moisture bubbles can decrease the tear evaporation, although these strategies are generally unacceptable to patients. The surface area available for evaporation can also be decreased simply by fitting the patient with spectacles, which can be further augmented with plastic side shields. Soft contact lenses are used with a high degree of risk in dry-eye patients, although gas-permeable lenses are frequently well tolerated. Scleral contact lenses may also be helpful in patients with severe dry-eye symptoms.

Dry-eye symptoms may be exacerbated by topical glaucoma medications. Chronic use of both topical β-blockers and miotic agents can decrease conjunctival goblet cell density. Topical β-blockers have been associated with an increased incidence of dry eye, possibly due to reduced corneal sensitivity. Oral administration of drugs such as the carbonic anhydrase inhibitors (eg, acetazolamide and methazolamide) can decrease tear production. See also BCSC Section 10, *Glaucoma*.

Many different systemic medications (diuretics, antihistamines, anticholinergics, and psychotropics) decrease aqueous tear production and increase dry-eye symptoms. These drugs should be avoided as much as possible in patients with symptoms of ATD (see Table 3-6).

The psychological problems associated with a highly symptomatic, incurable, chronic disease can require considerable support. Quality-of-life studies have shown that the impact of moderate to severe dry eye is similar to that of having moderate to severe angina. Organizations such as the Sjögren Syndrome Foundation (www.sjogrens.org) can provide valuable resources to these patients. In certain settings, consultation with physicians who specialize in pain management can be very useful.

SURGICAL MANAGEMENT Surgical treatment is generally reserved for patients with severe disease for whom medical treatment is either inadequate or impractical. Patients with moderate to severe dry eye may be helped by punctal occlusion. Tear drainage may be decreased with either reversible or irreversible punctal occlusion. Reversible punctal occlusion can be performed in a number of ways, with varying degrees of effectiveness, using light cautery of the puncta (Fig 3-10), collagen implants, or silicone punctal plugs

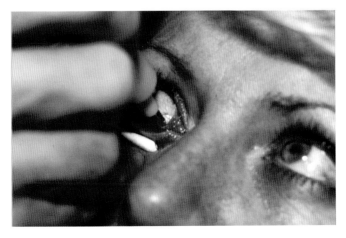

Figure 3-10 Use of cautery for punctal occlusion. *(Courtesy of Charles S. Bouchard, MD.)*

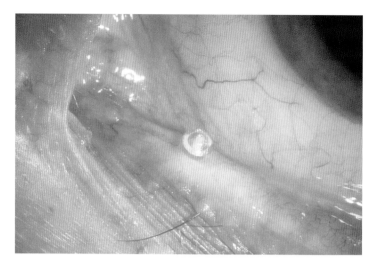

Figure 3-11 Silicone punctal plug. *(Courtesy of Vincent P. deLuise, MD.)*

(Fig 3-11). Collagen plugs usually dissolve within days and do not cause complete cana-licular occlusion. Reversible occlusion may be used as a trial measure before irreversible punctal occlusion is performed. Punctal plugs are available in a variety of sizes and shapes for easy insertion and removal. Instruments that assist in proper sizing of the punctal opening are commercially available. Excessive dilation of the puncta should be avoided. Silicone plugs will generally remain in place for months to years unless they fit loosely or are manually displaced. Once a plug has been displaced, subsequent plugs are more likely to be displaced. Most silicone plugs are continuously visible at the slit lamp, making it obvious if they become displaced. One disadvantage of punctal plugs is that they can be inadvertently inserted into the nasolacrimal system and require surgical removal. One type of plug is designed for intracanalicular placement. If the plug protrudes from the punctum, conjunctival abrasions may occur. Granuloma formation at the punctal open-ing has been observed and requires removal of the plug. In addition, punctual occlusion may lead to reduced tear flow. It appears that the effect of topical cyclosporine is additive to the effect of punctum plugs.

When patients have successfully tolerated reversible punctal occlusion, irreversible punctal occlusion can be performed in the most cost-effective manner with a disposable cautery, a hyfrecator, or a radiofrequency probe. Although the procedure is usually per-manent, the canaliculi and puncta may recanalize following thermal occlusion. The value of punctal occlusion for ocular surface disease other than dry eye is unproven. The proce-dure is recommended primarily for patients in whom basal tear secretion is minimal, with punctate keratopathy, and without significant ocular surface inflammation or infection; this includes especially older patients, in whom the risk of iatrogenically induced epiphora is minimal. Correction of eyelid malpositions such as entropion and ectropion may also be useful in managing patients with dry eye. Reduction of the palpebral aperture by means of lateral and/or medial tarsorrhaphy can be performed in severe KCS when more conser-vative measures have failed. Lateral tarsorrhaphy may limit the temporal visual field and produce a cosmetic defect.

The definition and classification of dry eye disease: report of the Definition and Classification Subcommittee of the International Dry Eye WorkShop. *Ocul Surf.* 2007;5(2):75–92.

Lemp MA. Advances in understanding and managing dry eye disease. *Am J Ophthalmol.* 2008;146(3):350–356.

Pflugfelder SC, Beuerman RW, Stern ME, eds. *Dry Eye and Ocular Surface Disorders.* New York: Informa Healthcare; 2004.

Preferred Practice Patterns Committee, Cornea/External Disease Panel. *Dry Eye Syndrome.* San Francisco: American Academy of Ophthalmology; 2008.

Stern ME, Pflugfelder SC. Inflammation in dry eye. *Ocul Surf.* 2004;2(2):124–130.

Sjögren Syndrome

Patients with ATD are considered to have *Sjögren syndrome (SS)* if they have associated hypergammaglobulinemia, rheumatoid arthritis, or antinuclear antibody. Involvement of the salivary glands is common, resulting in dry mouth and predisposing to periodontal disease. Mucous membranes throughout the body may be affected (ie, vaginal, gastric, and respiratory mucosae) and greatly impact patients' quality of life. Sjögren syndrome can be divided into 2 clinical subsets. *Primary SS* includes patients who either have ill-defined systemic immune dysfunction or lack any evidence of immune dysfunction or connective tissue disease. *Secondary SS* occurs in patients with a well-defined, generalized connective tissue disease. Secondary SS is most commonly associated with rheumatoid arthritis, although numerous other autoimmune diseases are also frequently encountered. The revised international classification criteria for Sjögren syndrome are in Table 3-5. Associated symptoms can include fever, fatigue, Raynaud phenomenon, arthralgias, and myalgias.

Although the precise cause(s) of ATD in SS is unknown, it is generally considered to be a T-cell–mediated inflammatory disease leading to destruction of the lacrimal glands. Pro-inflammatory cytokines (IL-1α and IL-1β, IL-6, IL-8, TGF-β_1, TNF-α), immune activation molecules (ICAM-1, HLA-DR, CD40, CD40 ligand), and proteolytic enzymes (MMP-2, MMP-3, MMP-9, MMP-13) have been reported to be expressed at elevated levels in both lacrimal and ocular surface tissue in patients with SS. These inflammatory mediators play a role in lacrimal tissue destruction, in part, by increasing the rate of programmed cell death (apoptosis).

Lacrimal gland histology provides many insights into the pathogenesis of SS. The histologic changes are usually identical to those noted in the salivary glands, with focal and/or diffuse lymphocytic infiltration associated with areas of glandular destruction. Experimental models of SS show progressive infiltration of autoreactive CD4$^+$ T cells, B cells, and smaller numbers of CD8$^+$ T cells consistent with a cell-mediated pathogenesis. As the disease advances, fibrous replacement of the glandular tissue may occur.

Sensory nerves in the cornea and conjunctiva make up the afferent branch of the lacrimal reflex arc. Sympathetic and parasympathetic nerves form the efferent limb of the reflex arc; these terminate in the lacrimal gland and, when stimulated, induce lacrimal production of water, electrolytes, and protein. Peripheral nervous system dysfunction may be present in as many as 20% of patients with SS and might contribute to ATD.

Androgenic hormones have an important influence on the functional activity of the lacrimal gland, as well as on its immunologic microenvironment. Androgenic receptors

Table 3-5 Criteria for the Classification of Sjögren Syndrome

1. **Ocular symptoms**
   Definition: A positive response to at least 1 of the following 3 questions:
   a. Have you had daily, persistent, troublesome dry eyes for more than 3 months?
   b. Do you have a recurrent sensation of sand or gravel in the eyes?
   c. Do you use tear substitutes more than 3 times a day?
2. **Oral symptoms**
   Definition: A positive response to at least 1 of the following 3 questions:
   a. Have you had a daily feeling of dry mouth for more than 3 months?
   b. Have you had recurrent or persistently swollen salivary glands as an adult?
   c. Do you frequently drink liquids to aid in swallowing dry foods?
3. **Ocular signs**
   Definition: Objective evidence of ocular involvement, determined on the basis of a positive
   result on at least 1 of the following 2 tests:
   a. Schirmer I test (<5 mm in 5 minutes)
   b. Rose bengal score (>4 van Bijsterveld score)
4. **Histopathologic features**
   Definition: Focus score >1 on minor salivary gland biopsy (*focus* defined as a conglomeration
   of at least 50 mononuclear cells; *focus score* defined as the number of foci in 4 mm² of
   glandular tissue)
5. **Salivary gland involvement**
   Definition: Objective evidence of salivary gland involvement, determined on the basis of a
   positive result on at least 1 of the following 3 tests:
   a. Salivary scintography: delayed uptake and/or secretion
   b. Parotid sialography: diffuse sialectasis without obstruction
   c. Unstimulated salivary flow (<1.5 mL in 15 minutes)
6. **Autoantibodies**
   Definition: Presence of at least 1 of the following serum autoantibodies:
   a. Antibodies to Ro/SS-A
   b. Antibodies to La/SS-B antigens

Exclusion criteria: Preexisting lymphoma, acquired immunodeficiency syndrome, sarcoidosis,
or chronic graft-vs-host disease, prior head and neck irradiation, hepatitis C, use of
anticholinergic medications

Primary Sjögren syndrome: Presence of 4 out of 6 items or presence of 3 of 4 objective criteria
(items 3–6)

Secondary Sjögren syndrome: A combination of a positive response to item 1 or 2 plus a positive
response to at least 2 items from among 3, 4, and 5

are found within the epithelial cell nuclei of the conjunctiva, cornea, and meibomian and
lacrimal glands. Deficiency of androgenic hormones may play a contributing role in the
progression of SS. The precise nature of this relationship requires further study.

Viral infections such as Epstein-Barr virus (EBV), type 1 human T-cell lymphotropic virus (HTLV-1), hepatitis C, and human immunodeficiency virus (HIV) have been
associated with the development of Sjögren-like syndromes in both animal models and
humans. Viral infection may contribute to chronic autoimmune destruction of lacrimal
and salivary glands.

Tuisku IS, Konttinen YT, Konttinen LM, Tervo TM. Alterations in corneal sensitivity and
nerve morphology in patients with primary Sjögren's syndrome. *Exp Eye Res.* 2008;86(6):
879–885.

Vitali C, Bombardieri S, Jonsson R, et al. Classification criteria for Sjögren's syndrome: a revised version of the European criteria proposed by the American-European Consensus Group. *Ann Rheum Dis.* 2002;61(6):554–558.

Non–Sjögren Syndrome

In *non–Sjögren syndrome,* ATD can be due to disease of the lacrimal gland, lacrimal gland obstruction, or reflex hyposecretion. Lacrimal disease may be primary, due to congenital conditions such as Riley-Day syndrome (familial dysautonomia); congenital alacrima, or absence of the lacrimal gland; anhidrotic ectodermal dysplasia; Adie syndrome; and idiopathic autonomic dysfunction (Shy-Drager syndrome). Secondary causes of lacrimal disease include sarcoidosis, chronic graft-vs-host disease, HIV, xerophthalmia, and surgical ablation of the lacrimal gland. Obstruction of lacrimal outflow may be caused by severe cicatricial conjunctivitis (trachoma, erythema multiforme, chemical burns, and cicatricial pemphigoid), in which the lacrimal excretory ducts present in the superior conjunctival fornix are destroyed.

Decreased lacrimal secretion can occur as a result of interruption of either the afferent or efferent limb of the reflex arc. Interruption of the afferent limb of the reflex arc can be caused by viral disease (eg, herpes simplex [HSV], varicella-zoster [VZV]), contact lens wear, peripheral neuropathies (eg, diabetes, Bell palsy), surgical disruption (eg, laser in situ keratomileusis [LASIK], photorefractive keratectomy [PRK], penetrating keratoplasty [PK], extracapsular cataract extraction [ECCE]), and aging. Decreased corneal sensation following either PRK or LASIK often results in dry-eye symptoms lasting several months. These symptoms typically resolve following the restoration of normal corneal sensitivity. The efferent limb of the reflex arc can be affected by numerous different systemic anticholinergic medications (Table 3-6).

[handwritten margin note: — ↓ corneal sensation]

[handwritten margin note: – anti-ACh meds can ↓ lacrimal secretion]

Evaporative Tear Dysfunction

Increased tear-film evaporation is most commonly caused by MGD but may also be caused by disease of the meibomian glands, poor apposition of the eyelids to the ocular surface, increase of the palpebral aperture, and contact lens wear. Symptoms consist of burning, foreign-body sensation, redness of the eyelids and conjunctiva, filmy vision, and recurrent chalazia. Signs of ETD include decreased TBUT, MGD, abnormal aqueous tear production, and a characteristic linear pattern of rose bengal/lissamine green staining of the inferior conjunctiva and cornea and eyelid margin.

Meibomian Gland Dysfunction

Meibomian gland dysfunction occurs as a result of progressive obstruction of the meibomian gland orifices due to keratinization. There is a subsequent reduction of lipid delivery to the ocular surface and increased inflammation of the eyelid characterized by hyperemia of the eyelid margin and tarsal conjunctival surface. Meibomian secretions may be clear, cloudy, or thickened. Meibomian orifices may be inspissated (plugged) and may become

Table 3-6 Medications With Anticholinergic Side Effects That Decrease Tear Production

Antihypertensives
Clonidine (α_1-blocker)
Prazosin (α_1-blocker)
Propranolol (β-blocker)
Reserpine
Methyldopa, guanethidine
Antidepressants and psychotropics
Amitriptyline, nortriptyline
Imipramine, desipramine, clomipramine
Doxepin
Phenelzine, tranylcypromine
Amoxapine, trimipramine
Phenothiazines
Nitrazepam, diazepam
Diuretics, sometimes in combination with other antihypertensive drugs
Cardiac antiarrhythmia drugs
Disopyramide
Mexiletine
Amiodarone
Parkinson disease medications
Trihexyphenidyl
Benztropine
Biperiden
Procyclidine
Antiulcer agents
Atropine-like agents
Metoclopramide, other drugs that decrease gastric motility
Muscle spasm medications
Cyclobenzaprine
Methocarbamol
Decongestants (nonprescription cold remedies)
Ephedrine
Pseudoephedrine
Antihistamines
Anesthetics
Enflurane
Halothane
Nitrous oxide
Bisphosphonates
Hormonal: estrogen replacement, androgen antagonists

posteriorly displaced as a result of scarring of the marginal and tarsal mucosa. A variable amount of meibomian gland dropout may also be present.

PATHOGENESIS   MGD is now recognized as a common yet frequently overlooked cause of ocular irritation. It can be broadly classified into obstructive, or hyposecretory, resulting from conditions such as anterior blepharitis, acne rosacea, and pemphigoid; and nonobstructive, or hypersecretory, resulting from meibomian seborrhea. Patients with MGD develop lipid tear deficiency, which results in tear-film instability, increased rate of tear-film evaporation, and elevated tear osmolarity.

CLINICAL PRESENTATION Symptoms consist of burning, foreign-body sensation, redness of the eyelids and conjunctiva, filmy vision, and recurrent chalazia. Inflammation is usually confined to the posterior eyelid margins, conjunctiva, and cornea, although patients may occasionally have associated seborrheic changes on the anterior eyelid margin (Fig 3-12). The posterior eyelid margins are often irregular and have prominent, telangiectatic blood vessels *(brush marks)* coursing from the posterior to anterior eyelid margins. The meibomian gland orifices may pout or show metaplasia, with a white plug of keratin protein extending through the glandular orifice. They also may become posteriorly displaced on the eyelid margin. Meibomian secretions in active disease may be turbid and have increased viscosity. Following years of meibomian gland inflammation, extensive atrophy of the meibomian gland acini may develop and eyelid compression no longer express the meibomian secretions. Atrophy of meibomian gland acini and derangement of glandular architecture can be shown by transillumination of the eyelid as well as infrared photography.

Foam may appear in the tear meniscus along the lower eyelid. Patients frequently have an unstable tear film with rapid TBUTs, particularly in long-standing disease with meibomian gland atrophy and reduced lipid production. Mild to severe ocular surface inflammation may accompany MGD, which may include the following manifestations:

- bulbar and tarsal conjunctival injection
- papillary reaction on the inferior tarsus
- episcleritis
- punctate epithelial erosions in the inferior cornea
- marginal epithelial and subepithelial infiltrates
- corneal neovascularization and scarring *(pannus)*
- corneal thinning

Patients with MGD are frequently noted as having one or more manifestations of rosacea, including facial telangiectasia in an axial distribution (forehead, cheeks, nose, and

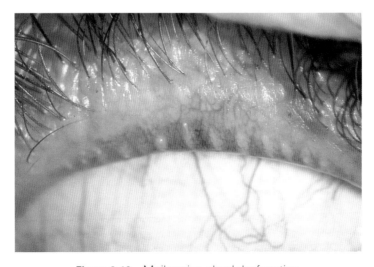

Figure 3-12 Meibomian gland dysfunction.

chin), persistent erythema, papules, pustules, hypertrophic sebaceous glands, and rhino-phyma (see Rosacea later in the chapter). Alterations of the chemical composition of the meibomian secretions have been observed in patients with MGD; however, the precise relationship between these changes and the disease process requires further elucidation.

MANAGEMENT   Eyelid hygiene is the initial treatment for patients with blepharitis. These measures include the application of warm compresses to the eyelids for several minutes in order to liquefy thickened meibomian secretions and soften adherent incrustations on the eyelid margins. The application of heat should be followed by gentle massage of the eyelids to express retained meibomian secretions. Eyelid massage can be followed by cleansing the closed eyelid margin with a clean washcloth, a cotton ball, or a commercially available pad. A diluted solution of a nonirritating shampoo, a commercially available solution designed for this purpose, or a dilute sodium bicarbonate solution (1 teaspoon of salt to 1 pint of boiled water), may facilitate cleansing. Routine performance of eyelid hygiene measures once or twice daily may improve the chronic symptoms of blepharitis. Short-term use of topical antibiotics to reduce the bacterial load on the eyelid margin may be helpful.

If the signs and symptoms of MGD are not adequately controlled with eyelid hygiene, systemic tetracyclines can be very effective. Treatment may be initiated with tetracycline 250 mg orally every 6 hours for the first 3–4 weeks, followed by a tapering dose guided by clinical response (usually 250–500 mg daily). Because tetracycline must be taken on an empty stomach and requires more frequent dosing, doxycycline and minocycline are now used with increasing frequency. The doses of doxycycline and minocycline are 100 mg and 50 mg, respectively, every 12 hours for 3–4 weeks, tapering to 50–100 mg per day, based on clinical response. Lower doses may be equally effective. It often takes 3–4 weeks to achieve a clinical response. Therapy must often be continued on a chronic basis. Erythromycin can be used as alternative therapy in patients with known hypersensitivity to tetracycline or in children. Patients with MGD should be informed that therapy may control but not eliminate their condition.

Side effects of the systemic tetracyclines include photosensitization, gastrointestinal upset, and, in rare instances, azotemia. Chronic use may lead to oral or vaginal candidiasis in susceptible patients. The use of tetracyclines is contraindicated during pregnancy, for women who are nursing, and in patients with a known hypersensitivity to these agents. These agents should be used with caution in women in the child-bearing age range, women with a family history of breast cancer, patients with a history of liver disease, and patients taking certain anticoagulants (eg, warfarin). Tetracyclines may also reduce the efficacy of oral contraceptives. These antibiotics should also be avoided in children younger than 8 years of age because they cause permanent discoloration in teeth and bones.

Topical corticosteroids may be required for short periods in cases with moderate to severe inflammation, particularly those with corneal infiltrates and vascularization. Patients treated with topical corticosteroids should be warned about the complications of chronic use, because this stubborn condition may prompt patients to become dependent.

Preliminary evidence has shown some benefit from the use of systemic omega-3 fatty acid supplements in some patients with MGD. The ultimate benefits and precise dosage required for a beneficial effect remain to be determined.

Bron AJ, Tiffany JM. The contribution of meibomian disease to dry eye. *Ocul Surf.* 2004;2(2): 149–165.

Driver PJ, Lemp MA. Meibomian gland dysfunction. *Surv Ophthalmol.* 1996;40(5):343–367.

Preferred Practice Patterns Committee, Cornea/External Disease Panel. *Blepharitis.* San Francisco: American Academy of Ophthalmology; 2008.

Rosacea

PATHOGENESIS *Rosacea* (sometimes called *acne rosacea*) is a chronic acneiform disorder that can affect both the skin and eyes. This disease has no proven cause. It is associated with cutaneous sebaceous gland dysfunction of the face, neck, and shoulders. Although rosacea has generally been thought to be more common in fair-skinned individuals, it may simply be more difficult to diagnose in persons with dark skin. It is infrequently diagnosed by ophthalmologists, in spite of its relatively frequent association with blepharitis and/or ATD. Diagnosis can be made difficult by dim lighting in ophthalmologic offices and may be made easier by asking about related symptoms. Although alcohol can contribute to a worsening of this disorder because of its effect on vasomotor stability, most patients with rosacea do not have a history of excessive alcohol intake. Experimental studies based on immunohistochemical staining of inflammatory cell infiltrates have shown this disease to represent a delayed hypersensitivity reaction. Dysfunction of the meibomian and other lipid-producing glands of the eyelids and skin of the face are believed to be responsible for these infiltrates.

CLINICAL PRESENTATION A skin condition that frequently involves the eyes, rosacea is characterized by excessive sebum secretion with a frequently recalcitrant chronic blepharitis. Eyelid margin telangiectasia is very common, as are meibomian gland distortion, disruption, and dysfunction, which can lead to recurrent chalazia. Ocular involvement can also progress, leading to chronic conjunctivitis, marginal corneal infiltrates, sterile ulceration, episcleritis, or iridocyclitis (Fig 3-13). If properly treated, these lesions can resolve with few sequelae. Repeated bouts of ocular surface inflammation can bring about corneal neovascularization and scarring, often in a characteristic triangular configuration (Fig 3-14).

This disorder is generally found in patients aged 30–60, with a slight female preponderance. However, ocular rosacea can be encountered in younger patients and is often underdiagnosed. Facial lesions consist of telangiectasias, recurrent papules and pustules, and midfacial erythema (Fig 3-15). Rosacea is characterized by a malar rash with unpredictable flushing episodes, sometimes associated with the consumption of alcohol, coffee, or other foods. *Rhinophyma,* thickening of the skin and connective tissue of the nose, is a characteristic and obvious sign associated with this disorder, but such hypertrophic cutaneous changes occur relatively late in the disease process.

MANAGEMENT The ocular and systemic diseases are managed simultaneously, with systemic tetracyclines as the mainstay of therapy. Tetracyclines have anti-inflammatory properties that include suppression of leukocyte migration, reduced production of nitric oxide and reactive oxygen species, inhibition of matrix metalloproteinases, and inhibition of phospholipase A2. In addition, tetracyclines may reduce irritative free fatty acids and diglycerides by suppressing bacterial lipases.

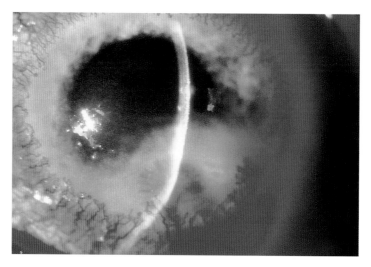

Figure 3-13   Marginal keratitis associated with rosacea.

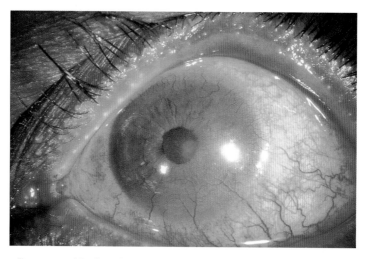

Figure 3-14   Rosacea with chronic superficial keratopathy and corneal neovascularization.

—topical metronidazole With time, oral therapy with doxycycline or minocycline can be tapered. In addition to oral therapy, application of topical metronidazole 0.75% gel (Metrogel) or 1% cream (Noritate) to the affected facial areas can significantly reduce facial erythema.

Ulcerative keratitis can be associated with infectious agents in rosacea, or it may have a sterile inflammatory etiology. Once it is ascertained that ulceration is noninfectious, topical corticosteroids, used judiciously, can play a significant role in reducing sterile inflammation and enhancing epithelialization of the cornea. In advanced cases with scarring and neovascularization, conservative therapy is generally recommended. Penetrating keratoplasty in rosacea patients is a high-risk procedure that may have a poor prognosis if the ocular surface is severely compromised.

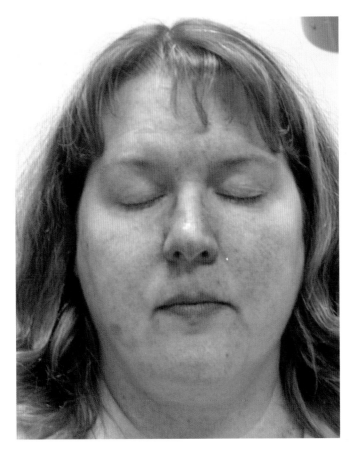

Figure 3-15 Facial characteristics of moderate acne rosacea. *(Courtesy of James J. Reidy, MD.)*

Bron AJ, Benjamin L, Snibson GR. Meibomian gland disease. Classification and grading of lid changes. *Eye.* 1991;5(Pt 4):395–411.

Stone DU, Chodosh J. Ocular rosacea: an update on pathogenesis and therapy. *Curr Opin Ophthalmol.* 2004;15(6):499–502.

Seborrheic Blepharitis

CLINICAL PRESENTATION   Seborrheic blepharitis may occur alone or in combination with staphylococcal blepharitis or MGD. Inflammation occurs primarily at the anterior eyelid margin; a variable amount of crusting, typically of an oily or greasy nature, may be found — *crusting on lids* on the eyelids, eyelashes, eyebrows, and scalp. Patients with seborrheic blepharitis often have increased meibomian gland secretions that appear turbid when expressed. Signs and symptoms include chronic eyelid redness, burning, and occasionally foreign-body sensation. A small percentage of patients (approximately 15%) develop an associated keratitis or conjunctivitis. The keratitis is characterized by punctate epithelial erosions distributed over the inferior third of the cornea. Approximately one third of patients with seborrheic blepharitis have ATD.

MANAGEMENT Eyelid hygiene is the primary treatment in patients with blepharitis. This regimen was detailed earlier, in the discussion of MGD. Concurrent treatment of scalp disease (eg, with coal tar–based shampoos) can also improve blepharitis.

If inflammation is a prominent component of the blepharitis, a brief course of topical corticosteroid applied to the eyelid margins may be helpful. If blepharitis involves primarily the posterior eyelid margin (eg, MGD), systemic antibiotics such as doxycycline are the mainstay of treatment. Blepharitis caused by bacteria (eg, staphylococcus) often responds to the use of a topical antibiotic ointment such as bacitracin or bacitracin–polymyxin B. (Staphylococcal blepharitis is discussed further in Chapter 5.)

Chalazion

CLINICAL PRESENTATION A *chalazion* is a localized lipogranulomatous inflammation involving either the meibomian or Zeis glands. It usually develops spontaneously as a result of obstruction of one or more of the glands. The nodules develop slowly and are typically painless. The overlying skin is erythematous (Fig 3-16). The lesion disappears in weeks to months when the contents drain either externally through the eyelid skin or internally through the tarsus, or when the extruded lipid is phagocytosed and the granuloma dissipates. A small amount of scar tissue may remain. Occasionally, patients with a chalazion may experience blurred vision secondary to astigmatism induced by its pressure on the globe.

PATHOGENESIS AND LABORATORY EVALUATION Sebaceous material trapped in a plugged Zeis or meibomian gland extrudes into adjacent tissues, where it elicits chronic granulomatous inflammation. A zonal granulomatous inflammatory response centered around lipid is seen histologically. As is typical of all granulomas, epithelioid cells are prominent. Also present are admixtures of other cells, including lymphocytes, macrophages, neutrophils, plasma cells, and giant cells. It must be emphasized that basal cell, squamous cell, and

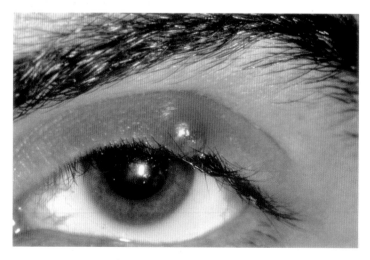

Figure 3-16 Chalazion. *(Courtesy of Vincent P. deLuise, MD.)*

sebaceous cell carcinoma can masquerade as chalazia or chronic blepharitis. The histopathologic examination of persistent, recurrent, or atypical chalazia is therefore quite important.

MANAGEMENT Because most chalazia are sterile, topical antibiotic therapy is of little or no value. Chalazia may be treated with hot compresses and attempted expression of the inflamed meibomian gland. Lesions that fail to respond to conservative therapy may be treated with intralesional injection of a corticosteroid (0.1–0.2 mL triamcinolone 10 mg/mL), incision and drainage, or a combination of both. In general, an intralesional corticosteroid injection works best with small chalazia, with chalazia on the eyelid margin, and with multiple chalazia. An intralesional corticosteroid injection in patients with dark skin may lead to depigmentation of the overlying eyelid skin and thus should be used with caution.

Larger chalazia are best treated with surgical drainage and curettage. Internal chalazia require vertical incisions through the tarsal conjunctiva along the meibomian gland to facilitate drainage and avoid horizontal scarring of the tarsal plates. Surgical drainage usually requires perilesional anesthesia. Recurrent chalazia should be biopsied to rule out meibomian gland carcinoma. Systemic tetracyclines can be of benefit in patients with associated rosacea.

Epstein GA, Putterman AM. Combined excision and drainage with intralesional corticosteroid injection in the treatment of chronic chalazia. *Arch Ophthalmol.* 1988;106(4):514–516.

Hordeolum

Hordeola are discussed in Chapter 5.

Sarcoidosis

Sarcoidosis is a multisystem disorder characterized by the development of noncaseating granulomatous inflammation in affected tissues. Evidence suggests that the etiology of systemic sarcoidosis is linked to a genetically predetermined enhancement of cellular immune responses (Th1/CD4+) to a limited number of microbial pathogens. Ocular involvement is seen in up to 50% of affected patients. Nontender small (millet seed) or large nodules may be seen in the eyelid skin and in the canthal region. Lacrimal gland involvement occurs in up to 25% of patients with ocular involvement, resulting in KCS. Concomitant enlargement of the lacrimal and salivary glands combined with the presence of dry eye is known as *Mikulicz syndrome*. Patients with *Lofgren syndrome* present with erythema nodosum, hilar adenopathy, and iridocyclitis. Patients presenting with uveitis, fever, and facial nerve palsy (uveoparotid fever) have *Heerfordt syndrome*.

Conjunctival granulomas have been observed in approximately 7% of patients with ocular involvement. Such granulomas are often small and easily overlooked, and they may be difficult to distinguish from normal conjunctival follicles. The most common corneal finding is calcific band keratopathy, often associated with chronic uveitis or elevated serum calcium levels. Nummular keratitis, thickening of Descemet's membrane, and deep stromal vascularization as a result of chronic intraocular inflammation can be seen. Granulomatous uveitis with mutton-fat keratic precipitates and iris nodules occurs in as many as two thirds of patients with ocular involvement. Periphlebitis is the most common fundus finding. Chronic cystoid macular edema and exudative retinal detachment are related to intense and long-standing inflammation. Granulomatous involvement of the optic nerve is also seen.

Moller DR, Chen ES. What causes sarcoidosis? *Curr Opin Pulm Med.* 2002;8(5):429–434.

See also BCSC Section 9, *Intraocular Inflammation and Uveitis,* for illustrations and further discussion of sarcoidosis.

Desquamating Skin Conditions: Ichthyosis

Ichthyosis represents a diverse group of hereditary skin disorders characterized by excessively dry skin and accumulation of scale. The disease is usually diagnosed during the first year of life. *Ichthyosis vulgaris,* an autosomal dominant trait, is the most common hereditary scaling disorder, affecting 1 in 250–300 people. Ocular involvement varies with the form of ichthyosis. Eyelid scaling, cicatricial ectropion, and conjunctival thickening are common. Primary corneal opacities are seen in 50% of patients with *X-linked ichthyosis* but are rarely seen in ichthyosis vulgaris. Dots or filament-shaped opacities appear diffusely in pre–Descemet's membrane or in deep stroma and become more apparent with age without affecting vision. Nodular corneal degeneration and band keratopathy have been described. Secondary corneal changes such as vascularization and scarring from severe ectropion-related exposure can develop.

Ichthyosis is a prominent feature in several genetic disorders, including Sjögren-Larsson, Rud, and Conradi syndromes, congenital *k*eratitis-*i*chthyosis-*d*eafness (KID) syndrome, Refsum disease, and *c*ongenital *h*emidysplasia with *i*chthyosiform eryth-roderma and *l*imb *d*efects (CHILD). Vascularizing keratitis is a prominent feature of KID syndrome; it may worsen with isotretinoin therapy. Treatment for the ichthyosis spectrum is aimed at hydrating the skin and eyelids, removing scale, and slowing the turnover of epidermis when appropriate. These disorders are not responsive to corticosteroids.

Ectodermal Dysplasia

Ectodermal dysplasia is a heterogeneous group of conditions characterized by the following:

- presence of abnormalities at birth
- nonprogressive course
- diffuse involvement of the epidermis plus at least one of its appendages (hair, nails, teeth, sweat glands)
- various inheritance patterns

Ectodermal dysplasia is a rare hereditary condition that displays variable defects in the morphogenesis of ectodermal structures, including hair, skin, nails, and teeth. It has been observed to be a component in at least 150 distinct hereditary syndromes.

Many ocular abnormalities have been described in the ectodermal dysplasias, including sparse lashes and brows, blepharitis, ankyloblepharon, hypoplastic lacrimal ducts, diminished tear production, abnormal meibomian glands, dry conjunctivae, pterygia, corneal scarring and neovascularization, cataract, and glaucoma. These changes may be due to limbal stem cell deficiency.

Anhidrotic ectodermal dysplasia is characterized by hypotrichosis, anodontia, and anhidrosis. Sweating is almost completely lacking, and hyperpyrexia is a common problem in childhood. Atopic disease is often an associated finding. The *ectodactyly-ectodermal dysplasial-clefting (EEC)* syndrome is an association of ectodermal dysplasia, cleft lip and/or palate, and a clefting deformity of the hands and/or feet ("lobster claw deformity").

Xeroderma Pigmentosum

Xeroderma pigmentosum (XP) is a recessively transmitted disease characterized by impaired ability to repair sunlight-induced damage to DNA. During the first or second decade of life, the patient's exposed skin develops areas of focal hyperpigmentation, atrophy, actinic keratosis, and telangiectasia—as though the patient had received a heavy dose of radiation. Many cutaneous neoplasms appear later, including squamous cell carcinoma, basal cell carcinoma, and melanoma.

Ophthalmic manifestations include photophobia, tearing, blepharospasm, and signs and symptoms of KCS. The conjunctiva is dry and inflamed with telangiectasia and hyperpigmentation. Pingueculae and pterygia often occur. Corneal complications include exposure keratitis, ulceration, neovascularization, scarring, and even perforation. Keratoconus, band-shaped nodular corneal dystrophy, and gelatinous dystrophy have also been reported. Ocular neoplasms occur in 11% of patients, most frequently at the limbus. Squamous cell carcinoma is the most frequent histologic type seen, followed by basal cell carcinoma and melanoma, similar to the cutaneous tumors. The eyelids can be involved with progressive atrophy, madarosis, trichiasis, scarring, symblepharon, entropion, ectropion, and sometimes even loss of the entire lower eyelid.

Mannis MJ, Macsai MS, Huntley AC, eds. *Eye and Skin Disease.* Philadelphia: Lippincott-Raven; 1996:3–12, 39–44, 131–145.

Noninflammatory Vascular Anomalies of the Conjunctiva

Causes of conjunctival hyperemia include the following:

- *inflammation:* infection, allergy, toxicity, neoplasia
- *direct irritation:* foreign body, aberrant eyelashes
- *reflex response:* eyestrain, emotional weeping
- *systemic or topical vasodilators:* alcohol, oxygen, carcinoid tumor
- *autonomic dysfunction:* sympathetic paresis, sphenopalatine ganglion syndrome
- *vascular engorgement:* venous obstruction, hyperviscosity

Conjunctival vascular tortuosity may result from trauma or from disorders such as rosacea and Fabry disease that cause chronic conjunctival vascular dilation. Systemic conditions that cause sludging and segmentation of blood flow in conjunctival vessels, as well as conjunctival varicosities and aneurysms, include

- hypertension
- diabetes mellitus
- sickle cell disease
- multiple myeloma
- polycythemia vera

Causes of subconjunctival hemorrhage and, less commonly, of bloody tears are listed in Table 3-7. Hereditary causes of conjunctival telangiectasia and hemorrhage are hereditary hemorrhagic telangiectasia and ataxia-telangiectasia.

Hereditary Hemorrhagic Telangiectasia

Spontaneous hemorrhage from telangiectatic vessels of the palpebral and bulbar conjunctiva may occur in individuals with hereditary hemorrhagic telangiectasia (Rendu-Osler-Weber disease), a vascular disorder that also involves the skin, nasal and oral mucous membranes, gastrointestinal tract, lungs, and brain. This dominantly inherited (but occasionally sporadic) disease is usually not apparent in early childhood, and its onset during early adult life may be subtle. Initial manifestations may be intermittent, painless gastrointestinal bleeding leading to iron deficiency anemia or recurrent epistaxis following minor trauma or occurring spontaneously.

Conjunctival hemorrhage may be associated with foreign-body sensation, and it usually occurs spontaneously or after minor trauma, such as rubbing of the eyelids. The hemorrhage may extend into the subepithelial connective tissues or may be external (bloody tears). Conjunctival bleeding can be copious, but in most instances it can be controlled with local pressure. The conjunctival telangiectasias appear sharply circumscribed, are slightly elevated, and are composed of arborizing dilated channels. Typically, they involve the palpebral region, although lesions of the bulbar conjunctiva have also been reported.

Histologic study has shown superficial, dilated, thin-walled vascular channels. Similar findings have been noted in telangiectatic lesions of the skin and nasal and oral mucous membranes. It is likely that hemorrhage results from minor trauma to these superficial vessels; however, intravascular factors affecting bleeding time may also play a role.

Lymphangiectasia

Lymphangiectasia may be a developmental anomaly or may occur in association with trauma or inflammation. Unlike lymphangiomas, which are cellular proliferations of lymphatic

Table 3-7 Causes of Subconjunctival Hemorrhage

Ocular	Systemic
Conjunctival, orbital, or cranial trauma	Sudden venous congestion (Valsalva maneuver)
Acute viral or bacterial conjunctivitis	Vascular fragility
	Thrombocytopenia and impaired clotting
	Systemic febrile illness
Pterygium, pinguecula	Ocular surface neovascularization

channel elements, lymphangiectasias are irregularly dilated, periodically hemorrhage-filled lymphatic channels of the bulbar conjunctiva. Surrounding conjunctival edema or subconjunctival hemorrhage may also be present, especially upon crying or exertion. Treatment is local excision or diathermy.

Lymphangiectasia must be distinguished from *ataxia-telangiectasia (Louis-Bar syndrome)*, in which the epibulbar and interpalpebral telangiectasia of the arteries lacks an associated lymphatic component. The conjunctival lesions of Louis-Bar syndrome are a marker for associated cerebellar and immunologic abnormalities (eg, hypogammaglobulinemia), which are conducive to sinopulmonary infection and lymphoreticular proliferations, particularly T-cell leukemias. The epibulbar vascular lesions do not acquire a tumefactive characteristic (hamartia) because they are simple telangiectasias that grow with the patient and the eyeball. No episodic events of hemorrhage or swelling are encountered. Ataxia-telangiectasia is discussed and illustrated in greater detail in BCSC Section 6, *Pediatric Ophthalmology and Strabismus.*

Nutritional and Physiologic Disorders

Vitamin A Deficiency

PATHOGENESIS Vitamin A is an essential fat-soluble vitamin. Human disease can be caused by too little or too much vitamin A intake. Table 3-8 presents an overview of vitamin A metabolism.

Vitamin A deficiency xerosis (dryness of the conjunctiva and cornea), associated with loss of mucus production by the goblet cells, can occur in epithelial cells of the gastrointestinal, genitourinary, and respiratory tracts. The ocular consequence is the *Bitôt spot*, a superficial foamy, gray triangular area on the bulbar conjunctiva that appears in the palpebral aperture (Fig 3-17). This spot consists of keratinized epithelium, inflammatory cells, debris, and *Corynebacterium xerosis.* These bacilli metabolize the debris and produce the foamy appearance.

Vitamin A deficiency leads to *xerophthalmia,* which is responsible for at least 20,000–100,000 new cases of blindness worldwide each year. At greatest risk of xerophthalmia are malnourished infants and babies born to vitamin A–deficient mothers, especially infants who have another biological stressor, such as measles or diarrhea. Superficial concurrent infections with herpes simplex, measles, or bacterial agents probably further predispose the child to keratomalacia and blindness. Although xerophthalmia usually results from

Table 3-8 Metabolism of Vitamin A

Level	Metabolite
Diet	Plant (carotenoids) and animal (retinyl-palmitate and retinol) foods
Intestine	Retinol-micelle
Portal circulation	Retinyl-palmitate
Liver	Retinol–retinol-binding protein
Target tissues	Retinoic acid (epithelium, epidermis, and lymphocytes)
	Retinal (rod photoreceptors)

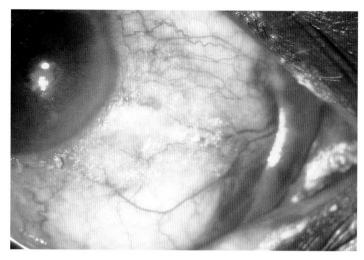

Figure 3-17 Conjunctival xerosis with focal keratinization (Bitôt spot) as a result of vitamin A deficiency. *(Courtesy of Vincent P. deLuise, MD.)*

low dietary intake of vitamin A, decreased absorption of vitamin A may also be responsible. When vitamin A deficiency and xerophthalmia occur in countries with a low rate of malnutrition, the condition is usually caused by unusual self-imposed dietary practices, chronic alcoholism, or lipid malabsorption (particularly cystic fibrosis, biliary cirrhosis, and bowel resection).

CLINICAL PRESENTATION *Nyctalopia* (night blindness) is often the earliest symptom of hypovitaminosis A, but retinal function does not always correlate with anterior segment findings. *Xerophthalmic fundus,* a rare associated abnormality, features yellow-white spots in the peripheral retina.

Prolonged vitamin A deficiency leads to involvement of the external eye, including xerosis, metaplastic keratinization of areas of the conjunctiva (Bitôt spots), corneal ulcers and scars, and eventually diffuse corneal necrosis (keratomalacia). The World Health Organization classifies the ocular surface changes into 3 stages:

1. conjunctival xerosis, without (X1A) or with (X1B) Bitôt spots
2. corneal xerosis (X2)
3. corneal ulceration, with keratomalacia involving less than one third (X3A) or more than one third (X3B) of the corneal surface

Patients with chronic alcoholism may present with persistent epithelial defect and corneal ulceration unresponsive to antimicrobial therapy. Night blindness with an abnormal electroretinogram, visual field constriction, and conjunctival xerosis or Bitôt spots may be the presenting manifestation of the chronic malabsorption syndromes just mentioned. Laboratory diagnosis of low serum level of vitamin A or retinol-binding proteins is usually used to confirm the clinical suspicion.

MANAGEMENT Systemic vitamin A deficiency, best characterized by keratomalacia, is a medical emergency with an untreated mortality rate of 50%. Although the administration of oral or parenteral vitamin A will address the acute manifestations of keratomalacia, these patients are usually affected by a much larger protein-energy malnutrition and should be treated with both vitamin and protein-calorie supplements. Problems with malabsorption may prevent oral administration from being effective in patients with acute vitamin A deficiency. Maintenance of adequate corneal lubrication and prevention of secondary infection and corneal melting are essential steps in treating keratomalacia, but identification and proper treatment of the underlying causes are vital to successful clinical management of the ocular complications.

As a result of the beneficial effects of systemic retinoids in xerophthalmia, studies were undertaken to determine if topical retinoids would be useful in reversing the squamous metaplasia and symptoms associated with dry-eye syndromes. Although double-blind, placebo-controlled studies failed to demonstrate the efficacy of topical therapy for patients with dry eye alone, subsequent studies revealed that topical retinoids were primarily useful in conditions with conjunctival keratinization, such as Stevens-Johnson syndrome, cicatricial pemphigoid, radiation-induced dry eye, drug-induced pseudopemphigoid, and toxic epidermal necrolysis. Currently, an ophthalmic preparation of topical retinoic acid is not commercially available in the United States.

Harris EW, Loewenstein JI, Azar D. Vitamin A deficiency and its effects on the eye. *Int Ophthalmol Clin.* 1998;38(1):155–161.

Sommer A, West KP Jr. *Vitamin A Deficiency: Health, Survival, and Vision.* New York: Oxford University Press; 1996.

Vitamin C Deficiency

Ascorbic acid, or vitamin C, is an essential vitamin for humans because we lack its synthetic enzyme, L-gulonolactone oxidase. A major action mechanism of ascorbic acid is its effect as a cofactor on the hydroxylation of lysine and proline in ribosomal collagen synthesis. Impairment of hydroxylation secondary to ascorbic acid deficiency results in unstable collagen fiber formation.

Following transport through the ciliary epithelium, ascorbic acid is about 15–20 times more concentrated in aqueous humor than in plasma. In scurvy, subconjunctival and orbital hemorrhage may occur. In a vitamin C–deprivation trial extending over approximately 3 months, some subjects developed xerosis. In animal studies, scorbutic guinea pig corneas subjected to injury showed impaired wound healing. Animal studies also suggest that the alkali-burned cornea represents a localized scorbutic state in which adequate collagen cannot be synthesized for stromal wound repair. In rabbit eyes, topical and parenteral ascorbate can restore the ascorbate level in aqueous humor after an alkali burn and significantly reduce the incidence of corneal ulcer and perforation. A well-controlled, prospective, case-controlled study proving the clinical efficacy of topical or systemic ascorbate in humans has yet to be done.

Pfister RR, Paterson CA. Ascorbic acid in the treatment of alkali burns of the eye. *Ophthalmology.* 1980;87(10):1050–1057.

Structural and Exogenous Disorders

Exposure Keratopathy

PATHOGENESIS   Exposure keratopathy can result from any disease process that limits eyelid closure. Lagophthalmos can be caused by the following:

- neurogenic diseases such as seventh nerve palsy
- degenerative neurologic conditions such as Parkinson disease
- cicatricial or restrictive eyelid diseases such as ectropion
- drug abuse
- blepharoplasty
- skin disorders such as Stevens-Johnson syndrome or xeroderma pigmentosum

Proptosis caused by thyroid eye disease or other inflammatory or infiltrative orbital diseases can also result in exposure keratopathy.

CLINICAL PRESENTATION   Exposure keratopathy is characterized by a punctate epithelial keratopathy that usually involves the inferior third of the cornea, although the entire corneal surface can be involved in more severe cases. Large, coalescent epithelial defects may result, which may lead to ulceration, melting, and perforation. Symptoms are similar to those associated with dry eye, including foreign-body sensation, photophobia, and tearing, unless there is an associated neurotrophic component resulting in corneal anesthesia.

MANAGEMENT   Therapy is similar to that described for severe dry eye. In the earliest stages, nonpreserved artificial tears during the day and ointment at bedtime may suffice. Taping the eyelid shut at bedtime can be helpful if the problem is primarily one of nocturnal exposure. The use of bandage contact lenses can be hazardous in these patients because of a high incidence of desiccation and infection. In cases where the problem is likely to be temporary or self-limited, a temporary tarsorrhaphy using tissue adhesive or sutures should be performed. However, if the problem is likely to be long-standing, definitive surgical therapy to correct the eyelid position is mandatory. Correction of any associated eyelid abnormalities, such as ectropion and/or trichiasis, is also indicated.

Most commonly, surgical management consists of permanent lateral and/or medial tarsorrhaphy. Insertion of gold or platinum weights into the upper eyelid is also an effective technique to promote eyelid closure. Implantation of an eyelid weight does not alter the dimension of the horizontal eyelid fissure and thus creates a less obvious cosmetic change than does a lateral tarsorrhaphy. Reported complications of gold weight implants include infection, shifting, extrusion, induced astigmatism, unacceptable ptosis, and noninfectious inflammatory response to the gold. The weights remain stable when exposed to MRI. In cases of paralytic ectropion of the lower eyelid, a horizontal tightening procedure may also be beneficial in correcting the flaccid lower eyelid.

See BCSC Section 7, *Orbit, Eyelids, and Lacrimal System,* for further discussion of lagophthalmos and proptosis.

Floppy Eyelid Syndrome

Floppy eyelid syndrome usually occurs in obese individuals who are often suffering from obstructive sleep apnea and consists of chronic ocular irritation and inflammation. Patients have a flimsy, lax upper tarsus that everts with minimal upward force applied to the upper eyelid. Clinical findings include small to large papillae on the upper palpebral conjunctiva, mucus discharge, and corneal involvement ranging from mild punctate epitheliopathy to superficial vascularization (Fig 3-18). Keratoconus has also been reported in patients with floppy eyelid syndrome. The problem may result from spontaneous eversion of the upper eyelid when it comes into contact with the pillow or other bedclothes during sleep. Direct contact of the upper eyelid with bed linens may traumatize the upper tarsal conjunctiva, inducing inflammation and chronic irritation. The condition may be unilateral if the patient always sleeps in the same position. Treatment consists of covering the affected eye(s) with a metal shield or taping eyelids closed at night or performing surgical eyelid-tightening procedures. Differential diagnosis includes vernal conjunctivitis, giant papillary conjunctivitis, atopic keratoconjunctivitis, bacterial conjunctivitis, and toxic keratopathy. See also BCSC Section 7, *Orbit, Eyelids, and Lacrimal System.*

Pham TT, Perry JD. Floppy eyelid syndrome. *Curr Opin Ophthalmol.* 2007;18(5):430–433.

Superior Limbic Keratoconjunctivitis

PATHOGENESIS   The pathogenesis of *superior limbic keratoconjunctivitis (SLK)* has not been established, although it is thought to result from mechanical trauma transmitted from the upper eyelid to the superior bulbar and tarsal conjunctiva. An association with autoimmune thyroid disease has been observed.

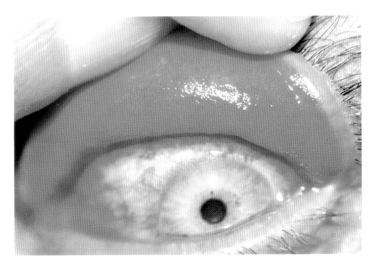

Figure 3-18   Floppy eyelid syndrome with papillary response on superior tarsus. *(Courtesy of Vincent P. deLuise, MD.)*

CLINICAL PRESENTATION   SLK is a chronic, recurrent condition of ocular irritation and redness. The condition typically develops in adult women 20–70 years of age, and may recur over a period of 1–10 years. The condition usually resolves spontaneously. It is often bilateral, although 1 eye may be more severely affected than the other. SLK can be associated with ATD or blepharospasm. Ocular findings may include the following:

- a fine papillary reaction on the superior tarsal conjunctiva
- injection and thickening of the superior bulbar conjunctiva (Fig 3-19A)
- hypertrophy of the superior limbus
- fine punctate fluorescein and rose bengal staining of the superior bulbar conjunctiva above the limbus and superior cornea just below the limbus (Fig 3-19B)
- superior corneal filamentary keratopathy

LABORATORY EVALUATION   Hyperproliferation, acanthosis, loss of goblet cells, and keratinization are seen in histologic sections of the superior bulbar conjunctiva. The condition can often be diagnosed by clinical signs; however, scrapings or impression cytology of the superior bulbar conjunctiva showing characteristic features of nuclear pyknosis with "snake nuclei," increased epithelial cytoplasm-to-nucleus ratio, loss of goblet cells, and keratinization may be helpful in diagnosing mild or confusing cases. Patients with SLK should have thyroid function tests, including T_4, TSH, and antithyroid antibody levels.

MANAGEMENT   A variety of therapies have been reported to provide temporary or permanent relief of symptoms. Treatments include topical anti-inflammatory agents, large-diameter bandage contact lenses, superior punctal occlusion, thermocauterization of the superior bulbar conjunctiva, resection of the bulbar conjunctiva superior to the limbus, topical cyclosporine, autologous serum eyedrops, and conjunctival fixation sutures.

Sahin A, Bozkurt B, Irkec M. Topical cyclosporine A in the treatment of superior limbic keratoconjunctivitis: a long-term follow-up. *Cornea.* 2008;27(2):193–195.

Theodore FH, Ferry AP. Superior limbic keratoconjunctivitis. Clinical and pathological correlations. *Arch Ophthalmol.* 1970;84(4):481–484.

Yamada M, Hatou S, Mochizuki H. Conjunctival fixation sutures for refractory superior limbic keratoconjunctivitis. *Br J Ophthalmol.* 2009;93(12):1570–1571.

Yang HY, Fujishima H, Toda I, Shimazaki J, Tsubota K. Lacrimal punctal occlusion for the treatment of superior limbic keratoconjunctivitis. *Am J Ophthalmol.* 1997;124(1):80–87.

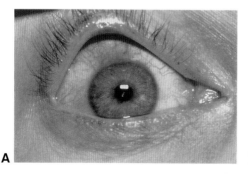 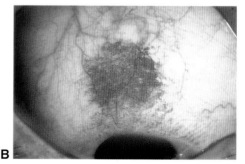

A   B

Figure 3-19   A, Superior limbic keratoconjunctivitis. **B,** Rose bengal dye staining pattern in superior limbic keratoconjunctivitis. *(Courtesy of Vincent P. deLuise, MD.)*

Recurrent Corneal Erosion

PATHOGENESIS   Recurrent erosions typically occur either in eyes that have suffered a sudden, sharp, abrading injury (fingernail, paper cut, tree branch) or in patients with pre-existing epithelial basement membrane dystrophy. This condition may also occur more commonly after PRK. The superficial injury produces an epithelial abrasion that heals rapidly, frequently leaving no clinical evidence of damage. After an interval varying from days to years, symptoms suddenly recur without any obvious precipitating event. Symptoms subside spontaneously in most cases, only to recur periodically. In contrast to shearing injuries, small superficial lacerating injuries involving the cornea rarely result in recurrent erosions. Poor adhesion of the epithelium is thought to be caused by underlying abnormalities in the epithelial basement membrane and its associated filament network. The precise nature of these abnormalities has yet to be fully determined.

Gelatinase activity (MMP-2 and -9) is up-regulated in the epithelium of patients with recurrent corneal erosions. Gelatinases alter the epithelial basement membrane during wound healing by cleaving collagen types IV, V, VII, and X. They also act on the adhesive macromolecules fibronectin and laminin, which are thought to mediate attachment of the basal epithelial cells to the basement membrane. Activation of MMPs on a chronic basis may be either a result of, or the cause of, poor epithelial adherence that leads to the symptoms of recurrent corneal erosion. Some patients with recurrent corneal erosions have been noted to have MGD, and increased levels of MMPs have been observed in the tear film of patients with MGD.

CLINICAL PRESENTATION   Recurrent corneal erosions are characterized by the sudden onset of eye pain, usually at night or upon first awakening, accompanied by redness, photophobia, and tearing. Individual episodes may vary in severity and duration. Minor episodes usually last from 30 minutes to several hours; typically the cornea has an intact epithelial surface at the time of examination. More severe episodes may last for several days and are often associated with greater pain, eyelid edema, decreased visual acuity, and extreme photophobia. Minor episodes resolve rapidly; often, when the patient is examined within hours of an acute recurrence, no abnormality is discernible on slit-lamp examination. Many patients seem to suffer from ocular discomfort that is out of proportion to the amount of observable pathology. However, slit-lamp examination using retroillumination can frequently reveal subtle corneal abnormalities (eg, epithelial cysts). The corneal epithelium is loosely attached to the underlying basement membrane and Bowman layer, both at the time of a recurrent attack and between attacks when the cornea appears to be entirely healed. During the acute attack, the epithelium in the involved area frequently appears heaped up and edematous. Although no frank epithelial defect may be present, significant pooling of fluorescein over the affected area is often visible.

LABORATORY EVALUATION   The key to making the distinction between posttraumatic erosion and dystrophic erosion in a patient who has no clear-cut history of superficial trauma lies in careful examination of the contralateral eye following maximal pupillary dilation. Occasionally, subtle areas of loosely adherent epithelium can be identified by gentle pressure with a surgical sponge following the instillation of topical anesthetics. The presence of basement membrane changes in the *unaffected* eye implicates a primary basement membrane defect in the pathogenesis, whereas the absence of such findings suggests a posttraumatic etiology. Other clinical conditions with associated abnormalities of the epithelial basement membrane include diabetes mellitus and dystrophies of the stroma and Bowman layer (see also Chapter 10 on corneal dystrophies).

MANAGEMENT   Traditional therapy for this condition in the acute phase consists of frequent lubrication with antibiotic ointments and cycloplegia, followed by use of nonpreserved lubricants or hypertonic saline solution (5% NaCl) during the day and ointment at bedtime for 6–12 months to promote proper epithelial attachment. Hypertonic agents provide lubrication and may transiently produce an osmotic gradient, drawing fluid from the epithelium and theoretically promoting the adherence of epithelial cells to the underlying tissue. Some patients find hypertonic medications unacceptably irritating, although many others do quite well with this therapy indefinitely. Systemic tetracyclines (doxycyline 50 mg bid) and topical corticosteroids (fluoromethalone 0.1% tid for 1 month) have been shown to be very efficacious. The mode of action is thought to be via localized inhibition of MMPs.

Although use of a therapeutic bandage contact lens may be helpful, proper patient education and judicious monitoring are crucial. The ideal therapeutic lens should have a flat base curve and high oxygen transmissibility (Dk). New-generation soft contact lenses with surface treatments that decrease bacterial adherence may offer a better safety profile. Concomitant use of a topical broad-spectrum antibiotic 3–4 times daily may reduce the possibility of secondary infection. Application of preservative-free topical ketorolac 4 times daily may improve patient comfort in the first 24 hours. Occasionally, judicious use of topical corticosteroids is necessary to treat associated secondary keratitis or uveitis.

Patients with recalcitrant disease should be treated by a stepwise sequence of interventions. When consistent conservative management fails to control the symptoms, more invasive surgical therapy may be indicated. In patients with posttraumatic recurrent erosions, *anterior stromal micropuncture* can be very effective (Fig 3-20). Using a specially designed 25-gauge needle with a bent top, the clinician makes numerous superficial puncture wounds in the involved area, producing a firm adhesion between the epithelium and the underlying stroma. This procedure should be used with caution in the visual axis. Rarely is a significant scar visible for more than a few months after this procedure. The treatment may need to be repeated in patients who were at first adequately controlled but later become symptomatic, usually because the area of treatment was inadequate. Histologic studies have revealed that the lesions produced by this procedure create subepithelial scars. Use of diathermy to create similar lesions in experimental animals has shown that the efficacy of these procedures is related to their ability to stimulate the formation of new basement membrane complexes.

In patients with dystrophic, degenerative, or other severe secondary basement membrane disorder–related recurrent erosions, the procedure of choice is *epithelial debridement,* which can easily be performed at the slit lamp. Following adequate application of topical anesthetic, loosely adherent epithelium is debrided using a surgical sponge, a spatula, or a surgical blade. Care must be taken not to damage the underlying Bowman layer. Light application of an ophthalmic diamond burr to Bowman layer in the affected area (outside the visual axis) may be effective in reducing recurrences in resistant cases.

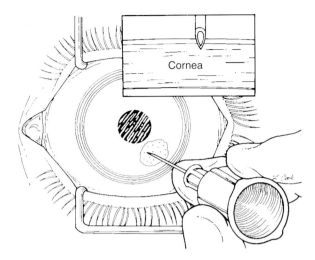

Figure 3-20 Anterior stromal puncture. The needle is used to encourage microcicatrization among epithelium, Bowman layer, and stroma. *(Reproduced with permission from Kenyon KR, Wagoner MD. Therapy of recurrent erosion and persistent defects of the corneal epithelium. Focal Points: Clinical Modules for Ophthalmologists. San Francisco: American Academy of Ophthalmology; 1991, module 9. Illustration by Laurel Cook.)*

Because a significant amount of discomfort can be expected for 3–4 days following this procedure, the patient will likely be more tolerant if debridement is performed at the time of a painful recurrent episode. Topical antibiotic ointment, cycloplegia, and, in some cases, bandage contact lenses are used until reepithelialization is complete. Oral analgesics are often necessary in the first 24 hours.

Excimer laser phototherapeutic keratectomy is an alternative modality for treating patients with recalcitrant recurrent erosions, particularly the dystrophic variant. By creating a large, shallow zone of ablation, this procedure can minimize the refractive effects; it can be used to correct an associated myopic refractive error as well. The mechanism of action of this procedure for this condition has yet to be established. (See BCSC Section 13, *Refractive Surgery,* for further discussion.)

Dursun D, Kim MC, Solomon A, Pflugfelder SC. Treatment of recalcitrant recurrent corneal erosions with inhibitors of matrix metalloproteinase-9, doxycycline and corticosteroids. *Am J Ophthalmol.* 2001;132(1):8–13.

Reidy JJ, Paulus MP, Gona S. Recurrent erosions of the cornea: epidemiology and treatment. *Cornea.* 2000;19(6):767–771.

Wang L, Tsang H, Coroneo M. Treatment of recurrent corneal erosion syndrome using the combination of oral doxycycline and topical corticosteroid. *Clin Experiment Ophthalmol.* 2008;36(1):8–12.

Persistent Corneal Epithelial Defect

PATHOGENESIS Persistent corneal epithelial defects are generally related to some underlying disease process. Common causes of these defects include

- herpetic corneal disease

- delayed postsurgical epithelial healing
- chemical burns
- toxicity from topically applied medications
- recurrent corneal erosions
- dry-eye syndromes
- infections
- neuroparalytic keratopathy
- neurotrophic keratopathy
- anterior segment necrosis

CLINICAL PRESENTATION   Persistent corneal epithelial defects are characterized by central or paracentral areas of chronic nonhealing epithelium that resist maximal therapeutic endeavors. They frequently have elevated, rounded edges and may be associated with significant underlying stromal inflammation. Corneal anesthesia is frequently an accompanying sign, and it should always be evaluated. Left untreated, this condition can progress to vascularization and corneal opacification or scarring. Alternatively, progressive inflammation can lead to necrosis and thinning of the stroma, occasionally resulting in perforation.

LABORATORY EVALUATION   The diagnosis is based on careful history taking, with particular attention to the preservatives present in any ophthalmic medications being administered. The lesions are frequently round or oval epithelial defects with grayish edges that are rolled under without heaped margins. The defects tend to be inferior or inferonasal and can be associated with an intense, coarse superficial keratitis. The inferonasal predilection of these lesions may be a result of the area's easy access and the protective effect of Bell phenomenon on the superior cornea. KCS is a frequently accompanying disease. Other associated conditions include corneal hypoesthesia as a result of previous cataract extraction or keratoplasty and prior herpes zoster or herpes simplex infections.

MANAGEMENT   Some medications used to treat ocular surface disease and glaucoma may impair epithelial wound healing and result in the formation of persistent corneal epithelial defects. The drugs most frequently implicated include topical anesthetics; topical nonsteroidal anti-inflammatory agents (NSAIDs); trifluridine; β-blockers; carbonic anhydrase inhibitors; and, in sensitive individuals, all drops containing the preservative benzalkonium chloride (BAK). Some authors refer to the condition as *toxic ulcerative keratopathy*. This clinical problem is frequently unrecognized and usually presents as a diffuse punctate keratopathy. In some instances, pericentral pseudodentritiform lesions and pseudogeographic defects may occur. These clinical findings are often misinterpreted as a worsening of the underlying disease and thus may lead to even larger doses of the offending medication. Frank ulceration and even corneal perforation can result.

   In addition to removing the offending stimulus or aggravating drugs or treating the underlying condition, a number of strategies have been used to manage persistent epithelial defects. Pharmacologic therapies have included systemic tetracycline, chosen for its anticollagenolytic effect, unrelated to the drug's antimicrobial properties.

   Generally, conventional therapies can be effective in promoting closure of the epithelial defect. These include frequent lubrication with nonpreserved ointments and, if necessary, temporary tarsorrhaphy or permanent lateral canthoplasty to encourage epithelial migration and minimize mechanical trauma from exposure and desiccation.

Persistent epithelial defects often occur in patients with diabetic retinopathy following epithelial debridement during vitreoretinal procedures. Diabetic neuropathy is thought to be a potential cause of neurotrophic keratopathy and nonhealing epithelial defects.

For more extensive insults, such as alkali injuries or other causes of devastating ocular surface trauma, damage to limbal stem cells cannot be overcome by conventional conservative therapies. Various strategies using healthy conjunctiva or limbal stem cells have been used with success in ocular surface reconstruction. (Limbal stem cell dysfunction is discussed at the end of this chapter; surgery of the ocular surface is covered in Chapter 14.)

Neurotrophic keratopathy

PATHOGENESIS   Neurotrophic keratopathy results from damage to CN V, which causes corneal hypoesthesia or anesthesia. The damage may be caused by surgical trauma (ablation of the trigeminal ganglion, PK, large limbal incisions, LASIK), cerebrovascular accidents, aneurysms, multiple sclerosis, tumors (eg, acoustic neuroma, neurofibroma, or angioma), herpes zoster ophthalmicus, herpes simplex keratitis, Hansen disease (leprosy), or the toxicity of certain topical medications (anesthetics, NSAIDs, β-blockers, and carbonic anhydrase inhibitors). Reduction of corneal sensation has been encountered with both type 1 and type 2 diabetes mellitus, presumably as a result of prolonged hypoglycemia. Hereditary causes include various types of hereditary sensory neuropathy and familial dysautonomia (Riley-Day syndrome).

Animal models have shown that tear-film osmolarity increases following corneal denervation. In addition to the ocular surface findings associated with a depressed tearing reflex, an additional mechanism for corneal disease was at work in these animal models, related to the trophic influence of CN V.

CLINICAL PRESENTATION   As a result of corneal denervation or damage to CN V, neurotrophic keratopathy generally involves the central or inferior paracentral cornea. Herpes zoster ophthalmicus can lead to a severe neurotrophic keratopathy. A patient showing other signs of herpes zoster ophthalmicus should undergo an assessment of corneal sensation to determine the relative level of risk. Corneal sensation may return to some extent during healing but usually remains permanently depressed. Neurotrophic keratopathy resulting from herpes simplex keratitis can result in persistent epithelial defects in the absence of replicating virus or active corneal inflammation. These epithelial defects stain intensely with fluorescein and are surrounded by raised, rolled-up gray edges (Fig 3-21). Progressive sterile ulceration or superinfection can result in perforation and loss of the eye.

Hereditary sensory and autonomic neuropathy, type 3 (familial dysautonomia, Riley-Day syndrome), is an autosomal recessive disorder that occurs almost exclusively in people of Ashkenazi Jewish descent. Clinical features include alacrima, vasomotor instability, decreased or absent deep tendon reflexes, absence of lingual fungiform papillae with impaired taste, and relative indifference to pain and temperature. Patients exhibit an increased sensitivity to adrenergic and cholinergic agents, suggesting functional autonomic denervation. This condition can lead to dramatic, persistent, nonhealing epithelial defects

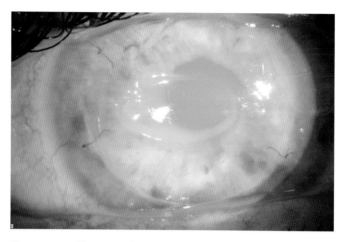

Figure 3-21 Neurotrophic ulcer. *(Courtesy of Kenneth M. Goins, MD.)*

in infants. Autonomic dysfunction diminishes aqueous tear production by the lacrimal gland and leads to secondary conjunctival xerosis. Affected individuals frequently develop keratitis ranging in severity from mild punctate stippling of the lower portion of the corneal epithelium to frank neurotrophic ulcerations.

MANAGEMENT   Management of persistent epithelial defects due to neurotrophic keratopathy includes treatment of the underlying disease and use of the full spectrum of approaches outlined earlier in the chapter for dry eye and exposure keratopathy. It is particularly important to choose ointments or eyedrops without potentially toxic preservatives, such as BAK, for patients with neurotrophic keratopathy. Management of toxic ulcerative keratopathy includes discontinuation of the offending agent, patching, and the use of nonpreserved medications. Medications with specific activity against MMPs, such as systemic tetracyclines and topical medroxyprogesterone, may help prevent or halt stromal melting in more severe cases. Corneal collagen cross-linking, early in the course of a melt, has been used in a small number of patients and has been very effective.

Autologous serum drops can be very useful in treating neurotrophic keratitis. Recent clinical studies of topically applied neuropeptides and neurotrophins to treat neurotrophic keratitis have shown promising results. However, these therapies remain experimental at this time.

Lateral and/or medial tarsorrhaphy is frequently required to prevent surface desiccation. Tarsorrhaphy decreases tear-film evaporation and tear-film osmolarity, presumably by reducing the surface area of corneal exposure. In rare cases, low-water-content, highly oxygen-permeable therapeutic contact lenses may be used. PK, although generally hazardous in cases of neurotrophic keratopathy, has been used with increasing success in patients with residual scarring from clinically inactive herpes zoster keratopathy. Concomitant lateral tarsorrhaphy and permanent punctal occlusion appear to improve the long-term survival of the corneal graft. Surgical fixation of preserved amniotic membrane has been reported to encourage healing of persistent epithelial ulcerations. Partial or total conjunctival flaps will prevent corneal melting, but they should be used as a last resort in order to preserve the eye.

Goins KM. New insights into the diagnosis and treatment of neurotrophic keratopathy. *Ocul Surf.* 2005;3(2):96–110.

Kojima T, Higuchi A, Goto E, Matsumoto Y, Dogru M, Tsubota K. Autologous serum eye drops for the treatment of dry eye diseases. *Cornea.* 2008;27(Suppl 1):S25–S30.

Müller LJ, Marfurt CF, Kruse F, Tervo TM. Corneal nerves: structure, contents and function. *Exp Eye Res.* 2003;76(5):521–542.

Schnitzler E, Spörl E, Seiler T. Irradiation of cornea with ultraviolet light and riboflavin administration as a new treatment for erosive corneal processes, preliminary results in four patients. *Klin Monatsbl Augenheilkd.* 2000;217(3):190–193.

Trichiasis and Distichiasis

Trichiasis refers to an acquired condition in which eyelashes emerging from their normal anterior origin are curved inward toward the cornea. Most cases are probably the result of subtle cicatricial entropion of the eyelid margin. Trichiasis can be idiopathic or secondary to chronic inflammatory conditions.

Distichiasis is a congenital (often autosomal dominant) or acquired condition in which an extra row of eyelashes emerges from the ducts of meibomian glands. These eyelashes can be fine and well tolerated or coarser and a threat to corneal integrity.

Aberrant eyelashes emerge from the tarsus as a result of chronic inflammatory conditions of the eyelids and conjunctiva such as trachoma, ocular cicatricial pemphigoid, Stevens-Johnson syndrome, chronic blepharitis, or chemical burns.

Aberrant eyelashes and poor eyelid position and movement should be corrected. Aberrant eyelashes may be removed by epilation, electrolysis, or cryotherapy. Mechanical epilation is temporary because the eyelashes will normally grow back within 2–3 weeks. Electrolysis works well only for removing a few eyelashes, although it may be preferable in younger patients for cosmetic reasons. Cryotherapy is still a common treatment for aberrant eyelashes, but freezing can result in eyelid margin thinning, loss of adjacent normal eyelashes, and persistent lanugo hairs that may continue to abrade the cornea. Treatment at –20°C should be limited to less than 30 seconds to minimize complications. The preferred surgical technique for aberrant eyelashes is a tarsotomy with eyelid margin rotation. For further discussion, see BCSC Section 7, *Orbit, Eyelids, and Lacrimal System.*

Factitious Ocular Surface Disorders

Factitious disorders include a spectrum of self-induced injuries with symptoms or physical findings intentionally produced by the patient in order to assume the sick role. Factitious conjunctivitis usually shows evidence of mechanical injury to the inferior and nasal quadrants of the cornea and conjunctiva. The areas of involvement show sharply delineated borders. Patients often have medical training or work in a medical setting, and they generally show an attitude of serene indifference. The detached conjunctival tissues usually show no evidence of inflammation by pathologic examination. Other types of noncorneal factitious ocular disorders include self-induced solar retinopathy, eyelid ulceration, and anisocoria.

Mucus-fishing syndrome

Mucus-fishing syndrome is characterized by a well-circumscribed pattern of rose bengal or lissamine green staining on the nasal and inferior bulbar conjunctiva. All patients have a history of increased mucus production as a nonspecific response to ocular surface damage. The inciting event is typically KCS. Patients usually demonstrate vigorous eye rubbing and compulsive removal of the mucus strands from the fornix (mucus fishing). The resultant epithelial injury heightens the ocular surface irritation, which, in turn, stimulates additional mucus production, resulting in a vicious cycle.

Topical anesthetic abuse

Clinical application of topical anesthetics has become an integral part of the modern practice of ophthalmology. However, indiscriminate use of topical anesthetics can cause serious ocular surface toxicity and complications. Local anesthetics are known to inhibit epithelial migration and division. Loss of microvilli, reduction of desmosomes and other intercellular contacts, and swelling of mitochondria and lysosomes have been reported in ultrastructural studies. The clinical features of anesthetic abuse are characterized by the failure of the presenting condition, such as corneal abrasions or infectious keratitis, to respond to appropriate therapy.

Initially, a punctate keratopathy is seen. As the abuse continues, the eye becomes more injected and epithelial defects appear or take on a neurotrophic appearance. As the process goes on, keratic precipitates and hypopyon develop, thus mimicking an infectious course. Diffuse stromal edema, dense stromal infiltrates, and large ring opacity are common presenting signs (Fig 3-22). Stromal vascularization may take place in chronic abuse, and secondary infection may ensue. Because of the presence of corneal infiltrates and anterior segment inflammation, infectious keratitis must be ruled out through corneal scraping, culture, or biopsy.

Differential diagnosis includes bacterial, fungal, herpetic, and amebic keratitis. Suspicion should be maintained in the face of negative cultures in any patient who is not responding to appropriate therapy. Often the diagnosis is made only when the patient is discovered concealing the anesthetic drops. Once the diagnosis is made and infectious keratitis is ruled out, corneal healing usually occurs if all exposure to anesthetics is removed. In advanced cases, permanent corneal scarring or perforation may occur. Occasionally, anesthetic abuse may continue after surgery. Psychiatric counseling is sometimes helpful.

Dellen

Desiccation of the epithelium and subepithelial tissues occurs at or near the limbus adjacent to surface elevations such as those produced by pterygia, large filtration blebs, or dermoids. Because the tear film is interrupted by these surface elevations, normal blinking does not wet the involved area properly. Clinically, *dellen* are saucerlike depressions in the corneal surface. The epithelium exhibits punctate irregularities overlying a thinned area of dehydrated corneal stroma. Treatment with frequent ocular lubrication or pressure patching accelerates the healing process and restores stromal hydration.

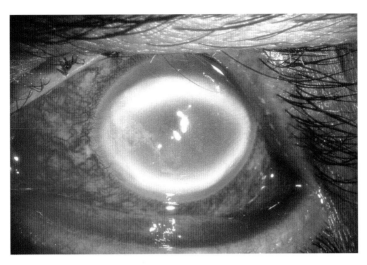

Figure 3-22 Topical anesthetic overuse with persistent corneal epithelial defect and necrotic ring opacity. *(Courtesy of Kirk R. Wilhelmus, MD.)*

The orbital and conjunctival tissues surrounding the sclera also play a role in maintaining scleral hydration. This function becomes especially evident during surgical procedures, when the conjunctiva and extraocular muscles are removed from the scleral surface. The exposed sclera becomes thinner and partially translucent unless it is continually remoistened. Removal of the perilimbal conjunctiva and interference with the wetting effect of the tear film (as after excision of a pterygium by the bare sclera technique) can cause the underlying sclera to become markedly thinned and translucent, forming a scleral delle.

Ocular Surface Problems Secondary to Contact Lens Wear

Metabolic epithelial damage

Contact lens overwear syndromes can be manifested in several forms. Central epithelial edema (Sattler veil) is found after many hours of wear, more commonly with hard contact lenses. This epithelial edema causes blurred vision that may persist for many hours or even progress to acute epithelial necrosis. Although acute epithelial necrosis is rarely seen, central epithelial edema can create epithelial erosions or frank ulceration. Physiologic stress as a result of hypoxia with lactate accumulation and impaired carbon dioxide efflux is responsible for these complications.

Microcystic epitheliopathy, another condition caused by impaired metabolic activities in epithelium, shows fine epithelial cysts best seen with retroillumination. This condition has been observed most commonly in patients using extended-wear soft contact lenses. The cysts may either be asymptomatic or cause recurrent brief episodes of pain and epiphora. It takes up to 6 weeks following discontinuation of contact lens wear for the cysts to resolve.

Toxic conjunctivitis

Conjunctival injection, epithelial staining, punctate epithelial keratopathy, erosions, and microcysts are all potential signs of conjunctival or corneal toxicity from contact lens solutions. Any of the proteolytic enzymes or chemicals used for cleaning contact lenses, or the preservative-containing soaking solution, can be the culprit. Cleaning agents such as BAK, chlorhexidine, hydrogen peroxide, and other substances used for chemical sterilization, if not properly removed from contact lenses, can cause an immediate, severe epitheliopathy with accompanying pain. See Chapter 13.

Allergic reactions

The preservative thimerosal can produce a delayed hypersensitivity response, resulting in conjunctivitis, keratitis with epithelial involvement, and even coarse epithelial and subepithelial opacities. Thimerosal may also be implicated in contact lens–induced SLK. The ocular signs of this disorder include injection of the superior bulbar conjunctiva, epitheliopathy of the cornea and conjunctiva, papillary conjunctivitis, and some superficial pannus. This condition has declined in prevalence, probably as a result of the replacement of thimerosal by other preservatives in contact lens solutions.

Neovascularization

Neovascular ingrowth into the peripheral cornea *(micropannus)* is common in soft contact lens wearers. Less than 2 mm of such growth is believed to be acceptable; contact lens wear should be discontinued if the neovascularization extends farther than 2 mm into the cornea. Superficial pannus is rarely associated with hard or rigid gas-permeable (RGP) contact lens wear but is encountered more frequently in patients using soft lenses. This type of neovascularization is probably caused by hypoxia and chronic trauma to the limbus, which leads to the release of angiogenic mediators. Other causes of pannus such as staphylococcal or chlamydial keratoconjunctivitis should be considered in the presence of appropriate accompanying signs.

Deep stromal neovascularization has been associated with extended-wear contact lenses, especially in aphakia. This condition is not usually symptomatic unless there is secondary lipid deposition. Deep neovascularization of the cornea is often irreversible and is best managed by discontinuing contact lens wear and resorting to other alternatives, such as spectacle correction.

Stein RM, Stein HA. Corneal complications of contact lenses. *Focal Points: Clinical Modules for Ophthalmologists.* San Francisco: American Academy of Ophthalmology; 1993, module 2.

Limbal Stem Cell Deficiency

PATHOGENESIS   The ocular surface is composed of permanently renewing populations of epithelial cells. These epithelial cells are replaced through proliferation of a distinct subpopulation of cells known as *stem cells*. The *corneal stem cells* are located in the basal cell layer of the limbus, whereas the *conjunctival stem cells* may be uniformly distributed throughout the bulbar surface or located in the fornices. Stem cells have an unlimited capacity for self-renewal and are slow cycling (low mitotic activity). Once stem cell differentiation begins, it is irreversible. The process of differentiation occurs by means of transit amplification. Transit-amplifying cells, which have a limited capacity for self-renewal, can be found at the limbus as well as at the basal layer of the corneal epithelium. Each of these cells is able to undergo a finite number of cell divisions. Corneal and conjunctival stem cells can be identified only by indirect means, such as clonal expansion and identification of slow cycling.

Approximately 25%–33% of the limbus must be intact to ensure normal ocular resurfacing. The normal limbus acts as a barrier against corneal vascularization from the conjunctiva and invasion of conjunctival cells from the bulbar surface. When the limbal stem cells are congenitally absent, injured, or destroyed, conjunctival cells migrate onto the ocular surface, often accompanied by superficial neovascularization. The absence of limbal stem cells reduces the effectiveness of epithelial wound healing, as evidenced by compromised ocular surface integrity with irregular ocular surface and recurrent epithelial breakdown.

See Table 3-9 for an etiologic classification of limbal stem cell deficiencies.

Table 3-9 Etiologic Classification of Limbal Stem Cell Deficiency

1. Idiopathic
2. Trauma
    Chemical/thermal burns
3. Iatrogenic
    A. Local
        i. Surgery
            Multiple ocular surface operations
            Cryotherapy
        ii. Radiation and radiotherapy
        iii. Contact lens use
        iv. Local chemotherapy (eg, antimetabolites such as 5-fluorouracil, mitocycin C)
    B. Systemic
        i. Medications: hydroxyurea
        ii. Graft-vs-host disease
4. Autoimmune
    Stevens-Johnson syndrome
    Ocular cicatrical pemphigoid
5. Eye disease
    Neoplasia and degeneration (eg, pterygium)
    Neurotrophic keratitis
    Infections (eg, herpetic, trachoma)
    Atopy
    Peripheral corneal ulcers (eg, Fuchs marginal keratitis)
    Anterior segment ischemic syndrome
6. Congenital and hereditary
    Aniridia
    Multiple endocrine neoplasia
    Ectodactyly-ectodermal dysplasia-clefting syndrome
    KID (keratitis-icthyosis-deafness) syndrome (due to mutations in the GJB2 gene coding for
        connexin-26
    Xeroderma pigmentosa
    LADD (lacrimo-auriculo-dento-digital) syndrome/Levy-Hollister syndrome)

CLINICAL PRESENTATION   Clinically, stem cell deficiency of the cornea can be observed in several ocular surface disorders. Patients usually suffer from recurrent ulceration and decreased vision as a result of the irregular corneal surface. Corneal neovascularization is invariably present in the involved cornea. A wavelike irregularity of the ocular surface emanating from the limbus can be more easily observed following the installation of topical fluorescein (Fig 3-23). In some cases, increased epithelial permeability can be observed clinically by diffuse permeation of topical fluorescein into the anterior stroma.

Stem cell deficiency states result from both primary and secondary causes. Primary causes include congenital aniridia, ectodermal dysplasia, sclerocornea, KID syndrome, and congenital erythrokeratodermia. Secondary causes include chemical burns, thermal burns, contact lens wear, ocular surgery, and chronic cicatricial conjunctivitis (cicatricial pemphigoid, trachoma, Stevens-Johnson syndrome), pterygia, and dysplastic or neoplastic lesions of the limbus.

LABORATORY EVALUATION   Impression cytology of the involved corneal surface usually shows the presence of goblet cells and conjunctival epithelium. There are no practical diagnostic tests for limbal stem cell deficiency at this time; however, it is likely that such tests will be developed in the future.

MANAGEMENT   Replacement of stem cells by limbal transplantation seems to be the logical choice for ocular surface reconstruction in diseases associated with limbal stem cell deficiency. When the limbus is focally affected in 1 eye, as with a pterygium, a limbal or conjunctival autograft can be harvested from the ipsilateral eye. For unilateral moderate or severe chemical injuries, a limbal autograft can be obtained from the healthy fellow eye. For bilateral limbal deficiency, as with Stevens-Johnson syndrome or bilateral chemical burns, a limbal allograft from an HLA-matched living related donor (or, if unavailable, an eye bank donor eye) can be considered. Systemic immune suppression is required following limbal allograft transplantation. Dramatic restoration of the ocular surface with limbal reconstruction has been reported in selected cases with desperate clinical situations. (See the discussion of ocular surface surgery in Chapter 14.)

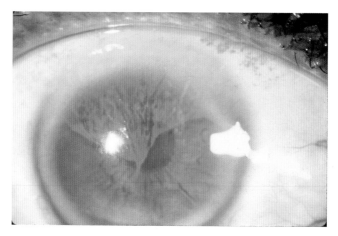

Figure 3-23   Stem cell deficiency. A wavelike irregularity of the ocular surface is seen following installation of topical fluorescein. *(Courtesy of James J. Reidy, MD.)*

CHAPTER 4

Infectious Diseases of the External Eye: Basic Concepts and Viral Infections

Defense Mechanisms of the External Eye

The external eye contains diverse tissues intricately linked to protect against infection. The ocular adnexa—periorbita, eyelids and lashes, lacrimal and meibomian glands—produce, spread, and drain the preocular tear film, physically protect the sensitive ocular mucosa, and cushion the globe. Lymphoid tissues within the conjunctiva, lacrimal glands, and lacrimal drainage tract furnish acquired immune defense.

The bony orbit and eyelids protect the eye from external injury. Normal eyelid position and function prevent desiccation of the ocular surface and promote tear turnover by periodic closure. Eyelid blinking pumps tears from the lacrimal gland onto the ocular surface and into the lacrimal sac. Tear turnover dilutes and removes microbes from the tear film. In addition, soluble macromolecules secreted by the lacrimal gland exert antimicrobial properties:

- Tear lysozyme degrades bacterial cell walls, while β-lysin in the tears disrupts bacterial plasma membranes.
- Tear lactoferrin inhibits bacterial metabolism by scavenging free iron, augments tear antibody function, and may influence complement activation.
- Immunoglobulins in the tear film, particularly secretory IgA, mediate antigen-specific immunity at the ocular surface. Components of both the classic and alternative complement pathways are also found in the tear film.
- Meibomian gland–derived lipids reduce evaporation of the tear film and indirectly protect the corneal epithelium from desiccation and injury.
- Mucin expression by ocular surface cells as well as goblet cell–derived mucin inhibits attachment of microbes to ocular surface epithelium.
- Cytokines, including epidermal growth factor (EGF), transforming growth factor betas (TGF-βs), and hepatocyte growth factor (HGF) are present in the tears. The contribution of these cytokines to ocular surface defense is a promising area of basic investigation.

BCSC Section 2, *Fundamentals and Principles of Ophthalmology,* discusses the biochemistry and metabolism of the tear film and cornea in detail.

Lamberts DW. Physiology of the tear film. In: Foster CS, Azar DT, Dohlman CH, eds. *Smolin and Thoft's The Cornea: Scientific Foundations and Clinical Practice.* 4th ed. Philadelphia: Lippincott Williams & Wilkins; 2005:577–599.

Pflugfelder SC, Solomon A, Stern ME. The diagnosis and management of dry eye: a twenty-five-year review. *Cornea.* 2000;19(5):644–649.

The epithelium of the ocular surface forms a mechanical barrier against microbial invasion. Phagocytosis and subsequent digestion of bacteria, combined with rapid cycling of epithelial cells, aid in the removal of microbes. Antigen-presenting cells such as Langerhans cells in the conjunctiva carry antigen to regional lymphatic tissue and facilitate an acquired immune response. In response to microbial invasion, ocular surface epithelial cells secrete interleukin-1 (IL-1) and other cytokines that boost the local immune response through the enhancement of immune-cell migration, adhesion, and activation.

Human conjunctiva contains a complete spectrum of immunologically competent cell types. Uninfected conjunctival epithelium possesses $CD8^+$ cytotoxic/suppressor T lymphocytes and Langerhans cells. Conjunctival substantia propria contains $CD4^+$ helper T cells and $CD8^+$ T cells in roughly equal numbers, along with natural killer T cells, mast cells, B lymphocytes, plasma cells, macrophages, and occasional polymorphonuclear leukocytes. Hyperplasia of conjunctival lymphoid follicles and painful swelling of draining preauricular lymph nodes accompany conjunctival infection by viruses, *Chlamydia,* and *Neisseria* species. The vascular and lymphatic channels of the conjunctiva transport humoral and cellular immune components to and from the eye. During an infection, inflammatory mediators promote vascular dilation, permeability, and diapedesis from conjunctival blood vessels.

The healthy cornea has classically been considered devoid of leukocytes, but activated Langerhans cells and other dendritic cells normally present in the peripheral corneal epithelium can migrate rapidly to the central cornea. Upon infection, the constitutive cells of the cornea, the keratocytes in particular, augment the inflammatory cascade by the secretion of proinflammatory cytokines. Lymphocytes and neutrophils are recruited into the cornea from the tear film, the limbal vascular arcades, and the anterior chamber.

For a more extensive, illustrated discussion of ocular immunology, see BCSC Section 9, *Intraocular Inflammation and Uveitis.*

Normal Ocular Flora

Bacterial colonization of the eyelid margin and conjunctiva is normal and beneficial for the eye. Interactions between ocular surface mucosa and resident nonpathogenic bacteria reduce opportunities for pathogenic strains to gain a foothold. The spectrum of normal ocular flora varies with the age and even the geographic locale of the host. Following vaginal birth, the infant's eye commonly harbors multiple bacterial species, including *Staphylococcus aureus, S epidermidis,* streptococci, and *Escherichia coli.* During the first 2 decades of life, streptococci and pneumococci predominate. With increasing age, gram-negative bacteria are more commonly isolated, but the most commonly isolated bacteria remain *S epidermidis* and other coagulase-negative staphylococci, *S aureus,* and diphtheroids

Table 4-1 Relative Prevalence of the Normal Flora of the Outer Eye

Microorganisms	Normal Conjunctiva	Normal Eyelid Margin
Staphylococcus epidermidis	+ + +	+ + +
Staphylococcus aureus	+ +	+ +
Micrococcus spp	+	+ +
Corynebacterium spp (diphtheroids)	+ +	+ +
Propionibacterium acnes	+ +	+ +
Streptococcus spp*	+	±
Haemophilus influenzae*	±	−
Moraxella spp	±	−
Enteric gram-negative bacilli	±	−
Bacillus spp	±	−
Anaerobic bacteria	+	±
Yeasts (Malassezia furfur, Candida spp, etc)	−	+
Filamentous fungi	±	−
Demodex spp	−	+ +

*More common in children.

(Table 4-1). Under the appropriate culture conditions, *Propionibacterium acnes, Malassezia furfur,* and *Candida* species may also be cultured from the eye. The parasites *Demodex folliculorum* and *Demodex brevis* are detected on the eyelid margins of normal healthy individuals and, with advancing age, become almost ubiquitous. Clinically, the use of antibiotics or topical corticosteroids, or a condition such as dry eye that prevents normal tear turnover, may alter the spectrum of eyelid and conjunctival flora.

> Osato MS. Normal ocular flora. In: Pepose JS, Holland GN, Wilhelmus KR, eds. *Ocular Infection and Immunity.* St Louis: Mosby; 1996:191–199.

Pathogenesis of Ocular Infections

Infection of the ocular surface can follow transplacental passage of the pathogen to the fetus; direct contact in the birth canal during delivery; exposure to fomites, fingers, airborne particles, or sexual contact; hematogenous seeding (rare); extension from contiguous adnexal disease; and spread from the upper respiratory tract through the nasolacrimal duct. The acquisition of infection is enhanced by circumstances that facilitate contact with the pathogen. Epidemic adenoviral conjunctivitis develops after mucosal contact with secretions from an infected person. Sexually transmitted ocular infections such as gonococcal and chlamydial conjunctivitis are spread through ocular contact with infected genital secretions during sexual activity. Zoonotic infections such as cat-scratch disease and Lyme disease are transmitted by contact with an infected animal host or vector. The risk of opportunistic infection by environmental pathogens may be enhanced by use of chemically disinfected but not fully sterilized surgical instruments *(Mycobacterium chelonei),* use of homemade saline or tap water for contact lens hygiene *(Acanthamoeba),* or trauma with soil or vegetable matter *(Bacillus cereus,* various fungi). The initiation, severity, and characteristics of subsequent infection are influenced by the interplay between the virulence of the pathogen, the size of the inoculum, and the competence and nature of host defense mechanisms.

Virulence

Successful infection of ocular tissues requires microorganisms to adhere, evade, invade, replicate, and, in some instances, persist. Microbial virulence factors represent evolutionary adaptations by each microorganism that increase the odds of infection and organism survival.

Adherence

For ocular surface infections acquired externally, adherence of organisms to ocular surface epithelium is the first step.

- Many bacteria express *adhesins,* which are microbial proteins that bind with high affinity to host cell surface molecules.
- *Candida albicans* expresses surface proteins that mimic mammalian *integrins* (transmembrane proteins that mediate cell–cell and cell–extracellular matrix interactions).
- Viruses typically express surface proteins or glycoproteins that attach to constitutive cell surface molecules such as heparan sulfate (herpes simplex virus) or sialic acid (adenovirus).

Evasion

Adherent bacteria evade interaction with unfavorable elements of their physical environment, such as immunologic cells or antibacterial molecules in the tears, by the expression of exopolysaccharides organized into a *biofilm,* a 3-dimensional structure that allows interbacterial communication and signaling and interferes with phagocytosis. For viruses, evasion of the immune response involves multiple strategies. For example, a herpes simplex virus (HSV)–encoded protein (eg, ICP47) successfully competes with antigenic viral peptides for transport into the endoplasmic reticulum, where peptides are loaded onto the major histocompatibility (MHC) complex. Thus, HSV-infected cells can be resistant to lysis by cytotoxic T cells.

Watnick P, Kolter R. Biofilm, city of microbes. *J Bacteriol.* 2000;182(10):2675–2679.

Invasion

Few bacteria can overcome intact epithelium. Those that can include

- *Neisseria gonorrhoeae*
- *Neisseria meningitidis*
- *Corynebacterium diphtheriae*
- *Shigella* spp

Most bacteria must rely on a break in the epithelial barrier function. Microbial invasion may be facilitated by microbial proteases that induce cell lysis and degrade the extracellular matrix. Bacterial exotoxins, such as those produced by streptococci, staphylococci, and *Pseudomonas aeruginosa,* can induce corneal cell necrosis. *Acanthamoeba* species and certain fungi secrete collagenases, whereas *Pseudomonas* elastase and alkaline protease destroy collagen and proteoglycan components of the cornea and degrade immunoglobulins, complement, interleukins, and other inflammatory cytokines. Microbial proteases also activate corneal matrix–derived metalloproteinases (MMPs) that in turn participate in autodigestion. For viruses, adherence interactions facilitate invasion by the appropriation of host cell mechanisms. For example, the interaction between adenovirus capsid proteins and host cell integrins mediates internalization of the adenovirus by means of an intracellular signaling cascade that culminates in actin polymerization and endocytosis of the virus.

Replication and persistence

Most organisms are cleared from the site of infection following acute infection. Some microorganisms persist in the host indefinitely. For example, following primary infection, HSV and varicella-zoster virus (VZV) establish latency in trigeminal ganglion cells. *Chlamydia* survives and causes local chronic disease by persistence within intracellular phagosomes. Biofilm formation by streptococci within the corneal stroma inhibits recognition of the bacteria by the immune system and accounts for the relative paucity of inflammation and the chronic nature characteristic of crystalline keratopathy, which is caused by this organism.

Inoculum

Different species and strains of microorganisms vary intrinsically in their capacity to induce infection in the host. For example, experimental bacterial keratitis in an animal model can be established with an inoculum of *P aeruginosa* smaller than that required of *S aureus*. The status of host defense mechanisms further determines the threshold of inoculum at which infection occurs.

Host Defense

Intrinsic anatomical mechanisms

Intrinsic anatomical mechanisms may predispose the eye to infection, including the following:

- Desiccation of the ocular surface epithelium may result from lagophthalmos, ectropion, exophthalmos, a reduced blink reflex due to parkinsonism, and keratoconjunctivitis sicca.
- Microtrauma to the epithelium occurs with trichiasis, contact lens wear, use of an ocular prosthesis, prolonged or intense administration of preservative-containing topical medications, and exposure to a free surgical suture.
- Acute traumatic abrasion, bullous keratopathy, recurrent corneal erosion, recurrent epithelial disruption secondary to corneal epithelial and anterior stromal dystrophies, retained foreign body, or corneal surgery similarly can predispose to infection.
- Persistent epithelial defects due to neurotrophic mechanisms such as postherpetic hypoesthesia, diabetic neuropathy, or traumatic injury to CN V also may precede microbial keratitis.

- Any surgery in which the conjunctival epithelium is disrupted, including strabismus and cataract surgery, can lead to infection of the conjunctiva and the underlying scleral wound.

Immunologic competence

Local or systemic immune compromise predisposes to ocular infection. The use of topical corticosteroids is a frequent contributing factor in the pathogenesis of postoperative infections. Preexisting corneal or conjunctival pathology may cause structural and functional alterations that affect normal tissue responses to injury, inflammation, or infection. The propensity for development of ocular infection also increases with systemic immune compromise in hosts with acquired immunodeficiencies such as those with AIDS and other chronic debilitating diseases or those on systemic chemotherapy; in such patients, normally nonpathogenic organisms may cause disease.

O'Brien TP, Hazlett LD. Pathogenesis of ocular infection. In: Pepose JS, Holland GN, Wilhelmus KR, eds. *Ocular Infection and Immunity.* St Louis: Mosby; 1996:200–214.

Ocular Microbiology

Of the many potentially pathogenic microorganisms capable of causing infectious external eye disease, those encountered most often are listed in Table 4-2.

Diagnostic Laboratory Techniques

The decision to procure clinical specimens for culture, antigen detection, or special chemical stains is based on the likelihood of benefit to the patient's condition. Interpretation of diagnostic specimens requires an understanding of the normal flora and cytology of the ocular surface. Appropriate materials should be available for optimal specimen collection (Table 4-3). The reader is encouraged to also review the discussion of specimen collection and handling in BCSC Section 4, *Ophthalmic Pathology and Intraocular Tumors.*

Specimen Collection and Culturing

Eyelid specimens

Eyelid vesicles or pustules may be opened with a sharp-pointed surgical blade or small-gauge needle. Material for cytology is smeared onto a glass slide and fixed in methanol or acetone for immunofluorescent staining. Collected vesicular fluid can be inoculated into a chilled viral transport medium for culture isolation in the laboratory. Microbial cultures are obtained by swabbing the abnormal area with a thioglycollate-moistened swab followed by direct inoculation of culture media.

Conjunctival specimens

Specimen collection must debride enough surface conjunctival epithelial cells so that intracellular microbes can be seen on chemical stains. Sterile Dacron swabs slightly

Table 4-2 Principal Causes of External Ocular Infections

Condition	Viruses	Bacteria	Fungi	Parasites
Dermatoblepharitis	Herpes simplex	*Staphylococcus aureus*		
	Varicella-zoster	*Streptococcus* spp		
Blepharitis	Herpes simplex	*Staphylococcus* spp		*Phthirus pubis*
	Molluscum contagiosum	*Moraxella* spp		
Conjunctivitis	Adenovirus	*Chlamydia trachomatis*		
	Herpes simplex	*Staphylococcus aureus*		
		Streptococcus spp		
		Neisseria gonorrhoeae		
		Haemophilus influenzae		
		Moraxella spp		
Keratitis	Herpes simplex	*Pseudomonas aeruginosa*	*Fusarium* spp	*Acanthamoeba* spp
		Staphylococcus aureus	*Aspergillus* spp	
		Staphylococcus epidermidis	*Candida albicans*	
		Streptococcus pneumoniae		
		Moraxella spp		
Dacryoadenitis	Epstein-Barr virus	*Staphylococcus aureus*		
	Mumps	*Streptococcus pneumoniae*		
Canaliculitis		Actinomycetes		
Dacryocystitis		*Staphylococcus* spp		
		Streptococcus spp		

Table 4-3 Materials for Collecting Eyelid, Conjunctival, and Corneal Specimens for Ocular Microbiology

Viral Infections	Chlamydial Infections	Microbial Infections
Topical anesthetic	Topical anesthetic	Topical anesthetic
Dacron swabs	Dacron swabs	Calcium alginate or Dacron swabs
Spatula	Spatula	Spatula
Glass slides	Glass slides	Glass slides
Acetone fixative	Methanol or acetone fixative	Methanol fixative
Viral transport medium	Chlamydial transport medium	Blood agar plate
Ice	Ice	Chocolate agar plate
		Sabouraud's dextrose agar plate

moistened with thioglycollate broth may be used to optimize recovery of microbial specimens. The swabbed material should initially be plated directly onto warmed solid media (blood, chocolate, and Sabouraud's). Then the "nonhandled" distal end of the swab may be broken off and placed directly into the remaining thioglycollate broth tube. If these media are not available, specimens should be harvested with any standard culterette tube system that contains appropriate transport media. The specimen should be sent immediately to any qualified microbiology laboratory for processing.

Conjunctival biopsy can also be performed to help in the diagnosis of conditions such as Parinaud oculoglandular syndrome or cicatricial pemphigoid.

Corneal specimens

A corneal culture is indicated in sight-threatening ulcers (>1–2 mm), in ulcers in which an atypical organism is suspected, and in any ulcer that is not responding to therapy. A microbial specimen can be collected from a corneal ulcer by scraping the lesion with a platinum Kimura spatula, sterile needle, surgical blade, or thioglycollate-moistened calcium alginate or Dacron swab. A blade or spatula is preferable for preparing smears for chemical staining, but either a spatula or swab is acceptable for inoculation of culture media; a combination of techniques may provide added benefit when few microorganisms are present. Furthermore, because growth patterns on culture media vary among different bacterial species, the material obtained from the corneal ulcer should be used to inoculate microscope slides for stained smears and several different culture media.

Specimens are best inoculated immediately onto microbiologic media that have been warmed to room temperature in anticipation of the culture procedure. To avoid contamination and false positives, care must be taken to avoid touching the blade or swab to the eyelids, and a sterile instrument or swab should be used for each row of C-shaped streaks on each agar plate (Fig 4-1) and for each type of broth culture. For a viral culture, a Dacron swab used to obtain viral-infected corneal or conjunctival cells is agitated in a

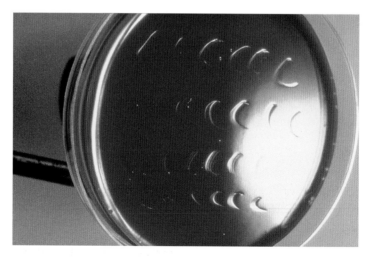

Figure 4-1   "C" streaks on a chocolate blood agar plate. *(Courtesy of James Chodosh, MD.)*

chilled viral transport medium and discarded. Calcium alginate and cotton swabs should be avoided as the calcium alginate and the wooden shaft of cotton swabs both may inhibit viral recovery.

Corneal biopsy may be necessary in cases of apparent and significant microbial infection when repeated corneal scrapings are negative. A small 2- to 3-mm trephine (disposable dermatologic skin punch) can be used to create a partial-thickness incision, and forceps and scissors are used to excise a lamellar flap of cornea. The specimen is generally split into 2 pieces, or separate biopsies are taken so that tissue can be evaluated by both histopathology and microbiology.

Isolation techniques

For viral and chlamydial infections, an appropriate tissue-culture cell line is selected for inoculation and examined for the development of cytopathic effects (CPE) and cellular inclusions. For bacterial and fungal infections, directly inoculated blood, chocolate, and Sabouraud's agar and thioglycollate broth are examined daily to detect visible growth. Microorganisms are studied by chemical staining, chemical reactions, and antimicrobial sensitivity testing. Acanthamoebae may be identified by trophozoite trails on blood agar, but nonnutrient agar with an overlay of killed *E coli* or *Enterococcus* spp is the optimal isolation medium.

> Alexandrakis G, Haimovici R, Miller D, Alfonso EC. Corneal biopsy in the management of progressive microbial keratitis. *Am J Ophthalmol.* 2000;129(5):571–576.

Staining Methods

See Table 4-4 for recommended stains and media in the setting of suspected microbial keratitis.

Table 4-4 Recommended Stains and Culture Media for Microbial Keratitis

Suspected Organism	Stain	Media
Aerobic bacteria	Gram Acridine orange	Blood agar Chocolate agar Thioglycollate broth
Anaerobic bacteria	Gram Acridine orange	Anaerobic blood agar Phenylethyl alcohol agar in anaerobic chamber Thioglycollate broth
Mycobacteria	Gram Acid-fast Lectin	Blood agar Lowenstein-Jensen agar
Fungi	Gram Acridine orange Calcofluor white	Blood agar (25°C) Sabouraud's agar (25°C) Brain–heart infusion (25°C)
Acanthamoeba	Acridine orange Calcofluor white	Nonnutrient agar with *E coli* overlay Blood agar Buffered charcoal–yeast extract agar

Public Health Ophthalmology

Nearly 150 million people worldwide are blind or have low vision. Corneal diseases, especially infection, are major causes of visual loss. In the absence of an available vaccine for these conditions, specific programs are designed to reduce the risk of communicable diseases. Examples of such efforts are the following:

- improved hygiene and mass distribution of antibiotics to interrupt hyperendemic trachoma
- eradication of the insect vector to control onchocerciasis
- vitamin A supplementation in communities with childhood xerophthalmia
- education about contact lens disinfection in industrialized countries

Schwab L. *Eye Care in Developing Nations.* 4th ed. London: Manson Publishing; 2007.

Virology and Viral Infections

Viruses are small (10–400 nm in diameter) infectious units consisting of a single- or double-stranded nucleic acid genome and a protein capsid shell, with or without an external lipid envelope. In generating a virus taxonomy, the International Committee on Taxonomy of Viruses (ICTV) considers multiple virus traits, including morphology, physical properties, nucleic acid type and strandedness, physical state of the genome, proteins expressed, antigenic properties, and serologic cross-reactivity, as well as the biologic effects of infection. Viruses lack the independent means for energy metabolism, molecular biosynthesis, or replication.

Viral nucleic acid consists of either RNA or DNA. RNA viral genome may be either single- or double-stranded and, in the case of single-stranded viruses, either positive-sense (same polarity as mRNA) or negative-sense (opposite polarity to mRNA). The transcription of viral nucleic acid to produce the enzymatic and structural proteins necessary for replication varies with the type of viral genome. Antiviral medications typically target viral gene transcription. Therefore, the clinical significance of the nucleic acid type lies principally in differences in susceptibility to antiviral medications.

The *viral capsid* is a protein shell that surrounds the nucleic acid. The capsid interacts internally with the genome to stabilize it, protects the genome from the external environment, and, in the case of nonenveloped viruses, expresses on its surface the ligand for virus–host cell binding. Viral capsid proteins also help in delivery of the viral genome to the intracellular site of viral replication. Thus, viral capsid structure is integrally related to many viral functions—in particular, transmission, attachment, and entry into host target cells, but also virion assembly and egress.

For some virus families, a host cell–derived lipid bilayer or envelope surrounds the protein capsid. Viral genome–encoded glycoproteins bound to the membrane act as ligands (antigens) for neutralizing antibodies directed against the virus. The viral envelope lipid bilayer is vulnerable to damage by ultraviolet light, detergents, alcohols, and general-use antiseptics.

Because of this vulnerability, *enveloped viruses* such as HSV and human immunodeficiency virus (HIV) are intrinsically susceptible to the external environment, and their infectivity is short-lived outside the host. Enveloped viruses are difficult to transmit via fomites or medical instruments, and alcohol treatment of medical instrumentation is generally sufficient to prevent iatrogenic infection.

In contrast, *nonenveloped viruses* such as adenoviruses are relatively resistant to environmental insult and, in some cases, can persist for weeks outside the human host. The application of dilute (1%) bleach to tonometer tips for at least 10 minutes is recommended to prevent transmission of adenoviruses, but care must be taken to clean residual bleach from the tonometer tip prior to use.

CDC, National Prevention Information Network. [website]. HIV/AIDS FAQs and Basic Facts. Available at www.cdcnpin.org/scripts/hiv/faq.asp.

Chodosh J, Stroop WG. Introduction to viruses in ocular disease. In: Tasman W, Jaeger EA, eds. *Duane's Foundations of Clinical Ophthalmology.* Philadelphia: Lippincott Williams & Wilkins; 1998:chap 85, pp 1–10

DNA Viruses: Herpesviruses

The structure of all herpesviruses includes a core of linear double-stranded DNA genome, surrounded by an icosahedral protein capsid, an amorphous-appearing protein tegument, and finally an envelope studded with viral glycoproteins. Of the 8 known human herpesviruses, those that affect the eye include herpes simplex virus (HSV) types 1 and 2, varicella-zoster virus (VZV), Epstein-Barr virus (EBV), cytomegalovirus (CMV), and Kaposi sarcoma–associated herpesvirus (KSHV)/human herpesvirus 8. The production of viral progeny invariably destroys the infected cell. All herpesviruses establish latency in their natural hosts, but the site of latency varies. For example, whereas HSV types 1 and 2 and VZV establish latent infections in dorsal root ganglia such as the trigeminal ganglion, Epstein-Barr virus latency occurs in B lymphocytes.

Knipe DM, Howley PM, eds. *Fields' Virology.* 5th ed. Philadelphia: Lippincott Williams & Wilkins; 2006.

Herpes Simplex Eye Diseases

PATHOGENESIS   HSV infection is ubiquitous in humans; nearly 100% of those older than 60 years of age harbor HSV in their trigeminal ganglia at autopsy. It has been estimated that one third of the world population suffers from recurrent infection. Therefore, HSV infections are a large and worldwide public health problem.

HSV type 1 (HSV-1) and type 2 (HSV-2) are antigenically related and may coinfect the same nerve ganglia. HSV-1 more commonly causes infection above the waist (orofacial and ocular infection) and HSV-2 below the waist (genital infection), but either virus can cause disease in either location. In industrialized societies, 40%–80% of adults have serum antibodies to HSV-1, which represents a decline in infection from previous decades, and the age at which individuals undergo serologic conversion is increasing; HSV is now more commonly acquired in adolescence than in childhood. HSV infection is spread by direct contact with infected lesions or their secretions but most commonly occurs as a result of exposure to viruses shed asymptomatically. HSV can be transmitted to neonates as they pass through the birth canal of a mother with genital infection and, in the newborn, can cause disease confined to the skin and mucous membranes or systemic infection, including encephalitis. BCSC Section 6, *Pediatric Ophthalmology and Strabismus,* discusses neonatal herpes infection in greater detail.

Primary HSV-1 infection in humans occurs most commonly on skin and mucosal surfaces innervated by CN V (trigeminal nerve). Primary infection frequently manifests as a nonspecific upper respiratory tract infection and is recognized as HSV less than 5% of the time. HSV spreads from infected skin and mucosal epithelium via sensory nerve axons to establish latent infection in associated sensory nerve ganglia, including the trigeminal ganglion. Latent infection of the trigeminal ganglion occurs in the absence of recognized primary infection, and reactivation of the virus may follow in any of the 3 branches of CN V, despite primary disease in the area of innervation of 1 particular branch. Approximately 0.15% of the US population has a history of external ocular HSV infection, and, of these, approximately one fifth develop stromal keratitis, the most common blinding manifestation of infection.

Liesegang TJ. Herpes simplex virus epidemiology and ocular importance. *Cornea.* 2001;20(1): 1–13.

Primary ocular infection

CLINICAL PRESENTATION Primary ocular HSV infection typically manifests as a unilateral blepharoconjunctivitis. The conjunctival inflammatory response is follicular and accompanied by a palpable preauricular lymph node. Vesicles on the skin (Fig 4-2) or eyelid margin (Fig 4-3) are important for diagnosis. Patients with primary ocular HSV infection can develop epithelial keratitis (discussed later in the chapter), but stromal keratitis and uveitis are uncommon.

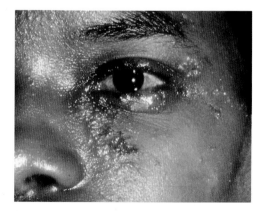

Figure 4-2 Skin vesicles of HSV dermatoblepharitis. *(Courtesy of James Chodosh, MD.)*

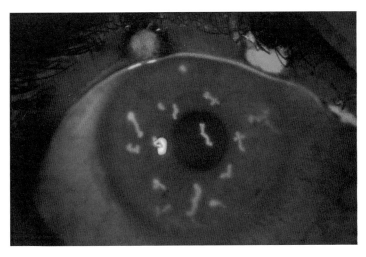

Figure 4-3 Fluorescein staining of an eye with primary HSV infection demonstrates character-istic lid margin ulcers and a coarse dendritic epithelial keratitis. *(Courtesy of James Chodosh, MD.)*

Signs that can be used to distinguish acute HSV ocular infection from that associated with adenovirus include

- cutaneous or eyelid margin vesicles, or ulcers on the bulbar conjunctiva (HSV)
- dendritic epithelial keratitis (HSV)
- conjunctival membranes or pseudomembranes (adenovirus)

Laterality is not a reliable distinguishing feature. Although adenoviral infections are more commonly bilateral, they can be unilateral, asymmetric, or bilateral with delayed involvement of the second eye. HSV ocular infection is typically unilateral, with only 3% of patients in the Herpetic Eye Disease Study (HEDS), a prospective multicenter clinical trial funded by the National Eye Institute in the 1990s, demonstrating bilateral disease (Table 4-5). The presence of bilateral disease should raise the question of immune dysfunction (eg, atopic dermatitis).

LABORATORY EVALUATION Demonstration of HSV is possible in productive epithelial infection with viral culture or antigen- or DNA-detection methodologies. Serologic tests for neutralizing or complement-fixing immunoglobulins may show a rising antibody titer during primary infection but are of no diagnostic assistance during recurrent episodes. As the majority of adults are latently infected with HSV, serologic testing generally is helpful only when negative.

Laboratory tests are indicated in complicated cases when the clinical diagnosis is uncertain and in all cases of suspected neonatal herpes infection. Vesicles can be opened with a needle, and vesicular fluid cultured. Scrapings from the vesicle base can be tested by cytology or for the presence of HSV antigen. Conjunctival scrapings or impression cytology specimens can be similarly analyzed by culture, antigen detection, or polymerase chain reaction (PCR).

Table 4-5 The HEDS Study

No.	Question	Study Design	Findings	Comment
1	Do topical corticosteroids treat stromal keratitis?	106 patients with stromal keratitis randomized to topical corticosteroids or placebo for 10 weeks. Treatment started with prednisolone 1% 8×/day and tapered to prednisolone 1/8% once a day. Both groups received topical trifluridine.	Yes. Topical corticosteroids significantly decreased stromal inflammation and shortened duration of keratitis.	The optimal corticosteroid regimen was not evaluated. Some patients respond to less corticosteroid and some may need a shorter/longer taper. Delaying corticosteroids for several weeks had no detrimental effect on vision.
2	Is oral acyclovir (in addition to treatment with trifluridine and corticosteroids) helpful in treating stromal keratitis?	104 patients with stromal keratitis randomized to oral acyclovir (400 mg 5×/day) vs placebo for a 10-week course. Both groups also received topical prednisolone and trifluridine.	No. Treatment of nonnecrotizing stromal keratitis with oral acyclovir was not beneficial.	Insufficient patients with necrotizing stromal keratitis to comment on effectiveness of acyclovir.
3	Is treatment-dose oral acyclovir helpful in treating HSV iritis?	50 patients with iritis treated with oral acyclovir (400 mg 5×/day) vs placebo for 10-week course.	Too few patients. A nonstatistically significant trend favoring the use of oral acyclovir.	Many clinicians favor use of oral acyclovir for treatment of HSV iridocyclitis.
4	Does oral acyclovir prevent patients with epithelial keratitis from developing stromal keratitis and iritis?	287 patients with epithelial keratitis received 3-week oral acyclovir (400 mg 5×/day) vs placebo; followed for 12 months.	No. No difference in development of stromal keratitis or iritis.	Best predictor for stromal keratitis is history of previous stromal keratitis.
5	Does acyclovir prophylaxis minimize HSV recurrences?	703 patients with inactive disease and off medications randomized to oral acyclovir (400 mg 2×/day) vs placebo for 12 months; followed for 18 months.	Recurrent ocular disease was less (approx 50%) in group on oral prophylaxis, especially those with recurrent stromal keratitis.	Long-term prophylaxis recommended for patients with recurrent HSV stromal keratitis.
6	What triggers HSV recurrences?	308 patients kept weekly log of stress, systemic infections, sunlight exposure, menstruation, CL wear, and eye injury.	No factors confirmed as triggers for recurrence.	

MANAGEMENT   Primary ocular HSV infection is a self-limited condition. Oral antiviral therapy speeds resolution of signs and symptoms. Table 4-6 summarizes the antiviral agents effective against HSV infections.

Recurrent ocular infection

PATHOGENESIS   Recurrent HSV infection is caused by reactivation of the virus in a latently infected sensory ganglion, transport of the virus down the nerve axon to sensory nerve endings, and subsequent infection of ocular surface epithelia. HSV latency in the cornea as a cause of recurrent disease remains a controversial concept.

Anecdotal reports that environmental factors act as triggers for the recurrence of HSV ocular disease were not confirmed by the HEDS Study Group. Psychologic stress, systemic infection, sunlight exposure, menstrual cycle, and contact lens wear were not shown to induce recurrent ocular HSV infection. An increased rate of recurrence for HSV keratitis was associated with HIV infection in a retrospective study. However, no difference was found in the severity of HSV keratitis between HIV-infected and uninfected persons, despite the observed discrepancy in recurrence rate.

> Psychological stress and other potential triggers for recurrences of herpes simplex virus eye infections. Herpetic Eye Disease Study Group. *Arch Ophthalmol.* 2000;118(12):1617–1625.

Table 4-6 Antiviral Agents in External/Corneal Infections With Herpes Simplex Virus

Agent	Mechanism of Action	Administration	Dosage for Acute Disease
Vidarabine	Purine analogue Inhibits DNA polymerase	3% ophthalmic ointment*	5×/day for 10 days
Trifluridine	Pyrimidine analogue Blocks DNA synthesis	1% ophthalmic solution	8×/day for 10 days
Acyclovir	Activated by HSV thymidine kinase to inhibit viral DNA polymerase	3% ophthalmic ointment† 200, 400, 800 mg; 200 mg/5 mL suspension 5% dermatologic ointment‡	5×/day for 10 days 400 mg 5×/day for 10 days 6×/day for 7 days
Famciclovir§	Pro-drug of penciclovir	125, 250, 500 mg	250 mg 3×/day for 10 days
Valacyclovir§	L-valyl ester of acyclovir	500, 1000 mg	1000 mg 2×/day for 10 days
Penciclovir	Inhibits viral DNA polymerase	1% dermatologic cream‡	8×/day for 4 days
Ganciclovir	Inhibits DNA polymerase	0.15% topical ophthalmic gel	5×/day until epithelium heals; then 3×/day for 7 days

*No longer manufactured; can be obtained through compounding pharmacies.
†Not commercially available in the United States.
‡Not for ophthalmic use.
§Optimal dose for ocular disease not determined.

CLINICAL PRESENTATION   Recurrent HSV can affect almost any ocular tissue, including the eyelid, conjunctiva, cornea, iris, trabecular meshwork, and retina. The most common presentations of clinically recognizable recurrent ocular HSV infection include

- blepharoconjunctivitis
- epithelial keratitis
- stromal keratitis
- iridocyclitis

Blepharoconjunctivitis   Eyelid and/or conjunctival involvement can occur in patients with recurrent ocular HSV infection, although it is clinically indistinguishable from primary infection. The condition is self-limited but can be treated with antivirals to shorten the course of illness.

Epithelial keratitis

CLINICAL PRESENTATION   Patients with epithelial keratitis complain of foreign-body sensation, light sensitivity, redness, and blurred vision. HSV infection of human corneal epithelium manifests as areas of punctate epithelial keratitis that may coalesce into 1 or more arborizing dendritic epithelial ulcers with terminal bulbs at the end of each branch. The cytopathic swollen corneal epithelium at the edge of a herpetic ulcer stains with rose bengal and lissamine green (Fig 4-4) due to loss of cell membrane glycoproteins and subsequent lack of mucin binding by the cells. The bed of the ulcer stains with fluorescein (Fig 4-5) due to loss of cellular integrity and absence of intercellular tight junctions. Particularly with use of topical corticosteroids, areas of dendritic keratitis may coalesce further and enlarge into a more expansive geographic epithelial ulcer (Fig 4-6). The swollen epithelium at the ulcer's edge will stain with rose bengal, and, frequently, dendritic morphology can be seen at the periphery of the ulcer.

Patients with HSV epithelial keratitis exhibit a ciliary flush and mild conjunctival injection. Mild stromal edema and subepithelial white blood cell infiltration may develop as well beneath the epithelial keratitis. Following resolution of dendritic epithelial keratitis, nonsuppurative subepithelial infiltration and scarring may be seen just beneath the area of prior epithelial ulceration, resulting in a ghost image, or ghost dendrite (Fig 4-7), reflecting the position and shape of the prior epithelial involvement.

Focal or diffuse reduction in corneal sensation develops following HSV epithelial keratitis. The distribution of corneal hypoesthesia is related to the extent, duration, severity, and number of recurrences of herpetic keratitis. Sectoral corneal anesthesia may be difficult to detect clinically and is not a reliable sign of herpetic disease.

Other conditions that may produce dendritiform epithelial lesions include

- varicella-zoster virus (see the discussion later in the chapter)
- adenovirus (uncommon)
- Epstein-Barr virus (rare)
- epithelial regeneration line
- neurotrophic keratopathy (postherpetic, diabetes mellitus)
- soft contact lens wear (thimerosal)

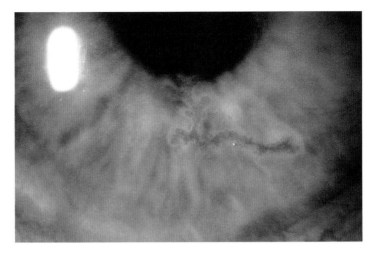

Figure 4-4 Rose bengal staining of herpetic epithelial keratitis outlines a typical dendrite. *(Courtesy of James Chodosh, MD.)*

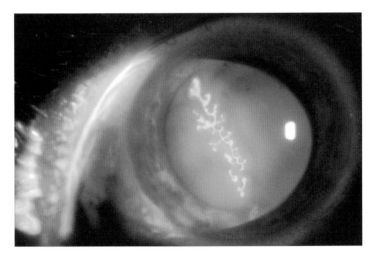

Figure 4-5 Fluorescein staining of herpetic dendritic keratitis. *(Courtesy of James Chodosh, MD.)*

- topical medications (antivirals, β-blockers)
- *Acanthamoeba*
- epithelial deposits (iron lines, Fabry disease, tyrosinemia type II, systemic drugs)

LABORATORY EVALUATION   A specific clinical diagnosis of HSV as the cause of dendritic keratitis can usually be made based on the presence of characteristic clinical features. Tissue culture and/or antigen detection techniques may be helpful in establishing the diagnosis in atypical cases.

MANAGEMENT   Most cases of HSV epithelial keratitis resolve spontaneously, and there is no evidence to suggest that the form of antiviral therapy influences the subsequent

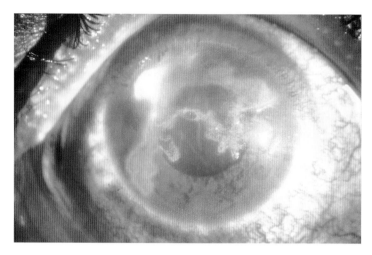

Figure 4-6 Herpetic geographic epithelial keratitis. *(Reprinted with permission from Chodosh J. Viral keratitis. In: Parrish RK, ed.* The University of Miami Bascom Palmer Eye Institute Atlas of Ophthalmology. *Boston: Current Medicine; 1999.)*

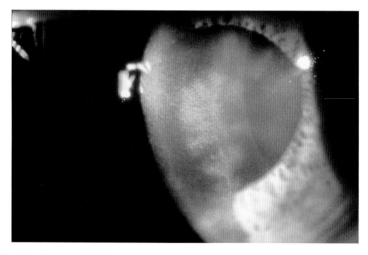

Figure 4-7 Residual stromal inflammation following dendritic epithelial keratitis may leave the impression of a ghost image of the dendrite. *(Reprinted with permission from Chodosh J. Viral keratitis. In: Parrish RK, ed.* The University of Miami Bascom Palmer Eye Institute Atlas of Ophthalmology. *Boston: Current Medicine; 1999.)*

development of stromal keratitis or recurrent epithelial disease. However, treatment shortens the clinical course and might conceivably reduce associated herpetic neuropathy. Minimal wiping debridement with a dry cotton-tipped applicator or cellulose sponge speeds resolution. Antiviral therapy can be used by itself or in combination with epithelial debridement. Topical trifluridine 1% solution 8 times daily is efficacious for both dendritic and geographic epithelial keratitis. Treatment of the disease with topical antivirals generally should be discontinued within 10–14 days to avoid unnecessary toxicity to the ocular surface. Acyclovir 3% ophthalmic ointment has been reported to be as effective as and less toxic than trifluridine and vidarabine, but the ophthalmic form is not available in the United States. Oral acyclovir has been reported to be as effective as topical antivirals for treating epithelial keratitis, and it has the advantage of no ocular toxicity. For this reason, oral therapy is preferred by an increasing number of physicians. Valacyclovir, a pro-drug of acyclovir likely to be just as effective for ocular disease, can cause thrombotic thrombocytopenic purpura/hemolytic uremia syndrome in severely immunocompromised patients such as those with AIDS; thus, it must be used with caution if the immune status is unknown. Topical corticosteroids are contraindicated in the presence of active herpetic epithelial keratitis; patients with this disease who are using systemic corticosteroids for other indications should be treated aggressively with systemic antiviral therapy.

Stromal keratitis   HSV stromal keratitis is the most common cause of infectious corneal blindness in the United States, and it is the form of recurrent herpetic external disease associated with the greatest visual morbidity. Each episode of stromal keratitis increases the risk of future episodes.

PATHOGENESIS   The pathogenesis of herpetic stromal keratitis in humans remains unknown but probably depends on the type of stromal inflammation (see the following section). Animal models of herpetic eye disease do not precisely replicate the human situation; studies of HSV stromal keratitis in mouse models have variously implicated HSV-specific CD4 and CD8 T lymphocytes and anti-HSV antibodies in keratitis pathogenesis. Studies also implicate cell-mediated immunity to corneal antigens up-regulated by HSV infection and the bystander effects of proinflammatory cytokine secretion by infected corneal cells.

> Streilein JW, Dana MR, Ksander BR. Immunity causing blindness: five different paths to herpes stromal keratitis. *Immunol Today.* 1997;18(9):443–449.

CLINICAL PRESENTATION   Herpetic stromal keratitis can be nonnecrotizing (interstitial or disciform) or necrotizing, and different forms may present simultaneously. *Herpetic interstitial keratitis* presents as unifocal or multifocal interstitial haze or whitening of the stroma in the absence of epithelial ulceration (Fig 4-8). Mild stromal edema may accompany the haze, but epithelial edema is not typical. In the absence of significant extracorneal inflammatory signs such as conjunctival injection or anterior chamber cells, it may be difficult to identify active disease in an area of previous scar and thinning. Long-standing or multiply recurrent HSV interstitial keratitis may be associated with corneal vascularization. The differential diagnosis of herpetic interstitial keratitis includes

- VZV keratitis
- *Acanthamoeba* keratitis
- syphilis
- EBV keratitis
- mumps keratitis
- Lyme disease
- sarcoidosis
- Cogan syndrome

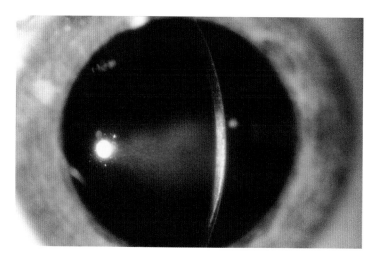

Figure 4-8 Herpetic interstitial keratitis (nonnecrotizing). *(Reprinted with permission from Chodosh J. Viral keratitis. In: Parrish RK, ed. The University of Miami Bascom Palmer Eye Institute Atlas of Ophthalmology. Boston: Current Medicine; 1999.)*

Herpetic disciform keratitis is a primary endotheliitis, which presents as corneal stromal and epithelial edema in a round or oval distribution, associated with keratic precipitates underlying the zone of edema (Fig 4-9). Iridocyclitis can be associated, and the disciform keratitis may be confused with uveitis with secondary corneal endothelial decompensation. However, in disciform keratitis, disc-shaped stromal edema and keratic precipitates appear out of proportion to the degree of anterior chamber reaction. Disciform keratitis due to HSV and that due to VZV are clinically indistinguishable.

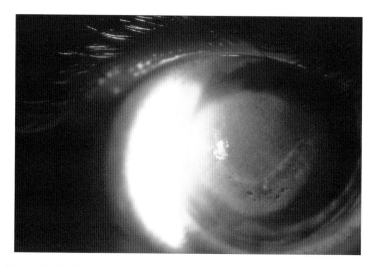

Figure 4-9 Herpetic disciform keratitis (nonnecrotizing). *(Reprinted with permission from Chodosh J. Viral keratitis. In: Parrish RK, ed. The University of Miami Bascom Palmer Eye Institute Atlas of Ophthalmology. Boston: Current Medicine; 1999.)*

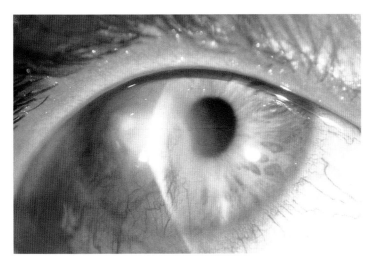

Figure 4-10 Necrotizing herpetic stromal keratitis.

Herpetic necrotizing keratitis appears as suppurative corneal inflammation (Fig 4-10). It may be severe, progress rapidly, and appear clinically indistinguishable from fulminant bacterial or fungal keratitis. Overlying epithelial ulceration is common, but the epithelial defect may occur somewhat eccentric to the infiltrate, and the edges of the epithelial ulcer do not stain with rose bengal dye. Corneal stromal vascularization is common. The differential diagnosis of herpetic necrotizing keratitis includes microbial keratitis due to bacteria, fungi, or acanthamoebae, retained foreign body, and topical anesthetic abuse.

MANAGEMENT Many past controversies regarding the optimal management of HSV stromal keratitis have been resolved by the HEDS trial (see Table 4-5). Most important, HEDS findings showed that topical corticosteroids given together with a prophylactic antiviral reduce persistence or progression of stromal inflammation and shorten the duration of HSV stromal keratitis; in addition, long-term suppressive oral acyclovir therapy reduces the rate of recurrent HSV keratitis and helps to preserve vision. Long-term antiviral prophylaxis is now recommended for patients with multiple recurrences of HSV stromal keratitis. The HEDS showed no additional benefit of oral acyclovir in treating active HSV stromal keratitis in patients receiving concomitant topical corticosteroids and trifluridine. When given briefly along with trifluridine during an episode of epithelial keratitis, acyclovir also did not appear to prevent subsequent HSV stromal keratitis or iritis.

The experimental protocol applied by HEDS investigators for patients with herpetic stromal keratitis is a useful starting point for a treatment algorithm. Visually significant herpetic interstitial keratitis is treated initially with 1% prednisolone drops every 2 hours accompanied by a prophylactic antiviral drug, either topical trifluridine qid or an oral agent such as acyclovir 400 mg bid or valacyclovir 500 mg once a day. The prednisolone drops are tapered every 1–2 weeks depending on the degree of clinical improvement. The antiviral is used to prevent severe epithelial keratitis should the patient shed HSV while on corticosteroid drops, and it is generally continued until the patient is completely off corticosteroids or using less than 1 drop of 1% prednisolone per day. Patients should be tapered to the lowest possible corticosteroid dosage that controls their inflammation.

Available topical antiviral medications are not absorbed by the cornea through an intact epithelium, but orally administered acyclovir penetrates an intact cornea and anterior chamber. In this context, anecdotal evidence suggests that oral acyclovir might benefit the deep corneal inflammation of disciform keratitis. The HEDS showed no additional benefit when acyclovir was added to trifluridine and prednisolone for the treatment of herpetic stromal keratitis, but disciform keratitis was not analyzed as a separate group. Some corneal specialists routinely substitute oral acyclovir for topical trifluridine in treating disciform keratitis.

Necrotizing herpetic stromal keratitis is probably the least common form of herpetic keratitis. The diagnosis is frequently one of exclusion following negative cultures for fungal and bacterial pathogens, but it is suggested by a history of HSV facial, conjunctival, and/or corneal infection. The toxicity of topical antiviral agents may be undesirable in patients with necrotizing inflammation and can confuse the clinical picture. Therefore, an oral antiviral such as acyclovir is preferred. Fortunately, necrotizing herpetic keratitis appears to be very sensitive to topical corticosteroids, and twice a day dosing may be sufficient to control inflammation in many patients.

Acyclovir for the prevention of recurrent herpes simplex virus eye disease. Herpetic Eye Disease Study Group. *N Engl J Med.* 1998;339(5):300–306.

Barron BA, Gee L, Hauck WW, et al. Herpetic Eye Disease Study. A controlled trial of oral acyclovir for herpes simplex stromal keratitis. *Ophthalmology.* 1994;101(12):1871–1882.

A controlled trial of oral acyclovir for the prevention of stromal keratitis or iritis in patients with herpes simplex virus epithelial keratitis. The Epithelial Keratitis Trial. The Herpetic Eye Disease Study Group. *Arch Ophthalmol.* 1997;115(6):703–712.

Oral acyclovir for herpes simplex virus eye disease: effect on prevention of epithelial keratitis and stromal keratitis. Herpetic Eye Disease Study Group. *Arch Ophthalmol.* 2000;118(8): 1030–1036.

Wilhelmus KR, Gee L, Hauck WW, et al. Herpetic Eye Disease Study. A controlled trial of topical corticosteroids for herpes simplex stromal keratitis. *Ophthalmology.* 1994;101(12): 1883–1895.

Iridocyclitis   Granulomatous or nongranulomatous iridocyclitis may accompany necrotizing stromal keratitis or occur independently of corneal disease. Elevated IOP caused by trabeculitis and/or patchy iris transillumination defects may be found in patients with HSV iridocyclitis. Infectious virus has been cultured from the anterior chamber of such patients and its presence positively correlated with ocular hypertension. Therefore, the diagnosis of HSV iridocyclitis is suggested by a unilateral presentation associated with an elevated IOP with or without focal iris transillumination defects. A history or clinical evidence of prior HSV ocular disease is suggestive. One HEDS trial suggested a statistical trend toward the benefit of oral acyclovir (400 mg, 5 times daily) in treating HSV iridocyclitis in patients also receiving topical corticosteroids, but the number of patients recruited was too small to achieve statistically conclusive results.

Complications of herpetic eye disease affect all layers of the cornea. *Epitheliopathy* is common when topical antiviral treatment is prolonged, and its severity and duration are directly related to the duration of antiviral use. Topical antiviral toxicity presents most commonly as diffuse punctate corneal epithelial erosions with conjunctival injection. *Neurotrophic keratopathy* may develop in patients with reduced corneal sensation secondary to past herpetic infection. Punctate epithelial erosions, sometimes with a vortex pattern of punctate fluorescein staining, chronic epithelial regeneration lines, and frank neurotrophic ulcers characterize neurotrophic keratopathy. These ulcers can be distinguished from herpetic epithelial keratitis by a relative absence of rose bengal staining. Neurotrophic ulcers are typically round or oval and located in the central or inferior cornea. Corneal epithelium at the edges of a neurotrophic ulcer may appear to roll under itself and typically has a gray, elevated appearance. Liberal use of nonpreserved lubricating drops, gels, and ointments combined with punctal occlusion are the mainstays of therapy. To prevent progressive stromal thinning and perforation, tarsorrhaphy is indicated for neurotrophic ulcers that fail to respond to conservative therapy. On occasion, active or resolving interstitial stromal keratitis due to HSV is associated with a chronic epithelial defect that does not stain with rose bengal. This so-called *metaherpetic ulcer* probably results from neurotrophic mechanisms or a devitalized corneal stroma.

Severe or long-standing disciform keratitis can result in *persistent bullous keratopathy.* Stromal inflammation in general, whether interstitial or necrotizing, commonly leads to permanent corneal scarring and irregular astigmatism. Both scarring and astigmatism may improve with time in some patients. Fitting with a gas-permeable contact lens usually improves visual acuity beyond that achieved with spectacle refraction. In patients with deep corneal stromal vascularization due to prior necrotizing herpetic inflammation, secondary lipid keratopathy may further impair the vision. Topical corticosteroids may suppress new vessel growth and halt additional lipid deposition.

A controlled trial of oral acyclovir for iridocyclitis caused by herpes simplex virus. Herpetic Eye Disease Study Group. *Arch Ophthalmol.* 1996;114(9):1065–1072.

SURGICAL TREATMENT Penetrating keratoplasty (PK) is indicated in selected patients with visually significant stromal scarring and astigmatism not correctable by spectacle or contact lens. Oral antiviral therapy may improve graft survival by reducing the risk of HSV recurrence and allow more liberal use of topical corticosteroids. Oral antivirals lack epithelial toxicity and are therefore generally preferable to topical antivirals in patients after PK. The prognosis for successful optical PK approaches 80% in eyes without signs of active inflammation for at least 6 months prior to surgery. Tectonic PK is indicated in impending or frank corneal perforation due to necrotizing or neurotrophic ulcers. Stromal inflammation, ulceration, and graft failure may develop in inflamed herpetic eyes undergoing tectonic PK. Therefore, small descemetoceles and perforations in inflamed eyes may best be treated by applying therapeutic tissue adhesive and a bandage contact lens and delaying PK until inflammation can be controlled. Amniotic membrane transplantation (AMT) may also be used for persistent epithelial defects with and without corneal thinning.

Varicella-Zoster Virus Dermatoblepharitis, Conjunctivitis, and Keratitis

PATHOGENESIS As with other herpesviruses, VZV causes a primary infection (varicella, or chickenpox) and subsequent latency, occasionally followed later by recurrent disease (zoster, or shingles). Primary VZV infection occurs upon direct contact with VZV skin lesions or respiratory secretions via airborne droplets and is highly contagious for naive individuals. VZV infection is usually a self-limited infection of childhood rarely associated with long-term sequelae. However, infection of adults or immunosuppressed individuals can be fatal. In children, VZV infection manifests with fever, malaise, and a vesicular dermatitis that lasts 7–10 days. Except for eyelid vesicles and follicular conjunctivitis, ocular involvement is uncommon during primary infection. As with HSV, VZV latency occurs in neural ganglia and, in approximately 20% of infected individuals, reactivates later. Of all cases with zoster, 15% involve the ophthalmic division of CN V (trigeminal). VZV infection, whether primary or recurrent, can usually be distinguished from HSV infection through a careful history and examination. Distinguishing features of each infection are listed in Table 4-7.

CLINICAL PRESENTATION   The rash of chickenpox begins as macules and progresses to papules, vesicles, and then pustules that dry, crust over, and may leave individual scars. Ocular involvement may include follicular conjunctivitis, occasionally associated with a vesicular lesion on the bulbar conjunctiva or eyelid margins. Punctate or dendritic epithelial keratitis is uncommon. Although subepithelial infiltrates, stromal keratitis, disciform keratitis, uveitis, and elevated IOP are rare, recurrent varicella keratouveitis may cause significant morbidity in some patients.

LABORATORY EVALUATION   Laboratory confirmation of acute or recurrent VZV infection is possible by immunodiagnostic methods, viral culture, and PCR. Serologic testing is used primarily to identify varicella-naive adults who might benefit from prophylactic vaccination. As with HSV, scrapings from a vesicle base can be tested by cytology, PCR, or culture, or for the presence of VZV antigen. Conjunctival scrapings or corneal impression cytology specimens can be similarly analyzed by culture, antigen detection, or PCR.

MANAGEMENT   Because infected individuals shed the virus in respiratory secretions before the onset of the characteristic rash, avoiding infected persons is not always possible.

Table 4-7 **Differentiating Features of Eye Disease Caused by Herpes Simplex Virus and Reactivation of Varicella-Zoster Virus**

	Herpes Simplex Virus	Varicella-Zoster Virus
Dermatomal distribution	Incomplete	Complete
Pain	Moderate	Severe
Dendrite morphology	Central ulceration with terminal bulbs; geographic in presence of corticosteroids	Smaller without central ulceration or terminal bulbs; dendritiform mucous plaques occur later
Skin scarring	No	Common
Postherpetic neuralgia	No	Common
Iris atrophy	Patchy	Sectoral
Bilateral involvement	Uncommon	No
Recurrent epithelial keratitis	Common	Rare
Corneal hypoesthesia	Sectoral or diffuse	May be severe

Vaccination against varicella is recommended for anyone older than 12 months of age without a history of chickenpox or with a negative serology. The severity of signs and symptoms may be reduced in clinically ill patients by the administration of oral acyclovir. Significant keratitis or uveitis can be treated with topical corticosteroids.

Herpes zoster ophthalmicus

PATHOGENESIS Following primary infection, VZV establishes latency in sensory neural ganglia. Zoster (shingles) represents endogenous reactivation of latent virus in people with a waxing level of immunity to infection. Most patients are in their sixth to ninth decades, and the majority are healthy, with no specific predisposing factors. However, zoster is more common in patients on immunosuppressive therapy; in those with a systemic malignancy, a debilitating disease, or HIV infection; and after major surgery, trauma, or radiation.

CLINICAL PRESENTATION Zoster manifests as a painful vesicular dermatitis typically localized to a single dermatome on the thorax or face. Patients may complain initially of fever and malaise, and warmth, redness, and increased sensation in the affected dermatome. The most commonly affected dermatomes are on the thorax (T3 through L3) and those supplied by CN V (trigeminal). The ophthalmic division of the trigeminal nerve is affected more often than the maxillary and mandibular branches, and its involvement is referred to as *herpes zoster ophthalmicus (HZO)* (Fig 4-11). A maculopapular rash, followed by vesicles and then pustules, is characteristic. Zoster dermatitis may result in large scabs that resolve slowly and leave significant scarring. Neurotrophic keratopathy and sectoral iris atrophy are characteristic. Inflammation of almost any ocular tissue can occur and recur in HZO.

Zoster dermatitis is accompanied by pain and dysesthesia. The pain usually decreases as lesions resolve; however, neuralgia in the affected dermatome can continue from months to years. The severity of pain ranges from mild to incapacitating. Ocular involvement occurs in more than 70% of patients with zoster of the first division of CN V and

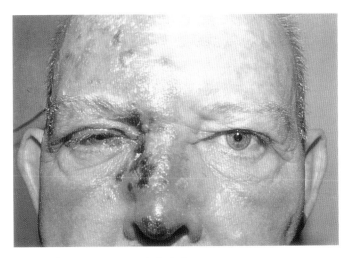

Figure 4-11 Herpes zoster ophthalmicus. *(Courtesy of Vincent P. deLuise, MD.)*

may appear in association with any branch, including the nasociliary, frontal, or lacrimal branches. Ophthalmic complications also may occur with zoster of the second (maxillary) division of CN V. In immunosuppressed patients, zoster may involve more than one branch of the trigeminal nerve at the same time, can chronically reactivate, and may be multiply recurrent.

Eyelid vesicular eruption can lead to secondary bacterial infection, eyelid scarring, marginal notching, loss of cilia, trichiasis, and cicatricial entropion or ectropion. Scarring and occlusion of the lacrimal puncta or canaliculi may occur. Episcleritis or scleritis associated with zoster may be nodular, zonal, or diffuse.

Both punctate and dendritic epithelial keratitis caused by viral replication in corneal epithelium are common manifestations of ophthalmic zoster. Dendrites may persist and remain chronically culture-positive for VZV in AIDS patients. Elevated dendritiform mucous plaques may occur weeks to months after resolution of the skin lesions. Diminished corneal sensation develops in up to 50% of patients. Nummular corneal infiltrates are said to be characteristic of zoster stromal keratitis (Fig 4-12), but the interstitial keratitis, disciform keratitis, and anterior uveitis with increased IOP in HZO are clinically indistinguishable from those caused by HSV infection. Chronic corneal stromal inflammation can lead to corneal vascularization, lipid keratopathy (Fig 4-13), and corneal opacity. Corneal anesthesia may be profound, and neurotrophic keratopathy due to HZO can be extremely difficult to manage.

Focal choroiditis, occlusive retinal vasculitis, and retinal detachment have been reported. Ipsilateral acute retinal necrosis (ARN) temporally associated with HZO is uncommon.

Orbital or CNS involvement as a result of an occlusive arteritis may lead to eyelid ptosis, orbital edema, and proptosis. Papillitis or retrobulbar optic neuritis may also develop. Cranial nerve palsies have been reported to occur in up to one third of cases of HZO, with CN III (oculomotor) most commonly affected. Cranial nerve involvement may occur

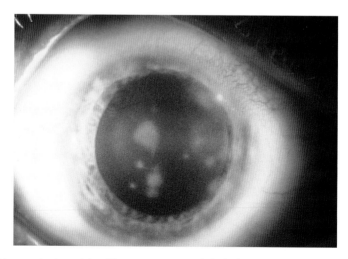

Figure 4-12 Nummular keratitis of herpes zoster ophthalmicus. *(Courtesy of Rhea L. Siatkowski, MD.)*

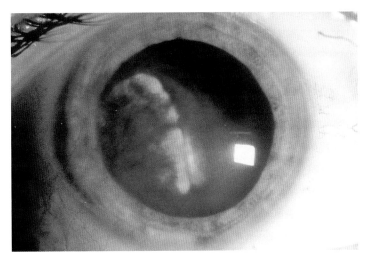

Figure 4-13 Lipid keratopathy following herpes zoster ophthalmicus. *(Reprinted with permission from Chodosh J. Viral keratitis. In: Parrish RK, ed. The University of Miami Bascom Palmer Eye Institute Atlas of Ophthalmology. Boston: Current Medicine; 1999.)*

within the orbit or the cavernous sinus. Systemic dissemination is unusual in immunocompetent patients but can occur in up to 25% of those who are immunocompromised.

MANAGEMENT   Oral antiviral therapy for HZO was found in randomized clinical trials to reduce viral shedding from vesicular skin lesions, reduce the chance of systemic dissemination of the virus, and decrease the incidence and severity of the most common ocular complications. Oral antiviral therapy may reduce the duration if not the incidence of postherpetic neuralgia if begun within 72 hours of the onset of symptoms. There are also reports to suggest that initiating antiviral therapy after 72 hours, especially in the presence of new vesicles, is beneficial. Amitriptyline has also been reported to decrease the duration of postherpetic neuralgia if given early on and continued until pain symptoms remit.

A varicella-zoster vaccine has recently been approved, after testing in 38,000 patients demonstrated a 50% reduction in incidence of zoster and a 66% reduction in postherpetic neuralgia. This vaccine is recommended for immunocompetent individuals over 60 years of age.

The current recommendation for HZO is oral famciclovir 500 mg 3 times per day, valacyclovir 1 g 3 times per day, or acyclovir 800 mg 5 times per day for 7–10 days, best if started within 72 hours of the onset of skin lesions. Topical antiviral medications are not effective. Intravenous acyclovir therapy is indicated in patients at risk for disseminated zoster due to immunosuppression. Cutaneous lesions may be treated with moist warm compresses and topical antibiotic ointment. Topical corticosteroids and cycloplegics are indicated for keratouveitis. Oral corticosteroids on a tapering dosage are recommended by some for treating patients with HZO over age 60 to reduce early zoster pain and facilitate a rapid return to a normal quality of life. However, the use of oral corticosteroids is controversial; their use does not seem to affect the incidence or duration of postherpetic neuralgia.

Postherpetic neuralgia (PHN) may respond to capsaicin cream applied to the involved skin, but low doses of amitriptyline, desipramine, clomipramine, or carbamazepine may be necessary to control severe symptoms. Gabapentin (Neurontin) and pregabalin (Lyrica) are also effective in managing PHN. Aggressive lubrication with nonpreserved tears, gels, and ointments, combined with punctal occlusion and tarsorrhaphy as necessary, may be indicated for neurotrophic keratopathy. In a patient with significant pain, early referral to a pain management specialist should be considered.

Liesegang, TJ. Herpes zoster virus infection. *Curr Opin Ophthalmol.* 2004;15(6):531–536.

Oxman MN, Levin MJ, Johnson GR, et al; Shingles Prevention Study Group. A vaccine to prevent herpes zoster and postherpetic neuralgia in older adults. *N Engl J Med.* 2005;352(22): 2271–2284.

Epstein-Barr Virus Dacryoadenitis, Conjunctivitis, and Keratitis

PATHOGENESIS   EBV is a ubiquitous herpesvirus that infects the majority of humans by early adulthood. Spread of EBV occurs by the sharing of saliva and results in subclinical infection in the first decade of life; if acquired later in life, it causes infectious mononucleosis. The virus remains latent in B lymphocytes and pharyngeal mucosal epithelial cells throughout life. Ocular disease is uncommon.

CLINICAL PRESENTATION   EBV is the most common cause of acute dacryoadenitis, characterized by inflammatory enlargement of 1 or both lacrimal glands. Acute follicular conjunctivitis, Parinaud oculoglandular syndrome, and bulbar conjunctival nodules have been reported in patients with acute infectious mononucleosis and may be the result of EBV infection. The 3 principal forms of EBV stromal keratitis are associated with EBV on the basis of a history of recent infectious mononucleosis and/or persistently high EBV serologic titers:

- *Type 1:* multifocal subepithelial infiltrates that resemble adenoviral keratitis
- *Type 2:* multifocal, blotchy, pleomorphic infiltrates with active inflammation (Fig 4-14) or granular ring-shaped opacities (inactive form) in anterior to mid stroma
- *Type 3:* multifocal deep or full-thickness peripheral infiltrates, with or without vascularization, that resemble interstitial keratitis due to syphilis

EBV-associated keratitis may be unilateral or bilateral and may, in select cases, appear similar to that induced by HSV, VZV, Lyme disease, adenovirus, or syphilis.

MANAGEMENT   Because of difficulty in isolating the virus, the diagnosis of EBV infection depends on the detection of antibodies to various viral components. During acute infection, first IgM and then IgG antibodies to viral capsid antigens (VCA) appear. Anti-VCA IgG may persist for the life of the patient. Antibodies to early antigens also rise during the acute phases of the disease and subsequently decrease to low or undetectable levels in most individuals. Antibodies to EBV nuclear antigens appear weeks to months later, providing serologic evidence of past infection. Acyclovir is not effective treatment for the clinical signs and symptoms of infectious mononucleosis, but the impact of antiviral

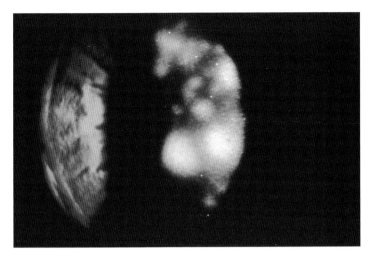

Figure 4-14 Epstein-Barr virus stromal keratitis. *(Reprinted with permission from Chodosh J. Viral keratitis. In: Parrish RK, ed.* The University of Miami Bascom Palmer Eye Institute Atlas of Ophthalmology. *Boston: Current Medicine; 1999.)*

therapy on the corneal manifestations of EBV infection remains unknown. Corticosteroids may be effective in patients with reduced vision due to apparent EBV stromal keratitis, but they should not be administered without a prophylactic antiviral if HSV infection is a possibility.

Chodosh J. Epstein-Barr virus stromal keratitis. *Ophthalmol Clin North Am.* 1994;7(4):549–556.

DNA Viruses: Adenoviruses

The Adenoviridae are double-stranded DNA viruses associated with significant human disease and morbidity. Forty-nine serotypes subdivide into 6 distinct subgroups (A–F) on the basis of genetic sequencing. Adenovirus subgroups associate broadly with specific clinical syndromes. For instance, subgroup D adenoviruses are strongly associated with epidemic keratoconjunctivitis. The nonenveloped protein capsid of the adenovirus forms a regular icosahedron. For most adenoviral subgroups, a projecting capsid protein serves as the ligand for the cellular adenovirus receptor, and the interaction of an adjacent capsid protein with cell surface integrins mediates internalization of the virus.

Knipe DM, Howley PM, eds. *Fields' Virology.* 5th ed. Philadelphia: Lippincott Williams & Wilkins; 2006.

PATHOGENESIS Originally isolated in 1953 from surgically removed human adenoids, adenoviruses cause a broad spectrum of diseases, including infections of the upper respiratory tract and ocular surface, meningoencephalitis, acute hemorrhagic cystitis of young boys, diarrhea of children, acute respiratory disease of children and military recruits, and respiratory and hepatic failure in an immunocompromised host. Adenoviruses are transmitted by close contact with ocular or respiratory secretions, fomites, or contaminated swimming pools. Transmission occurs more readily in populations living in close quarters, such as schools, nursing homes, military housing, and summer camps. Transmission of adenoviruses by contaminated instruments or eyedrops in physicians' offices may occur. For this reason, IOP measurements should be taken with an instrument with a disposable cover.

CLINICAL PRESENTATION   Each subgroup (A–F) of adenoviruses and, to a lesser degree, each serotype possesses unique tissue tropisms that reveal the association of specific adenoviruses with distinct clinical syndromes. Most adenoviral eye disease presents clinically as 1 of 3 classic syndromes:

1. simple follicular conjunctivitis (multiple serotypes)
2. pharyngoconjunctival fever (most commonly serotype 3 or 7)
3. epidemic keratoconjunctivitis (EKC; usually serotype 8, 19, or 37, subgroup D)

Different adenoviral syndromes are indistinguishable early in infection and may be unilateral or bilateral.

Adenoviral follicular conjunctivitis is self-limited, not associated with systemic disease, and often so transient that patients do not seek care. Epithelial keratitis, if present, is mild and fleeting. *Pharyngoconjunctival fever* is characterized by fever, headache, pharyngitis, follicular conjunctivitis, and preauricular adenopathy. The systemic signs and symptoms may mimic influenza. Any associated epithelial keratitis is mild.

Epidemic keratoconjunctivitis is the only adenoviral syndrome with significant corneal involvement. The infection is bilateral in a majority of patients and may be preceded by an upper respiratory infection. One week to 10 days after inoculation, severe follicular conjunctivitis develops, associated with a punctate epithelial keratitis. The conjunctival morphology is follicular but may be obscured by chemosis. Petechial hemorrhages and, occasionally, larger subconjunctival hemorrhages can occur. Preauricular adenopathy is prominent. Pseudomembranes or true membranes (Fig 4-15) occur predominantly on the tarsal conjunctiva and may be missed on cursory examination. Patients complain of tearing, light sensitivity, and foreign-body sensation. Large central geographic corneal erosions can develop and may persist for several days despite patching and lubrication. Within 7–14 days after onset of eye symptoms, multifocal subepithelial (stromal) corneal infiltrates become apparent on slit-lamp examination (Fig 4-16). Photophobia and reduced vision from adenoviral subepithelial infiltrates may persist for months to years.

Epithelial keratitis occurs due to adenovirus replication within the corneal epithelium. Subepithelial infiltrates are likely caused by an immunopathologic response to viral infection of keratocytes in the superficial corneal stroma. The evolution of keratitis in EKC is summarized in Figure 4-17. Chronic complications of conjunctival membranes include subepithelial conjunctival scarring, symblepharon formation, and dry eye due to alterations within the lacrimal glands or lacrimal ducts.

LABORATORY EVALUATION   Diagnosis of EKC is suggested in the setting of bilateral follicular conjunctivitis associated with petechial conjunctival hemorrhages, conjunctival pseudomembrane or frank membrane formation, or, later in the clinical course, the presence of bilateral subepithelial infiltrates. Other adenoviral ocular syndromes have less

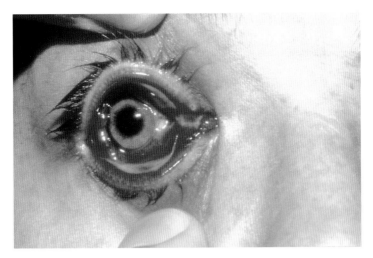

Figure 4-15 Conjunctival membranes in a patient with EKC. *(Courtesy of James Chodosh, MD.)*

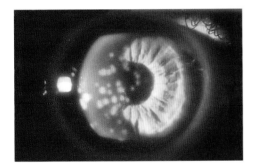
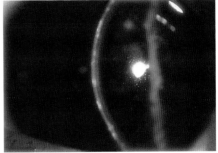

Figure 4-16 Subepithelial corneal infiltrates in a patient with EKC. *(Courtesy of Vincent P. deLuise, MD.)*

specific signs, but laboratory diagnosis is only rarely indicated. Although viral cultures readily differentiate adenovirus from HSV infection, the clinical disease typically subsides or resolves before results become available. A rapid immunodetection assay (RPS Adeno Detector [Rapid Pathogen Screening; South Williamsport, PA]) to detect adenovirus antigens in the conjunctiva is now available. Paired serologic titers 2–3 weeks apart allow confirmation of acute adenovirus infection, but this test is rarely performed.

MANAGEMENT   Therapy for adenoviral ocular infection is primarily supportive. Cool compresses and artificial tears may provide symptomatic relief. Topical antibiotics may be indicated only when the clinical signs, such as mucopurulent discharge, suggest an associated bacterial infection or when a viral cause is less certain.

For patients with conjunctival membranes due to EKC, manual removal by the physician with forceps or a cotton swab every 2–3 days, combined with judicious use of topical corticosteroids, may speed resolution and prevent scarring. Topical corticosteroids also reduce photophobia and improve vision impaired by adenoviral subepithelial infiltrates. Because corticosteroids may prolong viral shedding from adenovirus-infected patients

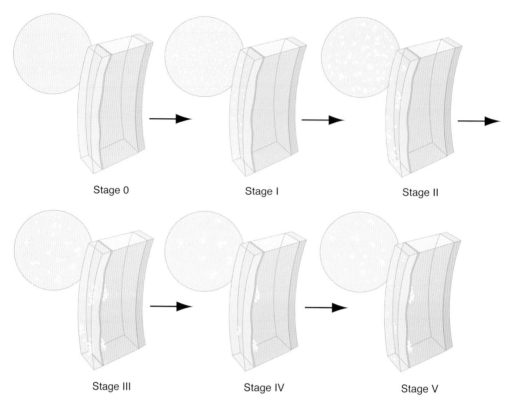

Stage 0   Stage I   Stage II

Stage III   Stage IV   Stage V

Figure 4-17 Schematic drawing illustrating the natural progression of specific corneal epithelial and stromal pathology in EKC. *Stage 0,* Poorly staining, minute punctate opacities within the corneal epithelium. *Stage I,* Fine punctate epithelial keratitis (PEK). *Stage II,* Fine and coarse PEK. Stains brightly with rose bengal. *Stage III,* Coarse granular infiltrates within deep epithelium, early subepithelial infiltrates, diminished PEK. *Stage IV,* Classic subepithelial infiltrates without PEK. *Stage V,* Punctate epithelial granularity adjacent to and distinct from the subepithelial infiltrates. *(Adapted from Jones DB, Matoba AY, Wilhelmus KR. Problem solving in corneal and external diseases. Course 626, presented at the American Academy of Ophthalmology. Atlanta, GA; 1995.)*

and can lead to worsening of HSV infections, their use should be reserved for patients with clinical signs of adenovirus infection who present with specific indications for treatment, including conjunctival membranes and reduced vision due to bilateral subepithelial infiltrates. The use of topical corticosteroids does not affect the natural course of the disease, and it may be difficult to wean patients from them. Nonsteroidal anti-inflammatory agents (NSAIDs) are ineffective therapy for adenoviral subepithelial infiltrates, but they may be helpful in preventing recurrence following tapering of the corticosteroids.

Actively infected people readily transmit adenoviruses. Viral shedding may persist for 10–14 days after onset of clinical signs and symptoms. Transmission can be prevented by personal hygiene measures, including frequent hand washing; cleaning of towels, pillowcases, and handkerchiefs; and disposal of contaminated facial tissues. Individuals who work with the public, in schools, or in health care facilities in particular should consider a temporary leave of absence from work to prevent infecting others, especially those who are already ill. Patients should be considered infectious if they are still hyperemic and tearing. It is more difficult to assess transmissibility in patients treated with topical corticosteroids, as they may appear quiet but still shed the virus.

DNA Viruses: Poxviruses

The Poxviridae encompass a large family of enveloped, double-stranded DNA viruses, with a distinctive brick or ovoid shape and a complex capsid structure. The best-known poxviruses are molluscum contagiosum, vaccinia, and smallpox (variola) virus.

Molluscum Contagiosum

PATHOGENESIS   Molluscum contagiosum virus is spread by direct contact with infected individuals. Infection produces 1 or more umbilicated nodules on the skin and eyelid margin and, less commonly, on the conjunctiva. Eyelid nodules release viral particles into the tear film.

CLINICAL PRESENTATION   A molluscum nodule is smooth with an umbilicated central core. It is smaller and associated with less inflammation than a keratoacanthoma. Punctate epithelial erosions and, in rare cases, a corneal pannus may occur. Any chronic follicular conjunctivitis should instigate a careful search for lid margin molluscum lesions (Fig 4-18).

LABORATORY EVALUATION AND MANAGEMENT   The molluscum contagiosum virus cannot be cultured using standard techniques. Histopathologic examination of an expressed or excised nodule shows eosinophilic, intracytoplasmic inclusions (Henderson-Patterson bodies) within epidermal cells. Diagnosis is based on detection of the characteristic eyelid lesions in the presence of a follicular conjunctivitis. Spontaneous resolution occurs but can take months to years. Treatment options include complete excision, cryotherapy, or incision of the central portion of the lesion. Extensive facial and eyelid molluscum lesions occur in association with AIDS (Fig 4-19).

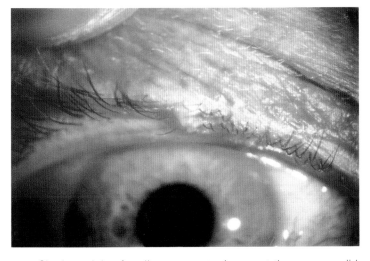

Figure 4-18   Single nodule of molluscum contagiosum at the upper eyelid margin.

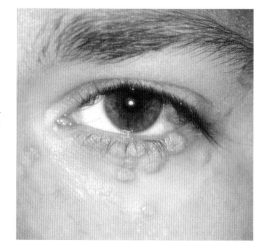

Figure 4-19 Multiple molluscum contagiosum lesions on the eyelid of a patient with AIDS. *(Courtesy of James Chodosh, MD.)*

Vaccinia

Discussion of another poxvirus, vaccinia, was previously removed from the BCSC series because of the eradication of smallpox. More recently, however, concerns of bioterrorism have prompted the reinstitution of a vaccination program, especially for military personnel. Ocular complications from self-inoculation have resulted, including potentially severe periorbital pustules, conjunctivitis, and keratitis. Treatment includes topical trifluridine. Use of vaccinia-immune globulin (VIG) is controversial but is indicated for severe disease. Concern about the use of VIG stems from limited rabbit studies that demonstrated a possible increase in corneal scarring. Individuals who are immunosuppressed, atopic, pregnant, breast-feeding, allergic to the vaccine, or living with a high-risk household contact should not receive the vaccine because of the risk of the possibly fatal, progressive vaccinia.

Fillmore GL, Ward TP, Bower KS, et al. Ocular complications in the Department of Defense Smallpox Vaccination Program. *Ophthalmology.* 2004;111(11):2086–2093.

Neff JM, Lane JM, Fulginiti VA, Henderson DA. Contact vaccinia—transmission of vaccinia from smallpox vaccination. *JAMA.* 2002;288(15):1901–1905.

DNA Viruses: Papovaviruses

Human papillomaviruses (HPV) are small, nonenveloped, double-stranded DNA viruses with an icosahedral capsid. Persistent viral infection of susceptible epithelial cells induces cellular proliferation and can lead to malignant transformation. Papillomavirus proteins can induce transformation of the cell and loss of senescence. HPV subtypes 6 and 11 are maintained in a latent state within basal epithelial cells as circular episomes with very limited viral gene transcription and low copy number. Early viral gene products stimulate cell growth and lead to a skin wart or a conjunctival papilloma. As HPV-containing basal epithelial cells mature and differentiate into superficial epithelial cells, they become permissive for complete viral gene expression and produce infectious virus. Neoplastic transformation due to HPV 6 or 11 is very rare. In contrast, HPV 16 and 18 stereotypically integrate their viral genome into host chromosomal DNA, and this in turn is associated with malignant transformation and squamous cell carcinoma. Recently developed immunization strategies specifically targeted against HPV oncogenes may result in a decreased incidence of these tumors in the future.

Verrucae and *papillomas* are caused by papillomavirus infection of the skin and conjunctival epithelium. Venereally acquired conjunctival papillomas resemble those on the larynx and urogenital tract. Papillomavirus associated conjunctival intraepithelial neoplasia and squamous cell carcinoma share many histologic features with similar lesions in the uterine cervix. Another neoplasm, Kaposi sarcoma of the skin or conjunctiva, is associated with infection by human herpesvirus type 8. These entities are discussed in greater detail in Chapter 8.

RNA Viruses

Picornaviruses are negative-sense, single-stranded RNA viruses with an icosahedral capsid and no envelope. Picornaviridae family members include the enteroviruses (poliovirus, coxsackievirus, echovirus, and enterovirus) and the rhinoviruses, the single most common etiology of the common cold.

Togaviruses are positive-sense, single-stranded RNA with no envelope. Togaviruses with general medical and ophthalmic importance include rubella, encephalomyelitis, yellow fever, and dengue viruses.

Orthomyxoviruses such as influenza virus are negative-sense, single-stranded RNA viruses with an enveloped helical icosahedral capsid. Structurally similar to the orthomyxoviruses, *paramyxoviruses* of ocular importance include mumps virus, measles (rubeola) virus, parainfluenza virus, respiratory syncytial virus, and Newcastle disease virus (a cause of follicular conjunctivitis in poultry handlers). The paramyxovirus envelope contains hemagglutinin-neuraminidase protein spikes and a hemolysin, which mediate viral fusion with the host cell membrane.

Eye infections due to RNA viruses present to the ophthalmologist less often than those due to DNA viruses, and they most commonly manifest as follicular conjunctivitis associated with an upper respiratory infection. However, certain RNA virus infections may cause pathologic changes in virtually any ocular tissue. For example, influenza virus can induce inflammation in the lacrimal gland, cornea, iris, retina, optic nerve, and other cranial nerves.

In *measles (rubeola) virus* (a paramyxovirus) infection, the classic triad of postnatally acquired measles—cough, coryza, and follicular conjunctivitis—can be observed. Mild epithelial keratitis may be present. Less common are optic neuritis, retinal vascular occlusion, and pigmentary retinopathy. Measles keratopathy, a major source of blindness in the developing world, typically presents as corneal ulceration in malnourished, vitamin A–deficient children. (For further information on the ocular effects of vitamin A deficiency, see Chapter 3.) A rare and fatal complication of measles virus infection, subacute sclerosing panencephalitis (SSPE), occurs in about 1 per 100,000 cases, often years after clinically apparent measles.

Mumps virus (a paramyxovirus) infection may result in dacryoadenitis, sometimes concurrent with parotid gland involvement. Follicular conjunctivitis, epithelial and stromal keratitis, iritis, trabeculitis, and scleritis have all been reported within the first 2 weeks after onset of parotitis.

Rubella virus (a togavirus), when acquired in utero, may cause microphthalmos, corneal haze, cataracts, iris hypoplasia, iridocyclitis, glaucoma, and salt-and-pepper pigmentary retinopathy. Congenital ocular abnormalities due to rubella are much worse when maternal infection ensues early in pregnancy. Measles, mumps, and rubella are all uncommon in places where childhood immunization is regularly performed.

Corneal biopsy and impression cytology have been useful in helping in the early diagnosis of *rabies virus* infection. Rabies virus can be transmitted via corneal transplant.

Zaidman GW, Billingsley A. Corneal impression test for the diagnosis of acute rabies encephalitis. *Ophthalmology.* 1998;105(2):249–251.

Acute hemorrhagic conjunctivitis (AHC), caused by *enterovirus* type 70 and *coxsackievirus* A24 variant, and, less commonly, adenovirus type 11, is one of the most dramatic ocular viral syndromes. Sudden onset of follicular conjunctivitis associated with multiple petechial hemorrhages of bulbar and tarsal conjunctiva characterizes AHC. The hemorrhages may become confluent and appear posttraumatic. Eyelid edema, preauricular adenopathy, chemosis, and punctate epithelial keratitis may be associated with infection. AHC is highly contagious and occurs in large and rapidly spreading epidemics. In approximately 1 out of 10,000 cases due to enterovirus type 70, a polio-like paralysis follows; neurologic deficits are permanent in up to one third of affected individuals.

Retroviruses are positive-sense, single-stranded enveloped RNA viruses that encode a viral enzyme, *reverse transcriptase,* that assists in conversion of the single-stranded RNA genome into a circular double-stranded DNA molecule. The viral nucleic acid then integrates into host cell chromosomal DNA.

The retrovirus of greatest medical importance is *human immunodeficiency virus (HIV),* the etiologic agent of AIDS. HIV enters the human host via sexual contact at mucosal surfaces, through breast-feeding, or via blood-contaminated needles. Sexually transmitted infection is facilitated by uptake of HIV by dendritic cells at mucosal surfaces. CD4$^+$ T lymphocytes are a primary target of the virus, as are dendritic cells and monocyte-macrophages. Infection of these cell types induces predictable defects of innate and acquired (both humoral and cellular) immunity. Primary viremia results in an infectious mononucleosis-like HIV prodrome, followed by seeding of the peripheral lymphoid organs and development of a measurable immune response. Infected patients may remain otherwise asymptomatic for several years, but CD4$^+$ T lymphocytes are progressively depleted. Clinical immunodeficiency eventually develops.

AIDS-related ocular disorders include herpes zoster ophthalmicus, molluscum contagiosum, keratoconjunctivitis sicca, microsporidial keratoconjunctivitis, HIV neuropathy, cryptococcal optic neuritis, retinal microvasculopathy, choroiditis and retinitis due to syphilis, mycobacteria, pneumocystosis, toxoplasmosis, cytomegalovirus, HSV, and VZV. For more information regarding HIV, see BCSC Section 1, *Update on General Medicine,* and Section 9, *Intraocular Inflammation and Uveitis.*

Cunningham ET Jr, Margolis TP. Ocular manifestations of HIV infection. *N Engl J Med.* 1998; 339(4):236–244.

Goedert JJ. The epidemiology of acquired immunodeficiency syndrome malignancies. *Semin Oncol.* 2000;27(4):390–401.

CHAPTER 5

Infectious Diseases of the External Eye: Microbial and Parasitic Infections

A detailed history and physical examination are essential to proper diagnosis of external eye infections. The patient's chief complaint and a complete systemic and ocular history, including the presence of risk factors for infections of the external eye, should be noted. A complete eye examination should include special attention to the skin of the face and eyelids, the preauricular lymph nodes, the globe–orbit relationship, ocular discharge, and conjunctival and corneal morphology. Diagnostic tests are chosen to differentiate between likely diagnostic entities and to assist in therapy (eg, antimicrobial sensitivity testing in microbial keratitis).

Bacteriology

In bacteria, round or rod-shaped cells with a wide range of sizes, the genetic material is not separated from the cytoplasm by a nuclear membrane; hence, these organisms are referred to as *prokaryotic* cells in contrast to *eukaryotic* cells, which have a membrane-bound nucleus. In prokaryotes, a plasma membrane encloses a single cytoplasmic compartment containing DNA, RNA, and protein in an amorphous matrix without membrane-bound cellular organelles. Most bacterial genes exist as part of a single circular chromosome, but other genes are present on smaller extrachromosomal circles called *plasmids*. Plasmid DNA typically determines inheritance of 1 or a few characteristics such as antibiotic resistance, and it represents an important mechanism by which traits are passed between different bacterial strains and sometimes between bacterial species. Bacterial classification is determined by the International Committee for Systemic Bacteriology (ICSB). Classification is based on microscopic and colony morphology, enzyme activity, biochemical tests, DNA fingerprinting, and genomic sequence (when known).

Prokaryote structure determines many aspects of infection pathogenesis. The protective coat or cell wall surrounding the plasma membrane of bacteria imparts shape and rigidity to the cell and mediates interactions with the environment, other bacteria, and bacterial viruses. The cell wall also forms the basis of Gram stain reaction. Bacteria stain violet (gram-positive) or red (gram-negative) based on the structure and biochemical composition of their cell wall. Some bacteria that stain poorly with Gram stain, including *Mycobacteria* and *Nocardia asteroides,* can be visualized with acid-fast stain.

Gram-positive bacterial cell walls contain predominantly peptidoglycan and teichoic acid. Gram-negative cell walls are complex and have a thin peptidoglycan layer and an external lipid membrane containing lipopolysaccharide, also referred to as *endotoxin*. Gram staining of clinical specimens is important not only because it helps to classify a pathogenic organism but also because gram-positive and gram-negative bacteria are typically susceptible to different classes of antibiotic drugs (Table 5-1).

Specialized structures external to the cell wall uniquely facilitate bacterial interactions with a diverse environment.

- *flagella*: enable some bacteria to negotiate a liquid environment
- *pili*: involved in bacterial conjugation (transfer of bacterial DNA from one bacterial cell to another)
- *fimbriae*: mediate adherence of one bacterium to another and to eukaryotic cells
- *adhesins*: specific surface-associated molecules or fimbriae that mediate attachment of bacteria to mucosal surfaces

Bacteria replicate by binary fission. A single bacterium can divide approximately every 20 minutes. This ability to replicate quickly allows rapid adaptation to environmental changes. The extreme variety of environmental niches also encourages bacterial survival strategies, including

- engagement of different enzymatic machinery (metabolic pathways)
- development of local bacterial ecosystems (biofilms)
- capacity to transmit genetic elements (plasmids) from one bacterial cell to another and, occasionally, from one bacterial species to another

Gram-positive Cocci

Staphylococcus *species*

Staphylococci inhabit the skin, skin glands, and mucous membranes of healthy mammals. They grow in grapelike clusters in culture but may be seen singly, in pairs, or in short chains on smears from ocular specimens. Staphylococci produce an external biofilm that interferes with phagocytosis and secrete a variety of extracellular proteins—including toxins, enzymes, and enzyme activators—that facilitate both colonization and disease.

Table 5-1 Bacterial Classification for Gram Staining

	Gram Positive	Gram Negative
Cocci	*Staphylococcus* spp *Streptococcus* spp *Enterococcus* spp	*Neisseria* spp
Rods	*Corynebacterium* spp *Propionibacterium* spp *Bacillus* spp	*Pseudomonas* spp *Enterobacter* spp *Haemophilus* spp *Bartonella henselae*
Filaments	*Mycobacterium* spp *Nocardia* spp *Actinomyces* spp	

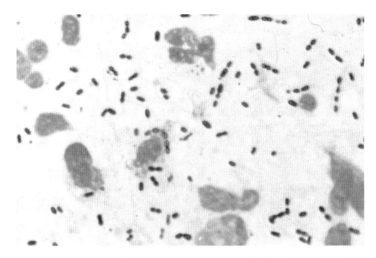

Figure 5-1 Gram-positive cocci *(Streptococcus pneumoniae).* (Gram ×1000). *(Courtesy of James Chodosh, MD.)*

Staphylococci also produce *lantibiotics,* small polypeptides that exert antibacterial effects on other bacteria competing for the same natural habitat. Staphylococci adapt quickly and effectively to administered antibacterial agents and may develop resistance to β-lactams, macrolides, tetracyclines, and quinolones.

Streptococcus *species*

Streptococci inhabit the mucous membranes of the normal upper respiratory tract and female genital tract (Fig 5-1). They grow in pairs and chains. The historical classification of streptococci based on their ability to hemolyze blood-containing agar media is useful for initial recognition of clinical isolates. Another historical means of classification was serologic grouping based on cell wall carbohydrates (Lancefield groups). These methods are used less today given the availability of genetic sequence data.

Disease-causing factors of the highly pathogenic β-hemolytic S *pyogenes* and other pyogenic streptococci include the M and M-like proteins, pyrogenic exotoxins, streptolysin, C5a peptidase, and hyaluronidase. M proteins anchor in the cytoplasmic membrane and extend externally through the bacterial cell wall to help the organism resist phagocytosis by neutrophils. Streptolysin lyses erythrocytes, platelets, and neutrophils. C5a peptidase cleaves and destroys the function of C5a, an important chemoattractant of neutrophils. Hyaluronidase is believed to act as a tissue invasion factor.

S *pneumoniae* appear in smears as lancet-shaped diplococci and express a polysaccharide capsule that resists phagocytosis by macrophages and neutrophils. The toxin pneumolysin is liberated by autolysis and inhibits neutrophil chemotaxis, phagocytosis, lymphocyte proliferation, and antibody synthesis.

Enterococcus *species*

Enterococci are gram-positive cocci that may be seen in pairs or in short chains. They are capable of survival in harsh environments but, in humans, are commensal in the gastrointestinal and genitourinary tracts. *E faecalis,* an important cause of endophthalmitis, uses a unique mechanism of plasmid exchange involving the expression of sex pheromones. These chemicals, when expressed on the surface of enterococci, induce a bacterial mating response and exchange of genetic material, a means by which enterococci acquire antibiotic resistance. Enterococci also produce a cytolysin with potent effects on eukaryotic cell membranes.

Gram-negative Cocci

Neisseria *species*

N gonorrhoeae causes urogenital, rectal, and pharyngeal infections, as well as hyperacute conjunctivitis, and can invade intact corneal epithelium, induce keratolysis of the corneal stroma, and perforate the cornea. *N gonorrhoeae* is always a pathogen, whereas the closely related species *N meningitidis* may be commensal in the pharynx without causing disease. *N gonorrhoeae* is a bean-shaped, gram-negative diplococcus usually seen within neutrophils on a clinical smear from ocular or genital sites (Fig 5-2).

Gram-positive Rods

Corynebacterium *species*

Corynebacterium species are pleomorphic bacilli that produce palisading or cuneiform patterns on smears. *C diphtheriae* is an exotoxin-producing cause of acute membranous conjunctivitis. Other *Corynebacterium* species are referred to as diphtheroids and are routinely isolated from the external eye in the absence of clinical infection. *C xerosis* is commonly seen on histologic sections of vitamin A deficiency–associated conjunctival Bitôt spots, but its significance in conjunctival xerosis is unknown.

Propionibacterium *species*

P acnes and related species are normal inhabitants of human skin. They are aerotolerant but prefer an anaerobic environment. These slender, slightly curved gram-positive rods

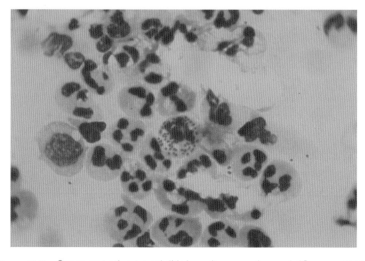

Figure 5-2 Gram-negative cocci *(Neisseria gonorrhoeae)*. (Gram ×1000).

sometimes have a beaded appearance (Fig 5-3). *P acnes* is a major cause of chronic postoperative endophthalmitis and a rare cause of microbial keratitis.

Bacillus *species*

Bacillus species are ubiquitous gram-positive or gram-variable rods commonly found in soil and characterized by the production of spores, a form of the bacteria that allows survival for extended periods of time under extremely harsh conditions. *Bacillus* species are typically motile, and this feature may play a role in the explosive character of *B cereus*–induced posttraumatic endophthalmitis. *B cereus* produces a number of toxins that may rapidly damage ocular tissues. The closely related genus *Clostridium* is anaerobic; *Bacillus* species are aerobes or facultative anaerobes.

Gram-negative Rods

Pseudomonas aeruginosa comprises slender gram-negative rods (Fig 5-4) commonly found as contaminants of water. *P aeruginosa* ocular infections are among the most fulminant. Permanent tissue damage and scarring are the rule following corneal infection. Structural virulence factors of *P aeruginosa* include polar flagella, adhesins, and surface pili. *P aeruginosa* organisms secrete a number of toxins that disrupt protein synthesis and damage cell membranes of ocular cells, as well as proteases that degrade the corneal stromal extracellular matrix.

Enterobacteriaceae

The Enterobacteriaceae family includes multiple genera of enteric non spore-forming gram-negative rods, including *Escherichia coli, Klebsiella, Enterobacter, Citrobacter, Serratia, Salmonella, Shigella,* and *Proteus.* In particular, *Klebsiella, Enterobacter, Citrobacter, Serratia,* and *Proteus* are important causes of keratitis. Pathogenetic factors include pili, adhesins, cytolysins, and toxins. Enteropathogenic *E coli* express a protein similar to cholera toxin.

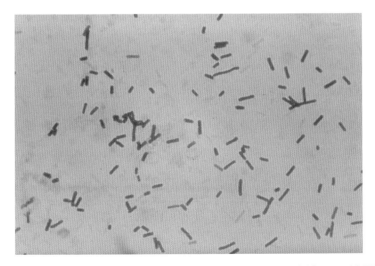

Figure 5-3 Gram-positive rods *(Propionibacterium acnes).* (Gram ×1000).

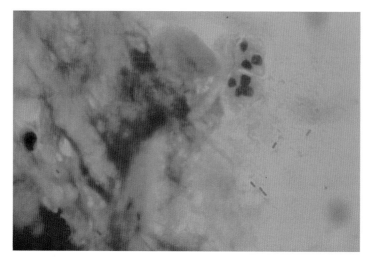

Figure 5-4 Gram-negative rods *(Pseudomonas aeruginosa).* (Gram ×1000).

Haemophilus *species*

Haemophilus species vary in morphology from coccobacilli to short rods. Culture isolation requires enriched media such as chocolate agar. These species are obligate parasites of mammalian mucous membranes and commonly inhabit the human upper respiratory tract and mouth. Along with streptococci, they are important agents of bleb infections following glaucoma filtering surgery. *H influenzae* can be divided into biotypes based on biochemical reactions; encapsulated strains are further divided into serotypes based on their capsular polysaccharides. *H influenzae* type B (Hib) is the primary human pathogen, and its capsule is a major virulence factor.

Bartonella henselae

The etiologic agent of cat-scratch disease, *B henselae* appear as gram-negative aerobic rods, best seen by Warthin-Starry staining of tissue biopsies. *B henselae* infection can be confirmed by culture, by polymerase chain reaction (PCR), by immunocytologic staining of histologic specimens, and by serology. Cats are the natural reservoir of *B henselae,* and infection may be transmitted by a cat scratch or by contact with fleas. (See Parinaud Oculoglandular Syndrome later in the chapter.)

Gram-positive Filaments

Mycobacterium *species*

Mycobacteria are nonmotile, aerobic, weakly gram-positive, but acid-fast; they appear on smears as straight or slightly curved rods. Löwenstein-Jensen medium is most commonly used for culture isolation. Mycobacteria are obligate intracellular pathogens and fall into 2 main groups based on growth rate. *M tuberculosis* and *M leprae* are slow growers. Ocular infection by *M tuberculosis* is uncommon, but it can manifest as a posterior uveitis. The fast-growing, atypical mycobacteria, including *M fortuitum* and *M chelonei,* more commonly cause ulcerative keratitis and are an important cause of keratitis following refractive surgery.

Nocardia *species*

N asteroides and related filamentous bacilli are gram-variable or gram-positive and weakly acid-fast. They may cause keratitis clinically similar to that caused by the atypical mycobacteria.

Actinomyces *species*

Actinomycetes are gram-positive, non–acid-fast anaerobic bacteria that colonize the mouth, intestines, and genital tract. They are an important cause of canaliculitis.

Chlamydia Species

Chlamydiae are spherical or ovoid obligate intracellular parasites of mucosal epithelium with a dimorphic life cycle. The infectious form is the *elementary body (EB),* which develops within an infected host eukaryotic cell into the intracellular replicating form, the *reticulate body (RB).* Only the EB survives outside the host, and only the EB is infectious. Reticulate bodies divide by binary fission to produce 1 or more EBs within a cytoplasmic vacuole, seen on light microscopy as a cellular inclusion.

Spirochetes

Spirochetes are characterized by the periplasmic location of their flagella *(endoflagella).* They are too narrow to be seen by light microscopy. Visualization in fresh clinical specimens requires dark-field illumination. Silver staining or immunocytology can aid identification in histopathologic specimens.

Treponema pallidum causes venereal syphilis. By dark-field illumination, *T pallidum* appear fine and corkscrew-shaped, with rigid, uniform spirals. For further discussion of syphilis, see BCSC Section 1, *Update on General Medicine,* and Section 9, *Intraocular Inflammation and Uveitis.*

Borrelia burgdorferi

Borrelia species are obligate parasites, best visualized with Giemsa stain. *B burgdorferi,* the etiologic agent of Lyme disease and associated Lyme uveitis, is transmitted to humans by tick bites. The preferred hosts for subadult ticks are rodents, whereas adult ticks feed on deer. *B burgdorferi* infection of migrating birds may account for the wide distribution of the organism. Pathogenetic factors of *B burgdorferi* include the expression of proteinases that facilitate tissue invasion, induction of proinflammatory cytokines on binding to phagocytes, and activation of the complement cascade. Although the organism can be cultured from biopsies of erythema migrans skin lesions, it is difficult to recover from blood or synovial fluid. In general, the diagnosis of Lyme disease is determined by serology and typical clinical findings. See also BCSC Section 1, *Update on General Medicine,* and Section 9, *Intraocular Inflammation and Uveitis.*

Mycology

Fungi are eukaryotes that develop branching filaments and reproduce by means of sexually or asexually produced spores. Fungal cell walls are rigid and contain chitin and polysaccharides. Fungi are classically divided into 2 groups: *yeasts* are round or oval fungi that reproduce by budding and sometimes form pseudohyphae by elongation during budding, and *molds* are multicellular fungi composed of tubular hyphae, either septate or nonseptate, that grow by branching and apical extension (Table 5-2). Yeasts may also form hyphae under certain circumstances. The branching hyphae of molds can form a *mycelium*, an interconnected network of hyphae. *Septate fungi* are distinguished by walls that divide the filaments into separate cells, each containing one or more nuclei (Fig 5-5). *Dimorphic fungi* grow in 2 distinct forms as a result of changes in cell wall synthesis in different environments. Such fungi may appear as yeast in the host and as molds in a room-temperature laboratory. Dimorphic fungi may be highly virulent pathogens. Fungal cell walls stain with Gomori methenamine silver but, except for *Candida*, do not take up Gram stain. Classification of filamentous fungi is based on microscopic features of *conidia* (fungal elements that form asexually) and *conidiophores* (the specialized hyphae where conidia are formed). Most antifungal medications target the sterol-containing cell membrane within the fungal cell wall.

Table 5-2 Fungus

| Yeasts | Molds (filamentous) | |
	Septate	Nonseptate
Candida spp	*Fusarium* spp	*Mucor*
Cryptococcus neoformans	*Aspergillus*	*Rhizopus*
Rhinosporidium	*Curvularia*	*Absidia*

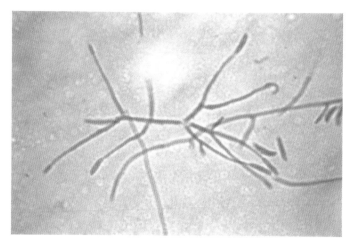

Figure 5-5 Septate hyphae of filamentous fungus *(Fusarium solani)*. (Gram ×1000). *(Courtesy of Vincent P. deLuise, MD.)*

Yeasts

The incidence of mycotic infections in general and yeasts in particular has risen concomitantly with the advent of extensive antibiotic usage in the general population and is closely associated with immunosuppression, whether due to disease or medical therapy. *Candida* species are ubiquitous in the environment and can be isolated in the absence of clinical disease from the gastrointestinal and genitourinary tracts, the oropharynx, and the skin. *C albicans* is the yeast most commonly isolated from each of these sites (Fig 5-6). Binding to host tissues is a prerequisite for infection; and the *C albicans* mannan protein, fibrinogen-binding protein, and a primitive, integrin-like protein facilitate adhesion to target tissues. The transformation to a hyphal form and the expression of aspartyl proteases and phospholipases (the latter at the hyphal tip) facilitate penetration of *C albicans* through tissue barriers.

Cryptococcus neoformans is acquired through inhalation and causes subclinical infection of the pulmonary tract. Clinical cryptococcal disease in the brain and optic nerve, eye, lung, skin, and prostate occur in immunosuppressed patients.

Rhinosporidium seeberi organisms are present in soil and groundwater and presumably infect humans through contact with these sources. Ocular rhinosporidiosis manifests as sessile or pedunculated papillomatous or polypoid lesions in the conjunctiva, which may be associated with similar lesions in the nose and nasopharynx.

Septate Filamentous Fungi

Fusarium species such as *F solani* and *F oxysporum* are encountered in warm, humid environments and can cause a fulminant keratitis. Most other filamentous fungal corneal infections are more indolent. Among the genera that have been isolated from the external eye are *Aspergillus*, *Curvularia*, *Paecilomyces*, and *Phialophora*. Most cases of oculomycosis follow trauma with vegetative matter.

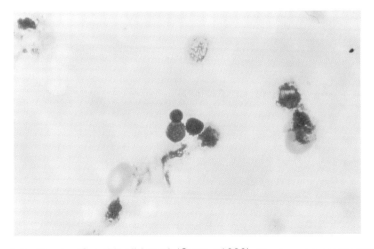

Figure 5-6 Yeasts *(Candida albicans)*. (Gram ×1000). *(Courtesy of James Chodosh, MD.)*

Nonseptate Filamentous Fungi

Nonseptate filamentous fungi include the *Mucor, Rhizopus,* and *Absidia* species in class Zygomycetes, order Mucorales, family Mucoraceae. These ubiquitous fungi cause life-threatening infections of the paranasal sinuses, brain, and orbit in immunocompromised patients, with particular predilection for those with failure of normal phagocytic responses due to acidosis from diabetes mellitus or renal failure. Fungal invasion of blood vessels results in ischemic necrosis of affected tissues.

Pneumocystis carinii was formerly classified as Protozoa, but gene sequencing has placed the organism firmly in the Fungi kingdom. *P carinii* remains one of the primary conditions associated with HIV infection and is an important cause of choroiditis in affected individuals.

Thomas PA, Geraldine P. Oculomycosis. In: Collier L, Balows A, Sussman M, eds. *Topley & Wilson's Microbiology and Microbial Infections.* 10th ed. *Medical Mycology,* ed Merz WG, Hay RJ. London: Hodder Arnold; 2005;chap 16.

Parasitology

Protozoa

Acanthamoeba species are aquatic protozoa (unicellular eukaryotes) that infect the human cornea and brain with potentially devastating results. The *Acanthamoeba* life cycle includes the motile trophozoite (15–45 µm in diameter) and the dormant cyst (10–25 µm in diameter) forms (Fig 5-7). Free-living amebae are found in both forms, but only the trophozoite is infectious. Both forms are found in infected human tissues. Cysts are double-walled and very resistant to environmental stressors. *Acanthamoeba* species are differentiated from one another on the basis of their cyst morphology and antigenic composition.

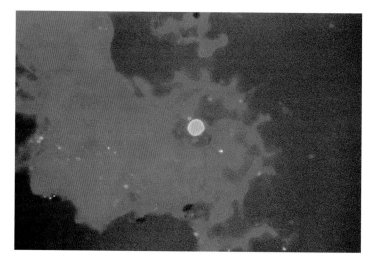

Figure 5-7 Amebic cyst *(Acanthamoeba polyphaga).* (Calcofluor white ×1000).

Microsporida are obligate intracellular parasites with a unique means of infection. *Microsporida* spores enter eukaryotic cells through a polar tube that opens a hole in the eukaryotic cell membrane. Growth and differentiation of the sporoplasm result in the formation of intracellular spores that may be liberated by lysis of the host cell. Of the phylum Microspora, the following genera have been implicated in human infection: *Nosema, Encephalitozoon, Pleistophora, Vittaforma* (formerly *Nosema corneum*), *Trachipleistophora, Enterocytozoon,* and unclassified microsporida.

Toxoplasma gondii causes one of the most common parasitic infections of humans and is a common cause of chorioretinitis (see BCSC Section 9, *Intraocular Inflammation and Uveitis*). Cats shed oocysts in their feces after ingestion of *T gondii*. Oocysts may be ingested by human food animals such as swine and the cyst-containing meat of these animals eaten by humans. Alternatively, cysts may be ingested directly by human contact with cat feces or feces-contaminated water. Transplacental transmission to the fetus of *T gondii* tachyzoites can result in a devastating fetal infection. See BCSC Section 6, *Pediatric Ophthalmology and Strabismus,* for discussion of the consequences of maternal transmission of toxoplasmosis.

Leishmania *species*

Cutaneous leishmaniasis is transmitted at the bite of its vector, the female sandfly, in endemic areas of tropical Asia, Africa, and Latin America. *Leishmania* organisms hide within the phagolysosomal system of macrophages. An infected eyelid ulcer may become granulomatous. Scrapings or biopsy material can show intracellular parasites by Giemsa or immunofluorescent stains. The parasites can sometimes be isolated on blood agar or insect tissue culture medium.

Helminths

Onchocercal filariae are transmitted by the bite of the blackfly of the genus *Simulium*. This fly lays its eggs on trailing vegetation in fast-flowing rivers (hence the common name *river blindness*) and is endemic in parts of sub-Saharan Africa, the Middle East, and Latin America. Microfilariae penetrate the skin and mature in nodules at the site of the fly bite. Maturation to the point of mating and microfilariae production takes approximately 1 year, and worms can live as long as 15 years in the human host. The adult female worm may grow to 100 cm long and liberates as many as 1500 microfilariae each day. Skin snips examined microscopically may show microfilariae of approximately 300 μm in length.

Migration of microfilariae to the skin and eye results in clinical onchocerciasis, and subsequent blackfly bites can carry the organism to others. Microfilariae may enter the peripheral cornea and reach the inner eye. Keratitis (including punctate keratitis and "snowflake" and sclerosing peripheral corneal opacities), anterior uveitis, and chorioretinitis occur upon death of the microfilariae. Onchocerciasis is cumulative; the severity of the disease depends on the degree of exposure to blackfly bites and the density of microfilariae in the tissues. Treatment by nodulectomy, oral ivermectin, and control of local blackfly populations has been successful in selected areas.

Loa loa larvae enter the skin at the bite of an infected *Chrysops* (mango horsefly). Adult worms may grow to 6 cm in length and migrate through the connective tissues, causing transient hypersensitivity reactions. *Loa loa* may appear beneath the conjunctiva.

Visceral larval migrans is a multisystem disease in young children caused by the migrating larvae of *Toxocara canis* and *Toxocara cati,* natural residents of dogs and cats, respectively. *Toxocara* larvae develop and mate in the intestines of their natural host; human ingestion of fertilized eggs in pet feces results in infection. *Toxocara* larvae in the human intestine do not receive the proper environmental signals and migrate throughout the body, invading and destroying tissues as they go. Ocular larval migrans occurs in older children, and the viscera are typically spared.

Taenia solium, the pork tapeworm, is transmitted to humans from ingestion of undercooked pork containing the cysticercus stage. In the stomach, proteolytic enzymes dissolve the cysticercus capsule. Adult worms attach to the intestinal wall by means of suckers at the head (scolex) and release eggs that then disseminate. A hydatid cyst can subsequently form in various tissues, including the eye and orbit, to cause cysticercosis.

Arthropods

Phthirus pubis

Phthiriasis is a venereally acquired crab louse *(P pubis)* infestation of coarse hair in the pubic, axillary, chest, and facial regions. Adult female crab lice (Fig 5-8) and immature nits on the eyelashes cause blepharoconjunctivitis.

Demodex *species*

D folliculorum and *D brevis* inhabit normal superficial hair and eyelash follicles and deeper sebaceous and meibomian glands, respectively. Eyelash colonization increases with age. The organism may be apparent as cylindrical sleeves around eyelash bases and is associated with blepharitis symptoms. (See Fungal and Parasitic Infections of the Eyelid Margin later in the chapter.)

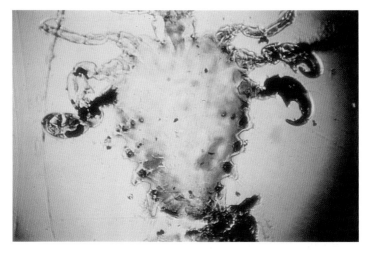

Figure 5-8 Crab louse *(Phthirus pubis).* (Wet mount ×200).

Fly larvae

Myiasis occurs when maggots invade and feed on the living or dead tissues of humans or animals. *Ophthalmomyiasis* (maggot infestation of the eye) can refer to external or internal infestation and involve almost any ocular tissue. Most myiasis occurs when a female fly lands on the host and deposits eggs or larvae. The larvae of some fly species can penetrate through healthy skin and migrate long distances to infest the eye. Extensive larval infestation of a compromised external eye can result in total destruction of orbital contents.

> Collier L, Balows A, Sussman M, eds. *Topley & Wilson's Microbiology and Microbial Infections.* 10th ed. *Parasitology,* ed Cox FEG, Wakelin D, Gillespie SH, Despommier DD. London: Hodder Arnold; 2005.

Prions

Prions are altered proteins that cause transmissible lethal encephalopathies, including Creutzfeldt-Jakob disease, scrapie in sheep, bovine spongiform encephalitis, and kuru. Transmission of Creutzfeldt-Jakob disease following corneal transplantation has been reported.

> Prusiner SB. Shattuck Lecture: neurodegenerative diseases and prions. *N Engl J Med.* 2001; 344(20):1516–1526.

Microbial and Parasitic Infections of the Eyelid Margin and Conjunctiva

Staphylococcal Blepharitis

PATHOGENESIS Inflammation of the eyelid margins, called *blepharitis*, is one of the most common causes of external ocular irritation. Blepharitis can have an infectious or inflammatory etiology; the most common causes of blepharitis are staphylococcal infection (usually caused by *Staphylococcus aureus* but occasionally other species) and irritation from oily meibomian gland secretions. The symptoms, signs, and treatment of infectious staphylococcal blepharoconjunctivitis and meibomian gland dysfunction overlap considerably. In general, the term *staphylococcal blepharitis* refers to cases in which bacterial infection of the eyelids (and frequently the conjunctiva) is predominant. *Meibomian gland dysfunction* and *seborrheic blepharitis* designate the presence of chronic abnormal oily secretions producing irritative effects in the eyelid margin and conjunctiva (these 2 latter conditions are discussed in Chapter 3). Clinical features that may help in the differential diagnosis of these entities are summarized in Table 5-3.

CLINICAL PRESENTATION Staphylococcal blepharitis is seen more commonly in younger individuals. Symptoms include burning, itching, foreign-body sensation, and crusting, particularly upon awakening. Symptoms of irritation and burning tend to peak in the

Table 5-3 Types of Blepharitis

	Staphylococcal	Meibomian Gland Dysfunction	Seborrheic
Location	Anterior eyelid	Posterior eyelid	Anterior eyelid
Loss and whitening of eyelashes	Frequent	(–)	Rare
Eyelid crusting	Hard, fibrinous scales; hard, matted crusts (often accompany ulcerative form)	+/–	Oily or greasy
Eyelid ulceration	Occasional	(–)	(–)
Conjunctivitis	Papillary (occasionally with mucopurulent discharge)	Mild to moderate injection, papillary tarsal reaction	Mild injection, follicular or papillary tarsal reaction
Keratitis	Inferior PEE, marginal infiltrates, vascularization, phlyctenulosis	Inferior PEE, marginal infiltrates, vascular pannus	Inferior PEE
Aqueous tear deficiency	Occasional	Occasional	Occasional
Rosacea	(–)	34%–66%	0%–33%

PEE = punctate epithelial erosions.

morning and improve as the day progresses, presumably as the crusted material that accumulates on the eyelid margin overnight dissipates.

Typical clinical manifestations include hard, brittle fibrinous scales and hard, matted crusts surrounding individual cilia on the anterior eyelid margin (Fig 5-9). Small ulcers of the anterior eyelid margin may be seen when the hard crusts are removed. Injection and

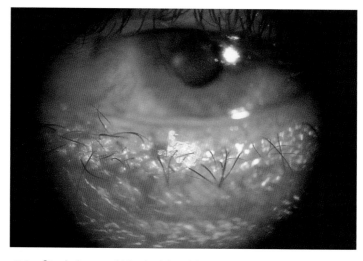

Figure 5-9 Staphylococcal blepharitis with collarettes surrounding eyelashes.

telangiectasis of the anterior and posterior eyelid margins, white lashes (poliosis), lash loss (madarosis), and trichiasis may be seen in varying degrees, depending on the severity and duration of the blepharitis.

Aqueous tear deficiency is found in some patients with staphylococcal blepharitis. Excessive secretion of bacterially modified lipid products into the tear film can increase instability and accentuate evaporative losses, thus further compounding any associated dry-eye state. (See additional dry-eye discussion in Chapter 3.)

Chronic conjunctivitis

A unilateral or bilateral conjunctivitis that persists for 4 or more weeks is considered chronic. When conjunctivitis accompanies blepharitis, as it frequently does, the condition is known as *staphylococcal blepharoconjunctivitis*. This association is marked by a chronic papillary reaction of the tarsal conjunctiva, particularly the inferior tarsal conjunctiva near the eyelid margin, as well as injection of the bulbar and tarsal conjunctivae. Chronic conjunctivitis tends to be associated with mild conjunctival injection and scant mucopurulent discharge.

Specific clinical signs are commonly seen in patients with chronic conjunctivitis caused by certain bacterial species. *S aureus* is often associated with matted golden crusts and ulcers on the anterior eyelid margin, inferior punctate keratopathy, marginal corneal infiltrates, and, in rare cases, conjunctival or corneal phlyctenules. *Moraxella lacunata* may produce a chronic angular blepharoconjunctivitis, with crusting and ulceration of the skin in the lateral canthal angle and papillary or follicular reaction on the tarsal conjunctiva. *Moraxella* angular blepharoconjunctivitis is frequently associated with concomitant *S aureus* blepharoconjunctivitis.

Conjunctival swabbings for culture and sensitivity should be performed in cases that do not respond to initial empiric antibiotic therapy. In cases of persistent chronic unilateral conjunctivitis refractory to therapy, masquerade syndrome (conjunctival malignancy) and factitious illness should be ruled out.

Keratitis

Several forms of keratitis may develop in association with staphylococcal blepharoconjunctivitis.

Punctate epithelial keratopathy manifests as erosions that stain with fluorescein. Frequently, the distribution of the keratopathy is mostly inferior, and it sometimes coincides with the contour of the eyelids across the corneal surface. Occasionally, a diffuse pattern may be observed, and asymmetric or unilateral keratopathy is not uncommon. The degree of corneal involvement can be markedly disproportionate to the severity of the eyelid disease, a circumstance that can lead to diagnostic confusion. Marginal corneal infiltrates may be the most distinctive clinical finding (Fig 5-10).

Phlyctenulosis is a local corneal and/or conjunctival inflammation that is believed to represent a cell-mediated, or delayed, hypersensitivity response induced by microbial antigens such as the cell wall components of staphylococcus. Phlyctenulosis is frequently associated with *S aureus* in developed countries and is classically associated with *Mycobacterium tuberculosis* in malnourished children in areas around the world with endemic tuberculosis.

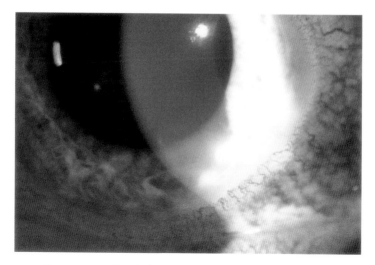

Figure 5-10 Staphylococcal marginal corneal infiltrate.

Phlyctenules typically present unilaterally at or near the limbus, on the bulbar conjunctiva or cornea, as one or more small, rounded, elevated, gray or yellow, hyperemic, focal inflammatory nodules accompanied by a zone of engorged hyperemic vessels (Fig 5-11). They typically become necrotic and ulcerate centrally and then spontaneously involute over a period of 2–3 weeks. With resolution of corneal phlyctenules, wedge-shaped fibrovascular scars form along the limbus. Conjunctival phlyctenules do not lead to scarring. Bilateral limbus-based fibrovascular corneal scarring, which tends to be greater inferiorly than superiorly, may indicate previous phlyctenulosis. Corneal involvement is recurrent, and centripetal migration of successive inflammatory lesions may develop. Occasionally, such inflammation leads to corneal thinning and, in rare cases, perforation.

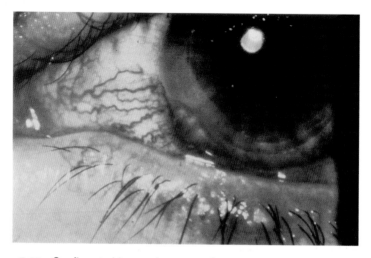

Figure 5-11 Confluent phlyctenules secondary to staphylococcal blepharitis.

LABORATORY EVALUATION   Eyelid and conjunctival cultures can be performed in suspected cases of staphylococcal blepharoconjunctivitis with a doubtful clinical diagnosis or a poor response to empiric treatment. If the infection is chronic or worsening, diagnostic cultures may be essential. If the patient is still on antibiotics or other topical therapeutic measures, then a brief washout period may be advantageous prior to culturing.

The characteristic laboratory finding in staphylococcal blepharoconjunctivitis is a heavy, confluent growth of *S aureus*. Nevertheless, the finding of a light to moderate growth of bacteria and/or the isolation of staphylococcal species other than *S aureus* does not exclude the diagnosis, particularly if a predominant manifestation of the disease is punctate epithelial keratopathy, marginal infiltrates, or phlyctenulosis. Susceptibility testing may be useful in guiding treatment in cases that have been refractory to empiric antibiotic therapy.

MANAGEMENT   Treatment consists of antibacterial and anti-inflammatory measures. Eyelid hygiene, using either commercially available eyelid scrub kits or warm water with diluted baby shampoo, may help reduce bacterial colonization and the accumulation of sebaceous secretions. Patient education should emphasize treatment directed toward the base of the lashes with a moistened cotton-tipped applicator or a small, soft facecloth sudsed with a dilute concentration of baby shampoo. Following scrubs, a thin film of antibiotic ointment may be applied to the eyelid margins. Topical bacitracin, erythromycin and azithromycin are commonly used. In addition, aqueous tear deficiency and/or lipid-induced tear-film instability is frequently present, and the use of artificial tears or other dry-eye remedies may be beneficial.

Cases with a prominent conjunctivitis component should be treated with an antibiotic solution. Treatment for staphylococcal blepharitis is frequently prolonged and repeated. This factors into the physician's selection of a topical antibiotic. To minimize toxicity and resistance, a well-tolerated, relatively narrow, spectrum antimicrobial agent effective against the majority of staphylococci should be selected. When possible, the agent should be shown to be efficacious by susceptibility testing data from the local or regional microbiology laboratory.

Anti-inflammatory therapy consists of limited and judicious use of mild doses of topical corticosteroids in selected cases. Corticosteroids should be reserved for patients who have a strong inflammatory component with little active infection. Patients with routine staphylococcal blepharitis or blepharoconjunctivitis may obtain more rapid symptomatic relief with the use of adjunctive topical corticosteroids, but the potential risks include prolonging or worsening the infection or inducing corticosteroid-related side effects. Therefore, corticosteroid use in routine cases is strongly discouraged.

Corticosteroids provide little therapeutic benefit for toxic-related punctate epithelial keratopathy. In contrast, marginal infiltrates and phlyctenulosis have a strong immunologic component and can thus respond to topical corticosteroid therapy. In the case of phlyctenulosis, corticosteroids are usually necessary early in the course of treatment. Conversely, in the case of marginal infiltrates, eyelid hygiene and antibiotic therapy alone may be sufficient. If the therapeutic effect is inadequate after a few days (in the case of marginal infiltrates), a time-limited course of low-dose corticosteroid can be prescribed.

If epithelial defects are noted over the infiltrates, diagnostic cultures should be obtained before instituting corticosteroid treatment. Chronic or indiscriminate use of corticosteroids should be avoided.

Hordeolum

PATHOGENESIS Hordeola are inflammatory or infectious nodules that develop in the eyelid. Most frequently, they result from inspissation and secondary infection of sebaceous glands. Those occurring on the anterior eyelid in the glands of Zeis or lash follicles are called *external hordeola*, or *styes*. Hordeola occurring at the posterior eyelid from meibomian gland inspissation are termed *internal hordeola*. Either type is associated with a localized purulent abscess, usually caused by *S aureus*.

CLINICAL PRESENTATION Hordeola present as painful, tender, red nodular masses near the eyelid margin. They may rupture, producing a purulent drainage. Hordeola are generally self-limited, improving spontaneously over the course of 1–2 weeks. Internal hordeola occasionally evolve into *chalazia*, which are chronic granulomatous nodules centered around sebaceous glands, usually the meibomian glands. (Chalazia are discussed further in Chapter 3.)

LABORATORY EVALUATION AND MANAGEMENT Cultures are not indicated for isolated, uncomplicated cases of hordeolum. Warm compresses with light massage over the lesion can facilitate drainage. Topically applied antibiotics are generally not effective and, therefore, not indicated unless an accompanying infectious blepharoconjunctivitis is present. Systemic antibiotics are generally indicated only in rare cases of secondary eyelid cellulitis; however, if the patient has a prominent and chronic accompanying meibomitis, oral doxycycline may be necessary. For large or persistent lesions, incision and drainage may be required.

Fungal and Parasitic Infections of the Eyelid Margin

Demodex is a genus of mites that are normal commensal acarian parasites of humans (see "*Demodex* species" earlier in the chapter). The human follicle mites, *D folliculorum* and *D brevis*, are obligate parasites that inhabit hair follicles and sebaceous/meibomian glands, respectively. They are commonly seen by slit-lamp biomicroscopy as waxy sleeves around eyelashes or as cylinders extending from sebaceous glands of the eyelid margin. The role of these parasites in the pathogenesis of blepharitis is unclear. Other organisms that survive on lipids of eyelid glands, such as *Malassezia furfur,* have also been incriminated in certain types of blepharitis.

A focal granuloma or dermatitis affecting the eyelid or conjunctiva can be caused by very rare infections, including

- blastomycosis
- sporotrichosis
- rhinosporidiosis
- cryptococcosis
- leishmaniasis
- ophthalmomyiasis

Lice infestation of the eyelids and eyelashes, also known as *phthiriasis palpebrum,* is an uncommon form of conjunctivitis or blepharitis affecting adolescents and young adults and is caused by the pubic louse and its ova. In rare instances, pediculosis involves the ocular region by localized extension of head or body lice (*Pediculus humanus capitis* or *Pediculus humanus corporis,* respectively). Mechanical removal of the lice and nits (eggs) can be performed with jewelers forceps, but pubic hairs are usually treated with a pediculicide. Any ointment can smother the lice and should be applied twice daily for at least 10 days, because the incubation period (of the nits) is 7–10 days. Periodic reexamination is recommended over 10–14 days to detect recurrence and remove any new nits. Bed linen, clothing, and any items of close contact should be washed and dried at the highest temperature setting (at least 50°C).

Bacterial Conjunctivitis in Children and Adults

PATHOGENESIS   A bacterial etiology is a less common cause of conjunctivitis in adults. Bacterial conjunctivitis is the result of bacterial overgrowth and infiltration of the conjunctival epithelial layer and sometimes the substantia propria as well. The source of infection is either direct contact with an infected individual's secretions (usually through eye–hand contact) or the spread of infection from the organisms colonizing the patient's own nasal and sinus mucosa. In an adult with unilateral bacterial conjunctivitis, the nasolacrimal system should be examined. Nasolacrimal duct obstruction, dacryosystitis, and canaliculitis may lead to unilateral bacterial conjunctivitis.

Although usually self limited, bacterial conjunctivitis can occasionally be severe and sight-threatening when caused by virulent bacterial species such as *N gonorrhoeae* or *S pyogenes.* In rare cases, it may presage life-threatening systemic disease, as with conjunctivitis caused by *N meningitidis.* Direct infection and inflammation of the conjunctival surface, bystander effects on adjacent tissues such as the cornea, and the host's acute inflammatory response and long-term reparative response all contribute to the pathology.

CLINICAL PRESENTATION AND MANAGEMENT   Bacterial conjunctivitis should be suspected in patients with conjunctival inflammation and a purulent discharge. The rapidity of onset and severity of conjunctival inflammation and discharge are suggestive of the possible causative organism. Table 5-4 shows the clinical classification of bacterial conjunctivitis based on these parameters.

Acute purulent conjunctivitis
Acute purulent conjunctivitis, a form of bacterial conjunctivitis, is characterized by an acute (less than 3 weeks' duration), self-limited infection of the conjunctival surface that evokes an acute inflammatory response with purulent discharge. Cases may occur spontaneously or in epidemics. The most common etiologic pathogens are *S pneumoniae, S aureus,* and *H influenzae.* The relative frequency with which each of these organisms is isolated depends in part on the patient's age and geographic location.

S pneumoniae is a common cause of acute purulent bacterial conjunctivitis. Moderate purulent discharge, eyelid edema, chemosis, conjunctival hemorrhages, and occasional inflammatory membranes on the tarsal conjunctiva are often associated

Table 5-4 Clinical Classification of Bacterial Conjunctivitis

Course of Onset	Severity	Common Organisms
Slow (days to weeks)	Mild–moderate	*Staphylococcus aureus* *Moraxella lacunata* *Proteus* spp Enterobacteriaceae *Pseudomonas*
Acute or subacute (hours to days)	Moderate–severe	*Haemophilus influenzae* biotype III* *Haemophilus influenzae* *Streptococcus pneumoniae* *Staphylococcus aureus*
Hyperacute (<24 hours)	Severe	*Neisseria gonorrhoeae* *Neisseria meningitidis*

*Previously referred to as *Haemophilus aegyptius*.

with acute conjunctivitis caused by *S pneumoniae*. Corneal ulceration occurs in rare instances.

H influenzae conjunctivitis occurs in young children, sometimes in association with otitis media, and in adults, particularly those chronically colonized with *H influenzae* (for example, smokers or patients with chronic bronchopulmonary disease). Acute purulent conjunctivitis caused by *H influenzae* biotype III (previously called *H aegyptius*) resembles that caused by *S pneumoniae*; however, conjunctival membranes do not develop, whereas peripheral corneal epithelial ulcers and stromal infiltrates occur more commonly. *H influenzae* preseptal cellulitis may predispose children to a fulminant meningitis in which up to 20% of patients who recover have long-term neurologic sequelae. The incidence of infection has been reduced by a vigorous program of vaccination against Hib.

S aureus may produce an acute blepharoconjunctivitis. The discharge tends to be somewhat less purulent than that seen in pneumococcal conjunctivitis, and the associated signs are generally less severe.

Gram-stained smears and culture of the conjunctiva are not necessary in uncomplicated cases of suspected bacterial conjunctivitis but should be performed in the following situations:

- certain compromised hosts, such as neonates or debilitated or immunocompromised individuals
- severe cases of purulent conjunctivitis, to differentiate it from hyperpurulent conjunctivitis, which generally requires systemic therapy
- cases unresponsive to initial therapy

MANAGEMENT   Most cases of acute purulent conjunctivitis can be managed with empiric antibiotic therapy. Uncomplicated cases that are equivocal or cases likely to represent a viral conjunctivitis should *not* be routinely treated with empiric antibiotics.

Initial medical therapy for acute nonsevere bacterial conjunctivitis includes the following topical agents: polymixin combination drops, aminoglycosides or fluoroquinolone (ciprofloxacin, ofloxacin, levofloxacin, moxifloxacin, or gatifloxacin) drops, or bacitracin or ciprofloxacin ointment. The dosing schedule is 4 times daily for approximately 5–7 days unless otherwise indicated. Cases with gram-negative coccobacilli on gram-stained smears are probably caused by *Haemophilus* species and should be treated with polymyxin B–trimethoprim. Supplemental oral antibiotics are recommended for patients with acute purulent conjunctivitis associated with pharyngitis, for conjunctivitis-otitis syndrome, and for *Haemophilus* conjunctivitis in children.

When empiric broad-spectrum antibiotic therapy is prescribed in cases of hyperacute conjunctivitis, the initial treatment should be weighted toward the results of the gram-stained morphology of the conjunctival smear, if available. Definitive treatment should be based on the culture results, if available, as smear results may sometimes be inconclusive as to the predominant category of organism responsible for the infection. Cultures of the nose or throat may be performed if an associated sinusitis or pharyngitis is present. Even if no overt sinusitis, rhinitis, or pharyngitis is present, nasal or throat swabs should be considered in cases of relapsing conjunctivitis, because the persistence of organisms colonizing the respiratory mucosa may be the source of infection.

Gonococcal conjunctivitis

Gonococcal conjunctivitis presents with explosive onset of severe purulent conjunctivitis: massive exudation; severe chemosis; and, in untreated cases, corneal infiltrates, melting, and perforation. The organism most commonly responsible for hyperpurulent conjunctivitis is *N gonorrhoeae* (Fig 5-12). Gonococcal conjunctivitis is a sexually transmitted disease resulting from direct genital–eye transmission, genital–hand–ocular contact, or maternal–neonate transmission during vaginal delivery.

The disease is characterized by rapid progression, copious purulent conjunctival discharge, marked conjunctival hyperemia and chemosis, and eyelid edema. Gonococcal conjunctivitis may be associated with preauricular lymphadenopathy and the formation

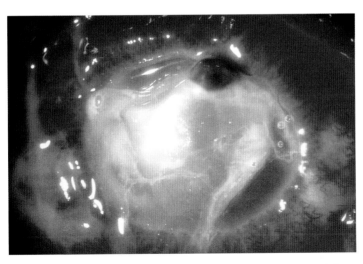

Figure 5-12 Peripheral corneal ulceration and perforation occurring several days after onset of hyperacute conjunctivitis caused by *N gonorrhoeae*.

of conjunctival membranes. Keratitis, the principal cause of sight-threatening complications, has been reported to occur in 15%–40% of cases. Corneal involvement may consist of diffuse epithelial haze, epithelial defects, marginal infiltrates, and peripheral ulcerative infectious keratitis that can rapidly progress to perforation.

LABORATORY EVALUATION   *N gonorrhoeae* grows well on chocolate agar and Thayer-Martin media.

MANAGEMENT   Gonococcal conjunctivitis should be treated with systemic antibiotics. Topical ocular antibiotics can supplement but not replace systemic therapy. Current treatment regimens for gonococcal conjunctivitis reflect the increasing prevalence of *penicillin-resistant N gonorrhoeae (PRNG)* in the United States. Ceftriaxone, a third-generation cephalosporin, is highly effective against PRNG. Gonococcal conjunctivitis without corneal ulceration may be treated on an outpatient basis with 1 intramuscular ceftriaxone (1 g) injection. Patients with corneal ulceration should be admitted to the hospital and treated with intravenous ceftriaxone (1 g IV every 12 hours) for 3 consecutive days. Patients with penicillin allergy can be given spectinomycin (2 g IM) or oral fluoroquinolones (ciprofloxacin 500 mg or ofloxacin 400 mg orally bid for 5 days).

Erythromycin ointment, bacitracin ointment, gentamicin ointment, and ciprofloxacin solution have been recommended for topical therapy. Just as important as systemic therapy for the treatment of severe cases is copious, frequent (every 30–60 minutes) irrigation of the conjunctival sac with normal saline. Such lavages help to remove inflammatory cells, proteases, and debris that may be toxic to the ocular surface and contribute to corneal melting.

Up to one third of patients with gonococcal conjunctivitis have been reported to have concurrent chlamydial venereal disease. Because of this frequent association, it is advisable to place patients on supplemental oral antibiotics for treatment of chlamydial infection. Treatment regimens for chlamydia are discussed later in this chapter. Patients should be instructed to refer their sex partners for evaluation and treatment.

Preferred Practice Patterns Committee, Cornea/External Disease Panel. *Conjunctivitis.* San Francisco: American Academy of Ophthalmology; 2008.

Bacterial conjunctivitis in neonates

N gonorrhoeae causes the most severe neonatal conjunctivitis. Fortunately, *N gonorrhoeae* is currently responsible for fewer than 1% of all cases of neonatal conjunctivitis in the industrialized countries. In order of decreasing prevalence, the causes of neonatal bacterial conjunctivitis are as follows:

- *Chlamydia trachomatis*
- *Streptococcus viridans*
- *Staphylococcus aureus*
- *Haemophilus influenzae*
- group D *Streptococcus*
- *Moraxella catarrhalis*
- *Escherichia coli* and other gram-negative rods
- *N gonorrhoeae*

Ophthalmia neonatorum is discussed in more detail in BCSC Section 6, *Pediatric Ophthalmology and Strabismus.*

Neonatal gonococcal conjunctivitis   The infrequency of neonatal gonococcal conjunctivitis has been attributed to effective prenatal screening for maternal gonococcal genital infection and prophylactic antimicrobial therapy for conjunctivitis in newborns. Infants with gonococcal conjunctivitis typically develop bilateral conjunctival discharge 3–5 days after parturition. The discharge may be serosanguineous during the first several days, and a copious purulent exudate may develop later. Corneal ulceration, corneal perforation, and endophthalmitis have been reported as complications of untreated neonatal gonococcal conjunctivitis. Infected infants may also have other localized gonococcal infections, including rhinitis and proctitis. Disseminated gonococcal infection with arthritis, meningitis, pneumonia, and sepsis resulting in death of the infant is a rare complication.

MANAGEMENT   Some strains of *N gonorrhoeae* are developing resistance to various antibiotics, including penicillin (PRNG), fluoroquinolones (quinolone-resistant *N gonorrhoeae,* or QRNG), and tetracycline. The currently recommended first-line treatment for neonatal gonococcal conjunctivitis is ceftriaxone. For *nondisseminated* infections, a single intramuscular or intravenous ceftriaxone injection (up to 125 mg or a dose of 25–50 mg/kg) or cefotaxime at a single dose of 100 mg/kg IV or IM is recommended. For *disseminated* infection, treatment should be augmented according to infectious disease consultation. Either of these regimens should be combined with hourly saline irrigation of the conjunctiva until discharge is eliminated. If corneal involvement is suspected, application of topical erythromycin or gentamicin ointment or frequent application of a topical fluoroquinolone should be considered. Topical cycloplegia may also prove beneficial. Systemic treatment is advised for infants born to mothers with active gonorrhea, even in the absence of conjunctivitis.

American Academy of Pediatrics. Gonococcal infections. In: Pickering LK, Baker CJ, Kimberlin DW, Long SS, eds. *2009 Red Book: Report of the Committee on Infectious Diseases.* 28th ed. Elk Grove Village, IL: American Academy of Pediatrics; 2009:305–313.

Centers for Disease Control and Prevention, Workowski KA, Berman SM. Sexually transmitted diseases treatment guidelines 2006. *MMWR Recomm Rep.* 2006;55(RR-11):1–94.

Neonatal chlamydial conjunctivitis   Chlamydial conjunctivitis in neonates differs clinically from adult chlamydial conjunctivitis in the following ways:

- There is no follicular response in newborns.
- The amount of mucopurulent discharge is greater in newborns.
- Membranes can develop on the tarsal conjunctiva in newborns.
- Intracytoplasmic inclusions are seen in a greater percentage of Giemsa-stained conjunctival specimens in newborns.
- The infection in newborns is more likely to respond to topical medications.

Both Gram and Giemsa stains of conjunctival scrapings are recommended in neonates with conjunctivitis to identify *C trachomatis* and *N gonorrhoeae,* as well as other bacteria, as causative agents. Other *Chlamydia*-associated infections, such as pneumonitis and otitis media, can accompany inclusion conjunctivitis in the newborn. Therefore, systemic erythromycin (12.5 mg/kg oral or IV qid for 14 days) is recommended, even though inclusion conjunctivitis in the newborn usually responds to topical erythromycin or sulfacetamide.

Chlamydial Conjunctivitis

PATHOGENESIS *C trachomatis* is an obligate intracellular bacterium that causes several different conjunctivitis syndromes; each is associated with different serotypes of *C trachomatis:*

- trachoma: serotypes A–C
- adult and neonatal inclusion conjunctivitis: serotypes D–K
- lymphogranuloma venereum: serotypes L1, L2, and L3

Rare cases of keratoconjunctivitis in humans have been reported caused by *Chlamydia* species that typically infect animals, such as *C psittaci,* an agent generally associated with disease in parrots, and the feline pneumonitis agent.

LABORATORY EVALUATION *C trachomatis* can be diagnosed by Giemsa stain, cell culture isolation, and PCR.

CLINICAL PRESENTATION AND MANAGEMENT Trachoma and adult inclusion conjunctivitis are discussed individually in the following sections.

Trachoma

Trachoma is an infectious disease that occurs in communities with poor hygiene and inadequate sanitation. It affects approximately 150 million individuals worldwide and is the leading cause of preventable blindness. Trachoma is currently endemic in the Middle East and in developing regions around the world. In the United States, it occurs sporadically among American Indians and in mountainous areas of the South. Most infections are transmitted from eye to eye. Transmission may also occur by flies and other household fomites. The fomites also spread other bacteria that cause secondary bacterial infections in patients with trachoma.

Solomon AW, Holland MJ, Alexander ND, et al. Mass treatment with single-dose azithromycin for trachoma. *N Engl Journal Med.* 2004;351(19):1962–1971.

CLINICAL PRESENTATION The initial symptoms of trachoma include foreign-body sensation, redness, tearing, and mucopurulent discharge. A severe follicular reaction develops, most prominently in the superior tarsal conjunctiva but sometimes appearing in the superior and inferior fornices, inferior tarsal conjunctiva, semilunar fold, and limbus. In acute trachoma, follicles on the superior tarsus may be obscured by diffuse papillary hypertrophy and inflammatory cell infiltration. Large tarsal follicles in trachoma may become necrotic and eventually heal with significant scarring. Linear or stellate scarring of the superior tarsus *(Arlt line)* typically occurs (Fig 5-13). Involution and necrosis of follicles may result in limbal depressions known as *Herbert pits* (Fig 5-14). Corneal findings in trachoma include epithelial keratitis, focal and multifocal peripheral and central stromal infiltrates,

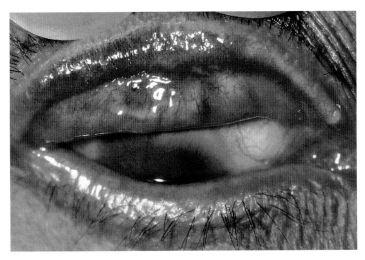

Figure 5-13 Linear scarring of the superior tarsal conjunctiva (Arlt line) in a patient with old trachoma. *(Courtesy of Vincent P. deLuise, MD.)*

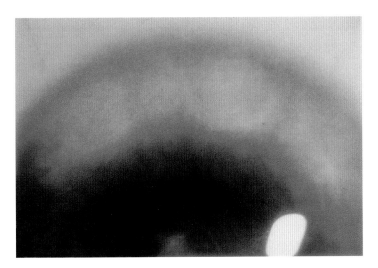

Figure 5-14 Trachoma exhibiting Herbert pits of the superior limbus (round to oval, relatively lucent areas within pannus).

and superficial fibrovascular pannus, which is most prominent in the superior third of the cornea but may extend centrally into the visual axis (Fig 5-15).

Clinical diagnosis of trachoma requires at least 2 of the following clinical features:

- conjunctival follicles on the upper tarsal conjunctiva
- limbal follicles and their sequelae (Herbert pits)
- typical tarsal conjunctival scarring
- vascular pannus most marked on the superior limbus

Severe conjunctival and lacrimal gland duct scarring from chronic trachoma can result in aqueous tear deficiency, tear drainage obstruction, trichiasis, and entropion.

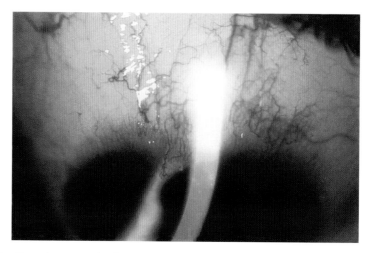

Figure 5-15 Superior corneal micropannus in a patient with adult chlamydial conjunctivitis.

The World Health Organization (WHO) has introduced a simple severity grading system for trachoma based on the presence or absence of 5 key signs:

1. follicular conjunctival inflammation
2. diffuse conjunctival inflammation
3. tarsal conjunctival scarring
4. aberrant lashes
5. corneal opacification

The WHO grading system was developed for use by trained personnel other than ophthalmologists to assess the prevalence and severity of trachoma in population-based surveys in endemic areas.

> Thylefors B, Dawson CR, Jones BR, West SK, Taylor HR. A simple system for the assessment of trachoma and its complications. *Bull World Health Organ.* 1987;65(4):477–483.

MANAGEMENT   Active trachoma is treated with topical and oral tetracycline or erythromycin. Topical tetracycline 1% or erythromycin ointment should be administered twice daily for 2 months. Oral tetracycline in a dosage of 1.5–2.0 g daily in divided doses should be administered for 3 weeks. Oral erythromycin is recommended for treatment of the rare cases of trachoma that are clinically resistant to tetracycline. A single dose of azithromycin, 1000 mg, is useful because of the long-term effectiveness of single doses. Management of the complications of trachoma may include tear substitutes for dry eye and eyelid surgery for entropion or trichiasis.

Adult chlamydial conjunctivitis

Adult chlamydial conjunctivitis is a sexually transmitted disease often found in conjunction with chlamydial urethritis or cervicitis. It is most prevalent in sexually active adolescents and young adults. Chlamydia is a systemic disease. The eye is usually infected by direct or indirect contact with infected genital secretions, although other modes of transmission may include shared eye cosmetics and inadequately chlorinated swimming pools. Onset of conjunctivitis is typically 1–2 weeks after ocular inoculation and is not as acute as with adenoviral keratoconjunctivitis. Often patients may complain of mild symptoms for weeks to months.

CLINICAL PRESENTATION   External signs of adult inclusion conjunctivitis include a follicular conjunctival response that is most prominent in the lower palpebral conjunctiva and fornix, scant mucopurulent discharge, and palpable preauricular adenopathy. Follicles in the bulbar conjunctiva and semilunar fold are frequently present, and these are a helpful and specific sign in patients who have not been using topical medications associated with development of bulbar follicles. Inflammatory conjunctival membranes do not develop in chlamydial keratoconjunctivitis.

Corneal involvement may consist of fine or coarse epithelial infiltrates, occasionally associated with subepithelial infiltrates. The keratitis is more likely to be found in the superior cornea but may also occur centrally and resemble adenoviral keratitis. A micropannus, usually extending less than 3 mm from the superior cornea, may develop.

MANAGEMENT   Left untreated, adult chlamydial conjunctivitis often resolves spontaneously in 6–18 months. Currently, one of the following oral antibiotic regimens is recommended:

- azithromycin 1000 mg single dose
- doxycycline 100 mg bid for 7 days
- tetracycline 250 mg qid for 7 days
- erythromycin 500 mg qid for 7 days

Patients with laboratory-confirmed chlamydial conjunctivitis and their sexual contacts should be evaluated for coinfection with other sexually transmitted diseases, such as syphilis or gonorrhea, before antibiotic treatment is started. Sexual partners should be concomitantly treated to avoid reinfection.

Centers for Disease Control and Prevention, Workowski KA, Berman SM. Sexually transmitted diseases treatment guidelines 2006. *MMWR Recomm Rep.* 2006;55(RR-11):1–94.

Parinaud Oculoglandular Syndrome

Granulomatous conjunctivitis with regional lymphadenopathy is an uncommon condition called *Parinaud oculoglandular syndrome. Cat-scratch disease (CSD),* which causes most cases of the syndrome, is estimated to affect approximately 22,000 people annually in the United States, with about 10% developing conjunctivitis. The primary causative agent is *B henselae.* Other, infrequent causes of Parinaud oculoglandular syndrome include

- *Afipia felis*
- *Bartonella clarridgeiae*
- tularemia
- tuberculosis
- sporotrichosis

- syphilis
- coccidioidomycosis

PATHOGENESIS *B henselae* lives on cats and their fleas. Most cases are transmitted by a scratch from a flea-infested kitten. Other modes of transmission include a cat's biting or licking the human skin. Local infection causes a granulomatous reaction.

CLINICAL PRESENTATION Unilateral granulomatous conjunctivitis with one or more raised or flat gelatinous, hyperemic, granulomatous lesions develops on the superior or inferior tarsal conjunctiva, fornix, or bulbar conjunctiva about 3–10 days after inoculation. Either concurrently or 1–2 weeks later, unilateral firm and tender regional preauricular and submandibular lymph nodes, and occasionally cervical nodes, develop. Approximately 10%–40% of the nodes enlarge and become suppurative. Mild systemic symptoms of fever, malaise, headache, and anorexia develop in about 10%–30% of patients, with severe, disseminated complications, including encephalopathy, encephalitis, thrombocytopenic purpura, osteolysis, hepatitis, and splenitis occurring in approximately 2% of CSD patients. Optic neuritis and neuroretinitis have been reported.

LABORATORY EVALUATION Serologic testing is the most cost-effective means for diagnosing typical CSD. Antibodies to *B henselae* can be detected by indirect fluorescent antibody testing or by enzyme immunoassay. The enzyme immunoassay for *B henselae* is more sensitive than the indirect fluorescent antibody test and is available from specialty laboratories. The skin test antigen for CSD is neither commercially available nor standardized. Atypical CSD is best approached by combining serologic testing with culture or PCR.

MANAGEMENT The ideal treatment has not yet been determined. Various antibacterial treatment regimens have reported success. Suggested agents generally include azithromycin, erythromycin, or doxycycline. Rifampin is often used as an adjuvant. Responses to trimethoprim-sulfamethoxazole and fluoroquinolones have also been reported but appear to be inconsistent.

Ormerod LD, Dailey JP. Ocular manifestations of cat-scratch disease. *Curr Opin Ophthalmol.* 1999;10(3):209–216.

Microbial and Parasitic Infections of the Cornea and Sclera

Bacterial Keratitis

Bacterial infection is a common sight-threatening condition. Some cases have explosive onset and rapidly progressive stromal inflammation. Untreated, it often leads to progressive tissue destruction with corneal perforation or extension of infection to adjacent tissue. Bacterial keratitis is frequently associated with risk factors that disturb the corneal epithelial integrity. Common predisposing factors include

- contact lens wear
- trauma
- contaminated ocular medications

- impaired defense mechanisms
- altered structure of the corneal surface

The most frequent risk factor for bacterial keratitis in the United States is contact lens wear, which has been identified as such in 19%–42% of patients who develop culture-proven microbial keratitis. Epidemiologic studies have estimated the annual incidence of cosmetic contact lens–related ulcerative keratitis at 0.21% for individuals using extended-wear soft lenses and 0.04% for patients using daily-wear soft lenses. The risk of developing microbial keratitis increases significantly (approximately 15 times) in patients who wear their contact lenses overnight and is positively correlated with the number of consecutive days lenses are worn without removal.

PATHOGENESIS Bacteria have multiple mechanisms of adherence. For example, S aureus uses adhesins to bind to collagen and other components of the exposed Bowman layer and stroma, whereas P aeruginosa can bind to molecular receptors exposed on injured epithelial cells. A clone of bacteria initially proliferates, then—within hours—invades the cornea between stromal lamellae. Corneal inflammation begins with the local production of cytokines and chemokines that enable diapedesis and migration of neutrophils into the peripheral cornea from the limbal vessels. Some microorganisms produce proteases that disrupt the extracellular matrix. Enzymes released by neutrophils and activation of corneal matrix metalloproteinases exacerbate inflammatory necrosis. With antimicrobial control of bacterial replication, wound healing processes begin that may be accompanied by neovascularization and scarring. Progressive inflammation, however, may lead to corneal perforation.

CLINICAL PRESENTATION Rapid onset of pain is accompanied by conjunctival injection, photophobia, and decreased vision in patients with bacterial corneal ulcers. The rate of progression of these symptoms depends on the virulence of the infecting organism. Bacterial corneal ulcers typically show a sharp epithelial demarcation with underlying dense, suppurative stromal inflammation that has indistinct edges and is surrounded by stromal edema. P aeruginosa typically produces stromal necrosis with a shaggy surface and adherent mucopurulent exudate (Fig 5-16). An endothelial inflammatory plaque, marked anterior chamber reaction, and hypopyon frequently occur.

Infections caused by slow-growing, fastidious organisms such as mycobacteria or anaerobes may have a nonsuppurative infiltrate and intact epithelium. *Infectious crystalline keratopathy,* an example of this type of infection, presents as densely packed, white, branching aggregates of organisms in the virtual absence of a host inflammatory response. It is believed to occur when a sequestered colony of slow-growing organisms develops after midstromal implantation in a cornea with compromised inflammatory responses. Corticosteroid use, contact lens wear, and infected corneal grafts can all create a predisposition to this infection. Infectious crystalline keratopathy has been reported with a number of bacterial species, most commonly α-hemolytic *Streptococcus* species (Fig 5-17).

LABORATORY EVALUATION The prevalence of a particular causative organism depends on the geographic location and risk factors for the infection. Common and uncommon organisms causing bacterial keratitis are listed in Table 5-5.

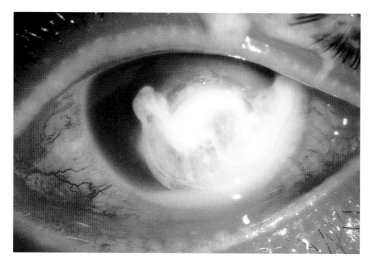

Figure 5-16 Suppurative ulcerative keratitis caused by *P aeruginosa.*

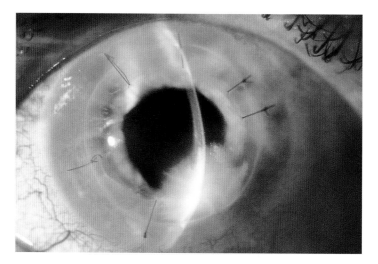

Figure 5-17 Infectious crystalline keratopathy in a corneal graft caused by α-hemolytic *Streptococcus* species.

Table 5-5 Causes of Bacterial Keratitis

Common Organisms	Uncommon Organisms
Staphylococcus aureus	*Neisseria* spp
Staphylococcus epidermidis	*Moraxella* spp
Streptococcus pneumoniae and other *Streptococcus* spp	*Mycobacterium* spp
	Nocardia spp
Pseudomonas aeruginosa (most common organism in soft contact lens wearers)	Non–spore-forming anaerobes
	Corynebacterium spp
Enterobacteriaceae *(Proteus, Enterobacter, Serratia)*	

By appearance alone, it can be difficult to determine whether a corneal ulcer has an infectious etiology. Before initiating antimicrobial therapy for cases of suspected bacterial keratitis, a clinician should consider conducting microbiologic diagnostic tests. (See Chapters 3 and 4 in this volume and BCSC Section 4, *Ophthalmic Pathology and Intraocular Tumors*, for specimen collecting, culturing, staining, and interpretation.)

If a patient has already been treated with topical antibiotics and is unresponsive to them, some advocate stopping the medication 12–24 hours prior to culturing in order to enhance recovery of viable organisms. This is controversial. Antimicrobial therapy should not be discontinued in severe or rapidly progressive corneal ulcers.

In addition to culturing the cornea, it may be helpful to culture contact lenses, contact lens cases, solutions, and any other potentially contaminating sources, such as inflamed eyelids, because any of these might provide a clue to the causative organism in the event that corneal cultures are negative. This approach can also help identify the source of the infection.

MANAGEMENT   Currently, no single antibiotic agent is effective against all bacterial species causing microbial keratitis. Initial broad-spectrum therapy is recommended until the offending microorganism is identified in culture. If 1 type of bacterium is prominently identified on a stained diagnostic smear, therapy may initially be weighted toward that class of microorganism. Broad-spectrum therapy, however, should not be eliminated, as cultures may reveal a different class of microorganism. Once the offending microbe is identified, or the clinical response suggests the change, appropriate monotherapy may be considered (Table 5-6).

The route of antibiotic administration should be based on the severity of the keratitis. Frequent (every 30–60 minutes) fortified topical antibiotics are now used for bacterial keratitis. Fortified antibiotic solutions produce therapeutic antibiotic concentrations in the corneal stroma, whereas commercially available antibiotic solutions may result in subtherapeutic concentrations. In severe cases, therapeutic stromal concentrations of antibiotic may be achieved more rapidly by initially administering the antibiotic drop every 5 minutes for 30 minutes as a loading dose. Oral antibiotics, especially the fluoroquinolones, which have excellent ocular penetration, and frequent use of topical antibiotics are indicated in cases with suspected scleral and/or intraocular extension of infection.

Modification of initial antimicrobial therapy should be based on clinical response, not on the results of antimicrobial sensitivity testing. Determination of antibiotic sensitivity or resistance in traditional antimicrobial sensitivity tests is based on antibiotic concentrations achievable in the serum by oral or parenteral administration. Often, antibiotic concentrations greatly exceeding the mean inhibitory concentrations of bacteria are achieved in the corneal stroma following frequent fortified antibiotic administration. An alternate antibiotic regimen should be considered in patients who do not show clinical response or who develop toxicity from the agent(s) used initially. Modification of antibiotic therapy in these cases should be based on antimicrobial sensitivity testing. Several clinical parameters are useful to monitor clinical response to antibiotic therapy:

- blunting of the perimeter of the stromal infiltrate
- decreased density of the stromal infiltrate

Table 5-6 Initial Therapy for Bacterial Keratitis

Organism	Antibiotic	Topical Dose	Subconjunctival Dose
Gram-positive cocci	Cefazolin	50 mg/mL	100 mg in 0.5 mL
	Vancomycin*	25–50 mg/mL	25 mg in 0.5 mL
	Moxifloxacin or gatifloxacin	5 or 3 mg/mL, respectively	Not available
Gram-negative rods	Tobramycin	9–14 mg/mL	20 mg in 0.5 mL
	Ceftazidime	50 mg/mL	100 mg in 0.5 mL
	Fluoroquinolones	3 mg/mL	Not available
No organism or multiple types of organisms	Cefazolin with	50 mg/mL	100 mg in 0.5 mL
	Tobramycin or	9–14 mg/mL	20 mg in 0.5 mL
	Fluoroquinolones	3 or 5 mg/mL	Not available
Gram-negative cocci	Ceftriaxone	50 mg/mL	100 mg in 0.5 mL
	Ceftazidime	50 mg/mL	
	Moxifloxacin or gatifloxacin	5 or 3 mg/mL, respectively	
Mycobacteria	Clarithromycin	10 mg/mL 0.03%	
	Moxifloxacin or gatifloxacin	5 or 3 mg/mL, respectively	

*For resistant *Staphylococcus* species.

Notes for Table 5-6: Preparation of topical antibiotics
Cefazolin 50 mg/mL
1. Add 9.2 mL of Tears Naturale artificial tears to a vial of cefazolin in 1 g (powder for injection).
2. Dissolve. Take 5 mL of this solution and add it to 5 mL of artificial tears.
3. Refrigerate and shake well before instillation.
Vancomycin 50 mg/mL
1. Add 10 mL of 0.9% sodium chloride for injection USP (no preservatives) or artificial tears to a 500-mg vial of vancomycin to produce a solution of 50 mg/mL.
2. Refrigerate and shake well before instillation.
Ceftazidime 50 mg/mL
1. Add 9.2 mL of artificial tears to a vial of ceftazidime 1 g (powder for injection).
2. Dissolve. Take 5 mL of this solution and add it to 5 mL of artificial tears.
3. Refrigerate and shake well before instillation.
Tobramycin 14 mg/mL
1. Withdraw 2 mL of tobramycin injectable vial (40 mg/mL).
2. Add 2 mL to a tobramycin ophthalmic solution (5 mL) to give a 14 mg/mL solution.
3. Refrigerate and shake well before instillation.

- reduction of stromal edema and endothelial inflammatory plaque
- reduction in anterior chamber inflammation
- reepithelialization
- cessation of corneal thinning

The frequency of topical antibiotic administration should slowly be tapered as the stromal inflammation resolves.

Combination therapy with an agent active against gram-positive bacteria (eg, vancomycin, bacitracin, Neosporin, cefuroxime, or cefazolin) and an agent active against gram-negative bacteria (eg, tobramycin, gentamicin, amikacin, ceftazidime, ciprofloxacin, levofloxacin, or ofloxacin) provides good initial broad-spectrum antibiotic coverage.

Single-agent therapy with a fluoroquinolone may also be considered. These antibiotics should initially be given every 30–60 minutes and then tapered in frequency according to the clinical response. Fortified antibiotics should generally be continued until substantial infection control has been achieved. Thereafter, a broad-spectrum, nonfortified antibiotic may be given 3–8 times daily according to the patient's clinical status.

Disadvantages of fortified antibiotics include ocular irritation, cost, and the inconvenience of extemporaneously preparing a solution that is not commercially available. Their chief advantage is their potential to save vision in aggressive infections. When irritation secondary to epithelial toxicity becomes a concern, lower-strength concentrations (eg, 25 mg/mL vancomycin) may be better tolerated.

An alternative to combination therapy is the use of fluoroquinolone monotherapy, which is most appropriate in compliant patients with less severe ulcers (eg, <3 mm in diameter, midperipheral or peripheral, and not associated with significant thinning). Fluoroquinolones (eg, levofloxacin, ciprofloxacin, ofloxacin, moxifloxacin, and gatifloxacin) must be administered at least every hour to maximize therapeutic effect. Because second-generation fluoroquinolones such as ciprofloxacin and ofloxacin typically have variable activity against streptococci, documented streptococcal infections should be treated with a cell wall–active agent (eg, bacitracin, cefazolin, vancomycin, or penicillin G) rather than a second-generation fluoroquinolone, regardless of in vitro testing that may suggest susceptibility.

The role of corticosteroid therapy for bacterial keratitis is controversial. It is well recognized that tissue destruction in microbial keratitis results from a combination of the direct effects of lytic enzymes and toxins produced by the infecting organism, as well as the damage caused by the inflammatory reaction directed at the microorganisms. An intense suppurative inflammatory reaction consisting predominantly of polymorphonuclear leukocytes causes significant tissue destruction by generating free radicals as well as liberating proteolytic enzymes, including collagenases and gelatinases. The rationale for using corticosteroids is to decrease this tissue destruction.

Several studies using animal models of bacterial keratitis have demonstrated that concurrent use of topical corticosteroids does not impair the killing effect of bactericidal antibiotics against susceptible microorganisms. Clinical series evaluating the effectiveness of corticosteroids for treatment of human bacterial keratitis have reported either no treatment effect or more rapid resolution of stromal inflammation than resulted from antibiotic therapy alone.

However, the use of topical corticosteroids following presumed resolution of gram-negative bacterial keratitis (especially that caused by *P aeruginosa*) has been documented to promote a relapse of the infection. If the immune system is impaired by administration of topical corticosteroids before complete clearance of virulent organisms, recurrent infection may result. Topical corticosteroids should therefore be used for treatment of bacterial keratitis with extreme caution. Following are recommended criteria for instituting corticosteroid therapy for bacterial keratitis:

- Corticosteroids should not be used in the initial phase of the treatment until an etiologic organism has been identified and the organism shows in vitro sensitivity to the antibiotic(s) being used for treatment.

- The patient must be able to return for frequent follow-up examinations and demonstrate compliance with appropriate antibiotic therapy.
- No other associated virulent or difficult-to-eradicate organism is found.

In addition, a favorable clinical response to antibiotic therapy is strongly advised before topical corticosteroids are initiated. Corticosteroid drops may be started in moderate dosages (prednisolone acetate or phosphate 1% every 4–6 hours), and the patient should be monitored at 24 and 48 hours after initiation of therapy. If the patient shows no adverse effects, the frequency of administration may be adjusted based on clinical response.

Penetrating keratoplasty (PK) for treatment of bacterial keratitis is indicated if the disease progresses despite therapy, descemetocele formation or perforation occurs, or the keratitis is unresponsive to antimicrobial therapy. The involved area should be identified preoperatively, and an attempt should be made to circumscribe all areas of infection. Peripheral iridectomies are indicated, because patients may develop seclusion of the pupil from inflammatory pupillary membranes. Interrupted sutures are recommended. The patient should be treated with appropriate antibiotics, cycloplegics, and intense topical corticosteroids postoperatively. See Chapter 16 for a more detailed discussion of PK.

Preferred Practice Patterns Committee, Cornea/External Disease Panel. *Bacterial Keratitis.* San Francisco: American Academy of Ophthalmology; 2008.

Schein OD, Glynn RJ, Poggio EC, Seddon JM, Kenyon KR. The relative risk of ulcerative keratitis among users of daily-wear and extended-wear soft contact lenses. A case-control study. Microbial Keratitis Study Group. *N Engl J Med.* 1989;321(12):773–778.

Atypical Mycobacteria

Atypical mycobacteria are important pathogens in post-LASIK infections. The most common pathogens are *M fortuitum* and *M chelonei,* which may be found in soil and water. These organisms should be suspected in delayed-onset postrefractive infections, classically with recalcitrant, nonsuppurative infiltrates. The diagnosis may be confirmed with acid-fast stain or culture on Lowenstein-Jensen media. Treatments include oral and topical clarithromycin, moxifloxacin, and gatifloxacin. Amikacin, previously the only treatment option, has been largely replaced by these newer treatment options.

Chang MA, Jain S, Azar DT. Infections following laser in situ keratomileusis: an integration of the published literature. *Surv Ophthalmol.* 2004;49(3):269–280.

Hyon JY, Joo MJ, Hose S, Sinha D, Dick JD, O'Brien TP. Comparative efficacy of topical gatifloxacin with ciprofloxacin, amikacin, and clarithromycin in the treatment of experimental Mycobacterium chelonae keratitis. *Arch Ophthalmol.* 2004;122(8):1166–1169.

Fungal Keratitis

PATHOGENESIS Fungal keratitis is less common than bacterial keratitis, generally representing less than 5%–10% of corneal infections in reported clinical series in the United States. Filamentous fungal keratitis occurs more frequently in warmer, more humid parts of the United States than in other regions of the country. Trauma to the cornea with plant or vegetable material is the leading risk factor for fungal keratitis. Especially predisposed are gardeners who use weed trimmers or other similar motorized lawn care equipment without wearing protective eyewear. Trauma related to contact lens wear is another common risk factor for the development of fungal keratitis. Topical corticosteroids are a major risk factor as well, as they appear to activate and increase the virulence of fungal organisms by reducing the cornea's resistance to infection. *Candida* species cause ocular infections in immunocompromised hosts and in corneas with chronic ulceration from other causes. The increasing use of topical corticosteroids during the past 4 decades has been implicated as a major cause for the rising incidence of fungal keratitis during this period. Furthermore, systemic corticosteroid usage may suppress the host's immune response, thereby predisposing to fungal keratitis. Other common risk factors include corneal surgery (eg, PK, radial keratotomy) and chronic keratitis (eg, herpes simplex [HSV], herpes zoster, or vernal/allergic conjunctivitis).

In early 2006, an outbreak of contact lens–associated fungal keratitis was observed, first in Singapore and the Pacific Rim and then in the United States. The epidemic occurred in association with the use of Renu with MoistureLoc solution (Bausch and Lomb, Rochester, New York). Bausch and Lomb withdrew the solution from the world market on May 15, 2006.

> Chang DC, Grant GB, O'Donnell K, et al; Fusarium Keratitis Investigation Team. Multistate outbreak of Fusarium keratitis associated with use of a contact lens solution. *JAMA.* 2006; 296(8):953–963.

CLINICAL PRESENTATION Patients with fungal keratitis tend to have fewer inflammatory signs and symptoms during the initial period than those with bacterial keratitis and may have little or no conjunctival injection upon initial presentation. Filamentous fungal keratitis frequently manifests as a gray-white, dry-appearing infiltrate that has irregular feathery or filamentous margins (Fig 5-18). Superficial lesions may appear gray-white, elevate

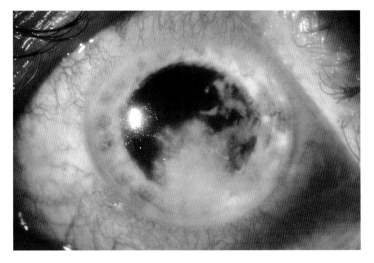

Figure 5-18 Fungal keratitis caused by *Fusarium solani* with characteristic dry white stromal infiltrate with feathery edges.

the surface of the cornea, and have a dry, rough, or gritty texture detectable at the time of diagnostic corneal scraping. Occasionally, multifocal or satellite infiltrates may be present, although these are less common than previously reported. In addition, a deep stromal infiltrate may occur in the presence of an intact epithelium. An endothelial plaque and/or hypopyon may also occur if the fungal infiltrate(s) is sufficiently deep or large.

As the keratitis progresses, intense suppuration may develop and the lesions may resemble bacterial keratitis. At this point, rapidly progressive hypopyon and anterior chamber inflammatory membranes may develop. Extension of fungal infection into the anterior chamber is often seen in cases with rapidly progressive anterior chamber inflammation. Occasionally, fungus may invade the iris or posterior chamber, and angle-closure glaucoma may develop from inflammatory pupillary block.

Yeast keratitis is most frequently caused by *Candida* species. This form of fungal keratitis frequently presents with superficial white, raised colonies in a structurally altered eye. Although most cases tend to remain superficial, deep invasion may occur with suppuration resembling keratitis induced by gram-positive bacteria.

LABORATORY EVALUATION   The fungal cell wall stains with Gomori methenamine silver but, except for *Candida,* does not take up Gram stain. Blood, Sabouraud's, and brain–heart infusion media are preferred media for fungal culture.

MANAGEMENT   Natamycin 5% suspension is recommended for treatment of most cases of filamentous fungal keratitis, particularly those caused by *Fusarium* species, which are the most common causative agents for exogenous fungal keratitis occurring in the humid areas of the southern United States. Most clinical and experimental evidence suggests that topical amphotericin B (0.15%–0.30%) is the most efficacious agent available to treat yeast keratitis; the majority of corneal yeast infections respond readily to the drug. Amphotericin B is also recommended for filamentous keratitis caused by *Aspergillus* species. Topical voriconazole is effective in treating fungal keratitis that is not responding to traditional treatment. Oral ketoconazole (200–600 mg/day) may be considered for adjunctive therapy in severe filamentous fungal keratitis and oral fluconazole (200–400 mg/day), for severe yeast keratitis. Oral itraconazole (200 mg/day) has broad-spectrum activity against all *Aspergillus* species and *Candida* but variable activity against *Fusarium*. Oral voriconazole (200–400 mg/day) is rapidly replacing other oral antifungals because of its excellent intraocular penetration and broad-spectrum coverage. Posaconazole may also be considered for treatment.

In the presence of a negative smear when fungal infection is suspected, repeated scrapings or biopsy may be necessary to identify fungal material. Furthermore, mechanical debridement may be beneficial for cases of superficial fungal keratitis. Fungal infiltration of the deep corneal stroma may not respond to topical antifungal therapy, because the penetration of these agents is reduced in the presence of an intact epithelium. Penetration of natamycin or amphotericin B has been shown to be significantly enhanced by debridement of the corneal epithelium, and animal experiments indicate that frequent topical application (every 5 min) for 1 hour can readily achieve therapeutic levels. Cases with progressive disease despite maximal topical and/or oral antifungal therapy may require therapeutic PK to prevent scleral or intraocular extension of the fungal infection. Both of these conditions carry a very poor prognosis for salvaging the eye.

Bunya VY, Hammersmith KM, Rapuano CJ, Ayres BD, Cohen EJ. Topical and oral voricon-azole in the treatment of fungal keratitis. *Am J Ophthalmol.* 2007;143(1):151–153.

Loh AR, Hong K, Lee S, Mannis M, Acharya NR. Practice patterns in the management of fungal corneal ulcers. *Cornea.* 2009;28(8):856–859.

Acanthamoeba Keratitis

PATHOGENESIS Acanthamoebae are free-living ubiquitous protozoa found in freshwater and soil. They are resistant to killing by freezing; desiccation; and the levels of chlorine routinely used in municipal water supplies, swimming pools, and hot tubs. They may exist as motile trophozoites or dormant cysts. The majority (70%) of reported cases of amebic keratitis have been associated with contact lens use. Homemade saline solution prepared by dissolving saline tablets in distilled water appeared to be a significant source of *Acanthamoeba* infection among contact lens wearers until saline tablets were taken off the US market in the 1980s.

Over the past 5 years, an increased number of *Acanthamoeba* cases have been observed in the United States, particularly on the East Coast and in the Midwest. The CDC conducted a multistate, retrospective review of cases, which found an association between *Acanthamoeba* keratitis and soft contact lens users who used Complete MoisturePlus multipurpose cleaning solution (Advanced Medical Optics; Santa Ana, CA). The solution was voluntarily removed from the market in May 2007. Unfortunately, initial reports have not found a dramatic decline in these cases since the removal.

Joslin CE, Tu EY, McMahon TT, Passaro DJ, Stayner LT, Sugar J. Epidemiological character-istics of a Chicago-area Acanthamoeba keratitis outbreak. *Am J Ophthalmol.* 2006;142(2): 212–217.

Joslin CE, Tu EY, Shoff ME, et al. The association of contact lens solution use and Acan-thamoeba keratitis. *Am J Ophthalmol.* 2007;144(2):169–180.

CLINICAL PRESENTATION Patients with amebic keratitis commonly have severe ocular pain, photophobia, and a protracted, progressive course. Frequently, they have shown no therapeutic response to a variety of topical antimicrobial agents. *Acanthamoeba* infection is localized to the corneal epithelium in early cases and may manifest as a diffuse punctate epitheliopathy or dendritic epithelial lesion. Cases with epithelial dendrites are often misdiagnosed as herpetic keratitis and treated with antiviral agents and/or corticosteroids. Stromal infection typically occurs in the central cornea, and early cases have a gray-white superficial, nonsuppurative infiltrate. As the disease progresses, a partial or complete ring infiltrate in the paracentral cornea is frequently observed (Fig 5-19). Enlarged corneal nerves, called *radial perineuritis,* may be noted, as well as limbitis or focal, nodular, or diffuse scleritis.

LABORATORY EVALUATION Diagnosis of *Acanthamoeba* keratitis is made by visualizing ame-bae in stained smears or by culturing organisms obtained from corneal scrapings. The

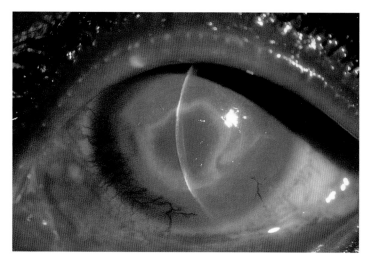

Figure 5-19 Ring infiltrate in *Acanthamoeba* keratitis.

highest diagnostic yield occurs relatively early in the course of the disease, when the organisms are localized to the epithelium. Later, the organisms penetrate into deeper layers and may be difficult to isolate from superficial scraping. Lamellar corneal biopsy may be required to establish the diagnosis in these cases. In contact lens–associated infections, the contact lenses and contact lens case can be examined.

Amebae are seen in smears stained with Giemsa or with periodic acid–Schiff (PAS), calcofluor white, or acridine orange stains. Nonnutrient agar with *E coli* or *E aerogenes* overlay is the preferred medium for culturing amebae, although the organisms frequently grow well on blood agar plates and on buffered charcoal–yeast extract agar. Characteristic trails form as the motile trophozoites travel across the surface of the culture plate. Confocal in vivo microscopy can also be used to show organisms, particularly the cyst forms.

MANAGEMENT   Early diagnosis of *Acanthamoeba* keratitis is the most important prognostic indicator of a successful treatment outcome. Unfortunately, many cases are treated initially for herpetic keratitis. Not only is the delay in diagnosis detrimental, but the use of corticosteroids early in the disease may also be correlated with a poor outcome due to compromise of the host's inflammatory response against *Acanthamoeba*. Late immunoinflammatory responses after the amebae have been killed may be reduced by corticosteroids, but this is controversial and remains an area for further investigation. Clinical features that suggest a diagnosis of *Acanthamoeba* keratitis rather than HSV keratitis include

- noncontiguous or multifocal pattern of granular epitheliopathy and subepithelial opacities (unlike the contiguous, dendritic pattern in HSV keratitis)
- disproportionately severe pain, probably secondary to perineural inflammation (unlike hypoesthesia and disproportionately mild pain secondary to trigeminal nerve involvement in HSV)

- presence of epidemiologic risk factors such as contact lens use or exposure to possibly contaminated freshwater
- failure to respond to initial antiviral therapy

Cases diagnosed during the early, epithelial stage of the disease respond well to epithelial debridement, followed by a relatively short (3–4 months) course of antiamebic therapy. The prognosis for visual recovery with only mild residual stromal involvement is very good. Once stromal infiltrates appear, however, eradication of organisms is more difficult, and treatment may be needed for 6–12 months.

A number of antimicrobial agents have been recommended for therapy of *Acanthamoeba* keratitis based on their in vitro amebicidal effects as well as their clinical effectiveness. Agents used for topical administration include

- *diamidines:* propamidine, hexamidine
- *biguanides:* polyhexamethylene biguanide (polyhexanide), chlorhexidine
- *aminoglycosides:* neomycin, paromomycin
- *imidazoles/triazoles:* voriconazole, miconazole, clotrimazole, ketoconazole, itraconazole

Most of these agents are effective against the free-living trophozoite form of the organism but have reduced efficacy in killing cysts. Although there is no consensus yet about the optimal therapeutic agent, successful resolution has been achieved with a biguanide with and without a diamidine. Recent reports favor the use of chlorhexidine 0.02% or polyhexamethylene biguanide (PHMB) 0.02% as initial therapy. Some specialists encourage the use of chlorhexidine or PHMB in combination with propamidine isethionate 0.1%. Treatment with topical corticosteroids is of uncertain long-term benefit and may contribute to prolonged persistence of viable cysts or potentiate mixed infections when a virus is present.

Penetrating keratoplasty is reserved for cases that are progressing despite maximal medical therapy and showing evidence of severe stromal melting with threatened perforation. The risk for recurrence in this setting is very high. Even in apparently quiet, treated eyes, optical PK procedures are associated with a high risk of recurrence if performed within the first year after the onset of infection. The presumed pathogenesis of such recurrences is the persistence of an occasional residual viable cyst in an eye with compromised immunity as the result of the presence of an allograft and the use of topical corticosteroids postoperatively. Therefore, it is advisable to perform any elective PK procedure only after a full course of amebicidal therapy has been completed and a minimum of 3–6 months of disease-free follow-up thereafter has been documented. There is some controversy about the timing of corneal transplantation, with some favoring earlier intervention.

Corneal Stromal Inflammation Associated With Systemic Infections

Nonsuppurative stromal keratitis can be caused by the following:

- reactive arthritis
- congenital or acquired syphilis

- Lyme disease
- tuberculosis
- Hansen disease (leprosy)
- onchocerciasis

Most of these conditions are discussed in BCSC Section 9, *Intraocular Inflammation and Uveitis.*

Microsporidiosis

Microsporida are intracellular protozoa that may cause ocular infection and have emerged in the literature because of their opportunistic nature in individuals with AIDS. There are 2 distinct clinical presentations of microsporidial infections, depending on the immune status of the patient. In immunocompetent individuals, a corneal stromal keratitis may develop, and in AIDS patients, conjunctivitis and an epithelial keratopathy may be seen. The latter group may also have disseminated microsporidiosis involving the sinuses, respiratory tract, or gastrointestinal tract.

Patients present with symptoms that include ocular irritation, photophobia, vision decrease, and bilateral conjunctival injection with little or no associated inflammation. Stromal keratitis is caused by agents of the *Nosema* genus, whereas the *Encephalitozoon* and *Septata* genera have been associated with keratoconjunctivitis. In the keratoconjunctivitis variant, corneal findings include superficial nonstaining opacities described as "mucoid" in appearance, along with dense areas of fine punctate fluorescein staining. The corneal stroma remains clear, with no or minimal iritis.

Light microscopy using the Brown and Hopps stain may identify small gram-positive spores in the epithelial cells of the conjunctiva. Transmission electron microscopy is a sensitive means of identification. Tissue culture techniques may also be used, but immunofluorescent antibody techniques have greater clinical utility. Some authors have discouraged corneal biopsy or scraping because of its potential for promoting additional corneal compromise.

Although there is no definitive treatment, topical fumagillin has been used to successfully treat microsporidial keratoconjunctivitis with low toxicity. In severe cases of *Vittaforma corneae*, granulomatous inflammation may lead to necrotic thinning and perforation. PK may then become the only available treatment for severe stromal thinning. In general, medical regimens require long-term use, and recurrence is common after treatment discontinuation.

Joseph J, Sridhar MS, Murthy S, Sharma S. Clinical and microbiological profile of microsporidial keratoconjunctivitis in southern India. *Ophthalmology.* 2006;113(4):531–537.

Krachmer JH, Mannis MJ, Holland EJ, eds. *Cornea.* 2nd ed. Vol 1. Philadelphia: Elsevier/Mosby; 2005.

Weber R, Canning EU. Microsporidia. In: Murray PR, Baron EJ, Jorgensen JH, Landry ML, Pfaller MA, eds. *Manual of Clinical Microbiology.* 9th ed. Washington, DC: ASM Press; 2007.

Loiasis

Loa loa and other filarial nematodes can cause conjunctivitis as well as dermatologic manifestations. After the bite of an infected vector, such parasites can burrow subcutaneously to reach the eye area. The microfilarial stage is transmitted from human to human by the bite of an infected female deer fly (genus *Chrysops*) indigenous to West and Central Africa. A migrating worm moves under the skin at about 1 cm/min but is most conspicuous when it is seen or felt wriggling under the periocular skin or bulbar conjunctiva. Extraction of the filarial worm cures the conjunctivitis; that is followed by antiparasitic treatment for widespread infestation. Diethylcarbamazine is generally given 2 mg/kg tid for 3 weeks and repeated as necessary. Ivermectin 150 mg/kg may also be effective, but significant side effects have been reported in patients with prominent intravascular loiasis. Concurrent administration of corticosteroids and/or antihistamines may be necessary to minimize allergic reactions.

Microbial Scleritis

PATHOGENESIS   Bacterial and fungal infections of the sclera are very rare. Most cases result from the extension of microbial keratitis involving the peripheral cornea. Trauma and contaminated foreign bodies (including scleral buckles) are possible risk factors. Bacterial scleritis has also occurred in sclerae damaged by previous pterygium surgery, especially when beta irradiation or mitomycin has been used (Fig 5-20). Bacteria and fungi can also invade tissue of the eye wall surrounding a scleral surgical wound, but endophthalmitis is more likely in this setting. Scleral inflammation can also be a feature of syphilis, tuberculosis, nocardia, atypical mycobacteria, and leprosy. Diffuse or nodular scleritis is an occasional complication of varicella-zoster virus eye disease.

LABORATORY EVALUATION   Evaluating suppurative scleritis is similar to evaluating microbial keratitis. Smears and cultures are obtained before antimicrobial therapy is begun. The workup of nonsuppurative scleritis is guided by the history and physical examination, as described in Chapter 7.

MANAGEMENT   Topical antimicrobial therapy is begun just as for microbial keratitis. Because of the difficulty in controlling microbial scleritis, subconjunctival injections and intravenous antibiotics may also be used. Long-term oral therapy shows promise.

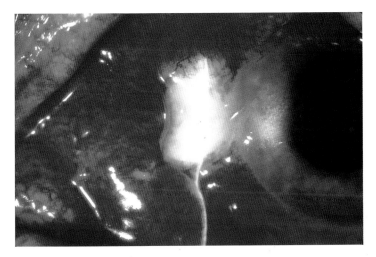

Figure 5-20 Bacterial scleritis occurring 2 weeks after pterygium surgery. *(Courtesy of Kirk R. Wilhelmus, MD.)*

CHAPTER 6

Ocular Immunology

Cellular Elements of the Ocular Immune Response

For an in-depth discussion of the various features of the innate and adaptive immune system, including the different types of hypersensitivity reactions with relevant ocular examples, see BCSC Section 9, *Intraocular Inflammation and Uveitis.* This chapter is an overview of the ocular immune response, which involves primarily the immune system and the lacrimal functional unit (LFU): lacrimal gland, ocular surface (conjunctiva, cornea, and meibomian glands), tear film, eyelids, and the sensory and motor nerves that connect these structures. (See also Chapter 4.)

Lacrimal Functional Unit

In addition to the normal secretory tissue, which produces tears, the lacrimal gland contains a variety of lymphocytes (plasma cells, T cells, B cells), macrophages, and dendritic cells, as well as soluble "immune" factors produced by the epithelial cells. These soluble and cellular elements play an important role in the innate and adaptive arms of the ocular immune response. The lacrimal gland is also an important component of the mucosa-associated lymphoid tissue (MALT). The plasma cells of the lacrimal gland, which produce secretory IgA (SIgA), a component of the humoral (antibody-dependent) immune system, circulate throughout the MALT and arrive in the lacrimal gland through specific homing receptors.

The Ocular Surface

The ocular surface comprises the conjunctiva, cornea, and meibomian glands.

The normal, uninflamed conjunctiva contains immunoglobulins and a few polymorphonuclear leukocytes (neutrophils), lymphocytes, macrophages, plasma cells, and mast cells within the subepithelial tissue. In addition, the conjunctival stroma has its own endowment of dendritic antigen-presenting cells (APCs). The epithelium contains a special subpopulation of dendritic APCs known as *Langerhans cells,* which are capable of both antigen uptake and priming (sensitizing) of naive antigen-inexperienced T lymphocytes. Hence, these dendritic cells serve as the sentinel cells of the immune system of the ocular surface. In addition to the presence of immune cells, the conjunctiva has a plentiful supply of lymphatic vessels, which facilitate the trafficking of immune cells and antigens to the draining lymph nodes, where the adaptive immune response is generated.

Table 6-1 summarizes the known distribution of certain immune and inflammatory cells in the ocular surface epithelium and substantia propria (stroma).

Table 6-1 Immunologic Components of the Ocular Surface

Cell	Epithelium	Substantia Propria
Dendritic cells	+	+
Helper T cells	+	+
Suppressor T cells	+	+
B cells and plasma cells	−	+
Neutrophils	+	+
Eosinophils	−	−
Mast cells	−	+

The normal, uninflamed cornea, like the conjunctiva, is endowed with dendritic cells. Like those in the conjunctiva, the dendritic cells in the corneal epithelium are also called *Langerhans cells.* They are located primarily in the corneal periphery and limbus. These APCs are in an activated, mature state (expressing class II major histocompatibility complex [MHC] antigens and costimulatory molecules) and hence capable of efficiently stimulating T cells. In addition to these dendritic cells (Fig 6-1), small numbers of lymphocytes are present in the peripheral epithelium and anterior stroma of the cornea. A highly regulated process, mediated by vascular endothelial adhesion molecules and cytokines, controls the recruitment of the various leukocyte subsets from the intravascular compartment into the limbal matrix.

Unlike the conjunctiva, the normal cornea is considered to be an immunologically privileged site, so called because the generation of immune responsiveness to foreign

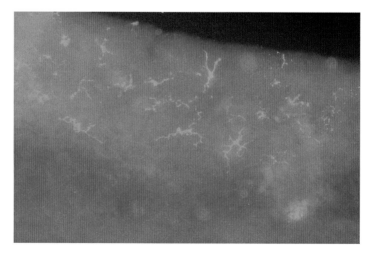

Figure 6-1 Langerhans cells represent a subpopulation of dendritic antigen-presenting cells of the ocular surface epithelium. As the sentinel cells of the immune system, they pick up, process, and present antigens to T cells. This micrograph shows the predominance of MHC class II⁺ Langerhans cells in the limbus of the uninflamed eye. *(Courtesy of the laboratory of M. Reza Dana, MD.)*

(including transplantation) antigens is relatively suppressed. The normal cornea's immune privilege is due to a multitude of factors, including

- absence of blood vessels, which impedes delivery of immune effector cells
- absence of lymphatics, which minimizes flow of antigens and APCs to the draining lymph nodes
- expression of immunosuppressive factors, including transforming growth factor βs (TGF-βs) and neuropeptides, such as α-melanocyte-stimulating hormone (α-MSH)
- expression of Fas ligand (CD95) by corneal cells, which is believed to play a critical role in inducing Fas-mediated apoptosis (programmed cell death) of activated lymphocytes

Hence, it has been postulated that the immune response generated to antigens located in the cornea and anterior chamber may lead to immune unresponsiveness or even immunologic tolerance.

The meibomian glands also contribute to the ocular inflammatory and immune response; these are regulated by a variety of local and systemic factors, including circulating androgens.

Dana MR, Qian Y, Hamrah P. Twenty-five-year panorama of corneal immunology: emerging concepts in the immunopathogenesis of microbial keratitis, peripheral ulcerative keratitis, and corneal transplant rejection. *Cornea.* 2000;19(5):625–643.

Streilein JW. Ocular immune privilege: therapeutic opportunities form an experiment of nature. *Nat Rev Immunol.* 2003;3(11):879–889.

Soluble Mediators of the Ocular Immune Response

Cellular elements of the ocular immune system function as a neuroregulatory unit comprising the ocular surface, the lacrimal gland, and the neuronal connections between them (Fig 6-2). Regulation (up- or down-modulation) of the expression of many molecules is a critical facet of ocular surface immunoinflammatory responses. For example, many immunoglobulins (primarily dimeric IgA) are normally present in the tear film. However, antibody levels may drop significantly with lacrimal gland atrophy (as protein synthesis in the gland decreases) in severe exocrinopathy, as seen in Sjögren syndrome. In contrast, immunoglobulin levels increase in patients with allergic disorders of the external eye or with other disorders that activate the humoral arm of the immune system, such as infections.

Tear Film

The normal tear film is a complex structure that contains a variety of elements, including components of the complement cascade, proteins, growth factors, and a variety of cytokines (see Chapter 3 for discussion of tear-film physiology and BCSC Section 9,

Zierhut Diagram

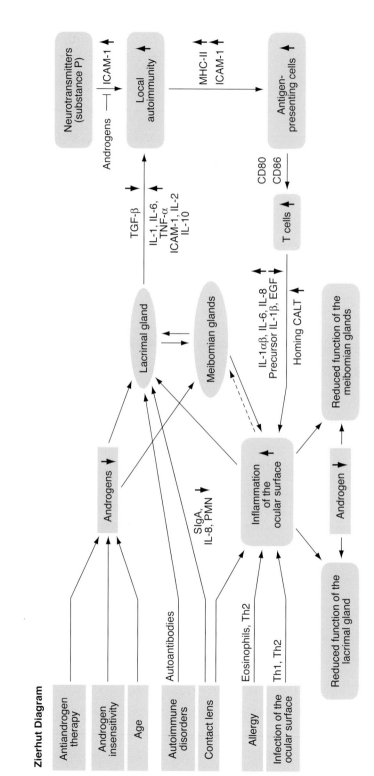

Figure 6-2 The lacrimal and meibomian glands might be influenced by various disorders, leading to stimulation of local autoimmunity, and activation of local antigen-presenting cells, followed by T-cell infiltration. This results in inflammation of the ocular surface and glandular structures with reduced exocrine function. Various factors (cytokines, chemokines, neurotransmitters, and androgen levels) can influence the intensity of the inflammatory response, which might result in blepharitis, conjunctivitis, keratitis, and the dry-eye syndrome. *CALT* = conjunctiva-associated lymphoid tissue, *EGF* = epidermal growth factor, *ICAM-1* = intercellular adhesion molecule 1, *IL* = interleukin, *MHC* = major histocompatibility complex, *PMN* = polymorphonuclear leukocyte, *TGF-β* = transforming growth factor βs, *TNF-α* = tumor necrosis factor α. *(Reproduced with permission from Zierhut M, Dana MR, Stern ME, and Sullivan DA. Immunology of the lacrimal gland and ocular tear film. Trends Immunol. 2002;23(7):333–335.)*

Intraocular Inflammation and Uveitis, for more in-depth discussion and illustrations of the immune system). Cytokines such as interleukin-1 (IL-1) and tumor necrosis factor α (TNF-α) are significantly up-regulated in a variety of corneal inflammatory disorders, such as corneal graft rejection and dry eye. Similarly, an increased expression of growth factors, prostaglandins, neuropeptides, and proteases has been shown in a wide array of immune disorders of the cornea and ocular surface.

Effective immune responses to foreign antigens require cells to "traffic" through tissues. Critical mediators that provide the trafficking signals to immune cells are called *chemokines* (*chemo*tactic cyto*kines*). These are small molecular-weight proteins, of which more than 50 have been identified to date; they have been classified into different subgroups based on their amino acid sequence. Although there is some overlap in the function of these cytokine species, they can also be classified functionally into those that promote neutrophil recruitment (eg, IL-8), T helper-1 (Th1) lymphocyte recruitment and activation (MIP-1 β), monocyte/macrophage recruitment (MCP-1), and eosinophil recruitment (eotaxin). As a better understanding of these critical mediators evolves, the possibility is emerging of molecularly targeting those chemokines that specifically regulate a pathologic function (eg, eotaxin, or its receptor CCR3, in allergy). To date, many chemokines have been identified as playing important roles in corneal inflammation. A brief tabulation of some important soluble mediators involved in corneal and ocular surface immune and inflammatory responses is given in Table 6-2.

Akpek EK, Gottsch JD. Immune defense at the ocular surface. *Eye.* 2003;17(8):949–956.

Zierhut M, Dana MR, Stern ME, Sullivan DA. Immunology of the lacrimal gland and ocular tear film. *Trends Immunol.* 2002;23(7):333–335.

Table 6-2 Soluble Mediators of Ocular Inflammation

Group	Example	Example of Action
Cell adhesion molecules	ICAM-1	Promotes leukocyte recruitment
Chemokines	RANTES	Directs leukocyte traffic
Clotting and fibrinolytic systems	Fibrin	Enhances leukocyte activity
Complement	C5a	Promotes leukocyte recruitment
Corneal proteases	Collagenase	Degrades protein in stromal matrix
Cytokines	Interleukin-1	Promotes leukocyte recruitment
Eicosanoids	TNF-α	Promotes inflammation and breakdown of
	Leukotriene B_4	blood–ocular barriers
Growth factors	VEGF	Promotes angiogenesis and vascular
	TGF-βs	permeability
Kinin-forming system	Bradykinin	Increases vascular permeability
Leukocyte oxidants	Hydrogen peroxide	Oxidizes free radicals
Neuropeptides	Substance P	Promotes inflammation and pain
	α-MSH	Suppresses inflammation and T-cell responses
Vasoactive amines	Histamine	Dilates blood vessels

Hypersensitivity Reactions of the Ocular Surface

Hypersensitivity responses typically involve normal adaptive protective mechanisms that, because of increased antigenic exposure and/or heightened immune status, become so amplified that they lead to pathologic changes. Hypersensitivity reactions are classified into several basic mechanisms grouped as types I–V (type V is not discussed in this Section; see BCSC Section 9, *Intraocular Inflammation and Uveitis*). Most clinically relevant ophthalmic diseases are probably not due exclusively to a single type of hypersensitivity reaction. Nevertheless, a basic understanding of the mechanisms of hypersensitivity, as shown in Figure 6-3, can be useful in explaining the pathogenesis of several immune-mediated disorders of the cornea and ocular surface (Table 6-3). In the following sections,

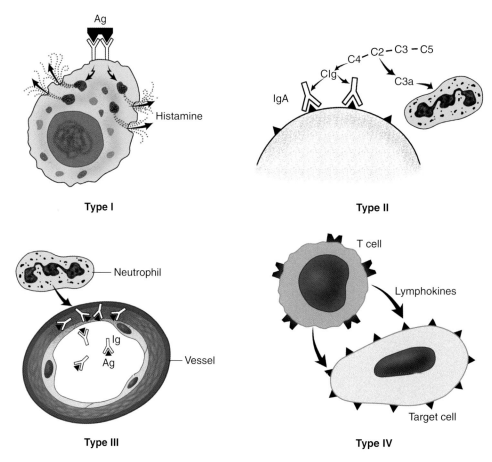

Figure 6-3 Classifications of hypersensitivity reactions. Type I anaphylactic reactions are mediated by IgE antibodies bound to mast cells. Type II cytolytic or cytotoxic reactions are mediated by immunoglobulins against membrane antigens that activate complement. Type III immune-complex reactions occur when antigen–antibody complexes accumulate in a tissue and activate the complement cascade to attract leukocytes. Type IV delayed hypersensitivity immune reactions are mediated by T cells that release lymphokines to attract macrophages. *(Illustration by Christine Gralapp.)*

Table 6-3 Hypersensitivity Reactions and Selected Ocular Disease

Type	Ocular Disease
I	Allergic conjunctivitis
II	Ocular cicatricial pemphigoid
III	Scleritis
	Stevens-Johnson syndrome
IV	Contact dermatitis
	Phlyctenulosis
	Corneal graft rejection

each type of hypersensitivity response is put in the context of common corneal and ocular surface inflammatory pathologies. See BCSC Section 9, *Intraocular Inflammation and Uveitis,* for a full discussion of basic immunopathogenic mechanisms.

Anaphylactic or Atopic Reactions (Type I)

The pathogenesis of allergic reactions begins with APCs interacting with CD4$^+$ T helper-2 (Th2) cells that release interleukin-4 (IL-4) and other Th2 cytokines. In type I reactions, antigens combine with IgE antibodies bound to receptors on mast cells, resulting in the release of histamine and other preformed mediators, as well as a new synthesis of prostaglandins and leukotrienes (Table 6-4).

Atopy is associated with an inherited mutation in the receptor for IL-4 that is associated with enhanced IgE production by B cells and increased numbers of T helper cells. Other features associated with atopy are decreased levels of putative suppressor (or regulatory) T cells. These cells play a role in down-modulating immune responses to common

Table 6-4 Selected Soluble Mediators Released by Mast Cells and Eosinophils

Substance	Action
Released by mast cells	
Histamine	Vasodilation and increased capillary permeability
Heparin	Anticoagulation
Tryptase	Complement activation
Eosinophil chemotactic factor	Eosinophil chemotaxis
Neutrophil chemotactic factor	Neutrophil chemotaxis
Platelet-activating factor	Vasodilation and increased capillary permeability
Prostaglandins (PGD$_2$)	Vasodilation
Leukotrienes (LTB$_4$)	Leukocyte chemotaxis
Released by eosinophils	
Major basic protein	Mast cell degranulation
Cationic protein	Epithelial cytotoxicity
Peroxidase	Epithelial cytotoxicity
Eotaxin	Eosinophil chemotaxis
Platelet-activating factor	Vasodilation and increased capillary permeability
Leukotrienes (LTC$_4$)	Increased capillary permeability
Slow-reacting substance of anaphylaxis	Increased capillary permeability

antigens in the environment. Treatment strategies include the use of topical mast-cell in-hibitors, antihistamines, vasoconstrictors, cyclooxygenase inhibitors, and, occasionally, systemic corticosteroids in severe disease.

Cytotoxic Hypersensitivity (Type II)

A type II reaction involves interaction of immunoglobulins with foreign or autoantigens closely associated with cell membranes. Cell lysis may result from complement activation (and development of membrane attack complexes) and from recruitment of leukocytes, including neutrophils, lymphocytes, and macrophages. So-called killer lymphocytes may be involved in antibody-dependent, cell-mediated cytotoxicity (ADCC). In general, most investigators maintain that type II responses do not play a major role in corneal and ocu-lar surface morbidities. However, one disease in which type II responses are likely to be relevant is ocular cicatricial pemphigoid (discussed in Chapter 7). In this condition, sev-eral antigens along the conjunctival basement membrane zone can react with IgG or IgA antibodies. Treatment of type II responses usually requires systemic immunosuppression or immune modulation.

Immune-Complex Reactions (Type III)

A type III reaction results from the deposition of antigen–antibody (immune) complexes in tissue with secondary complement and effector cell activation and recruitment. Im-mune complexes can fix complement that attracts polymorphonuclear leukocytes. The typical *Arthus reaction* involves vasculitis from immune-complex deposition in small blood vessels. Similarly, the pathophysiology of scleritis and ocular syndromes second-ary to vasculitis (eg, peripheral ulcerative keratitis) has been related to immune-complex deposition. However, a basic understanding of mechanisms is still deficient, because the inciting factors remain largely unknown.

Delayed Hypersensitivity (Type IV)

Type IV, or cell-mediated, immunity involves sensitized CD4+ Th1 lymphocytes. Anti-gens interact with receptors on the surface of T lymphocytes, resulting in the release of lymphokines. Contact dermatitis is a common delayed hypersensitivity response caused by lipid-soluble, low-molecular-weight haptens. These penetrate the skin and gain entry into the epidermal layer, where they may be picked up by Langerhans APCs. These cells can then process the antigen and prime (sensitize) naive T cells by coexpressing the pro-cessed antigen with the MHC class II antigens to them. A similar process is thought to be responsible for corneal graft rejection.

Patterns of Immune-Mediated Ocular Disease

Conjunctiva

The conjunctiva is the part of the MALT that involves many mucosal tissues in the body, including the lacrimal gland. Humoral immunity in the conjunctiva largely involves IgA, and cellular immunity is dominated by CD4+ T cells. Serosal mast cells that contain neutral proteases are normally present in the conjunctiva, and mucosal mast cells with granules containing only tryptase are increased in the conjunctiva of atopic patients. Mast-cell degranulation produces conjunctival redness, chemosis, mucus discharge, and itching.

Cornea

The normal cornea can have neither an acute allergic reaction (as it contains no mast cells) nor a typical Arthus reaction (as there are no blood vessels). However, the cornea does participate in immune reactions by way of humoral and cellular immune elements that enter the periphery from the limbal blood vessels. These anatomical features may explain why so many immune-mediated disorders of the cornea occur primarily in the corneal periphery and limbus. Alternatively, ingress of leukocytes through the ciliary body/iris root and ingress of plasma proteins through breakdown of the blood–ocular barrier (as occurs in uveitis syndromes) are other internal pathways for immune effectors to the cornea.

The cornea can act as an immunologic blotter, soaking up antigens from the ocular surface. This phenomenon was first described by Wessely in 1911, when foreign antigen was injected into the cornea of a previously sensitized animal and a ring-shaped infiltrate formed in the corneal stroma concentric to the injection site, much like an antigen–antibody complex in an immunodiffusion test. Still called a *Wessely immune ring,* this infiltrate contains complement factors and/or neutrophils. Circulating antibodies are not required if sufficient local antibody production is stimulated by antigens deposited in the cornea. The antigen may be a drug, as in the peripheral corneal infiltrates associated with a neomycin reaction; a foreign body; or an unknown substance, as in the corneal infiltrates that can occur in contact lens wearers. Wessely rings may persist in corneas traumatized with a foreign body for some time, even after the foreign body is removed.

Sclera

Nearly one half of patients with scleritis have an associated systemic immunologic or connective tissue disease. Immune-complex deposition, granulomatous inflammation, and occlusive vasculitis have been implicated in the pathogenesis of scleral inflammation.

Diagnostic Approach to Immune-Mediated Ocular Disorders

Many, but not all, immune-mediated ocular disorders are secondary to a systemic disease. As with most medical problems, diagnostic investigations need to begin with a complete history, including a review of systems, and a general physical examination, as indicated. Some of the more common laboratory diagnostic tests that are selected to further narrow the differential diagnosis are listed in Table 6-5. In general, except for rheumatoid arthritis, which has a strong predilection for scleral and corneal involvement, the workup for patients with immune-mediated corneal disease in whom an underlying disease is suspected is quite similar to that for the uveitis patient. Diagnosing systemic vasculitis in a patient presenting with ocular inflammation with tests, including ANCA (see Table 6-5), may have a profound effect in instituting early life-saving therapy.

Table 6-5 Common Laboratory Tests for Suspected Systemic Immune-Mediated Disease

Test	Assay
Rheumatoid factor (RF)	Autoantibody (IgG, IgA, or IgM) against epitopes of the Fc portion of IgG
Antinuclear antibody (ANA)	Antibodies against cell nuclear antigens (DNA-histone, double-stranded DNA, single-stranded DNA, histone, RNA, nuclear ribonucleoprotein, etc)
Antineutrophil cytoplasmic antibodies (ANCA)	c-ANCA generally sensitive for Wegener granulomatosis p-ANCA generally indicative of small-vessel vasculitis (microscopic angiitis), either generalized or related to inflammatory bowel disease, especially ulcerative colitis
Urinalysis	Rule out active nephritis by checking for casts, red blood cells, etc
Complete blood count	Abnormally high or low blood counts are indicative of systemic disease
Erythrocyte sedimentation rate or C-reactive protein	High values indicate systemic inflammation

See BCSC Section 9, *Intraocular Inflammation and Uveitis,* for the diagnostic workup of patients with uveitis. Table 6-6 provides the clinical interpretation of ocular surface cytology for immune-mediated keratoconjunctivitis. Finally, it should be noted that corneal and ocular surface morbidities may result from underlying autoimmune disease. Generally, when a systemic disease is suspected, it is also advisable to coordinate care with an internist or rheumatologist, especially if systemic immune suppression is contemplated.

Niederkorn JY, Kaplan HJ, eds. *Immune Response and the Eye.* 2nd, rev ed. Basel: Karger AG; 2007.

Pflugfelder SC, Beuerman RW, Stern ME. *Dry Eye and Ocular Surface Disorders.* New York: Informa Healthcare; 2004.

Zierhut M, Rammensee H-G, Streilein JW. *Antigen-Presenting Cells and the Eye.* New York: Informa Healthcare; 2007.

Zierhut M, Stern ME, Sullivan DA. *Immunology of the Lacrimal Gland, Tear Film and Ocular Surface.* New York: Informa Healthcare; 2005.

Table 6-6 Clinical Interpretation of Ocular Surface Cytology for Immune-Mediated Keratoconjunctivitis

Finding	Examples
Significant neutrophils	Severe acute/subacute ocular surface inflammation
Predominance of lymphocytes and monocytes	Chronic toxic or allergic conjunctivitis
Eosinophils	Acute allergic conjunctivitis
Basophils or mast cells	Vernal conjunctivitis
Keratinized epithelial cells	Ocular cicatricial pemphigoid Stevens-Johnson syndrome Severe keratoconjunctivitis sicca Graft-vs-host disease

CHAPTER 7

Clinical Approach to Immune-Related Disorders of the External Eye

Immune-Mediated Diseases of the Eyelid

Contact Dermatoblepharitis

PATHOGENESIS Topical ophthalmic medications, cosmetics, and environmental substances can occasionally trigger a local allergic reaction. This may occur acutely as an anaphylactic reaction, which results from a type I IgE-mediated hypersensitivity reaction, or it may begin 24–72 hours after exposure to the sensitizing agent, as with contact blepharoconjunctivitis, a type IV T-cell–mediated, or delayed, hypersensitivity reaction.

CLINICAL PRESENTATION Type I immediate hypersensitivity reactions typically occur within minutes after exposure to an allergen. These reactions are associated with itching, eyelid erythema and swelling, and conjunctival redness and chemosis (Fig 7-1). In rare cases, patients may develop signs of systemic anaphylaxis. Ocular anaphylactic reactions can follow instillation of topical anesthetics and antibiotics such as bacitracin, cephalosporins, penicillin, sulfacetamide, and tetracycline but often resolve spontaneously.

Delayed, type IV, hypersensitivity reactions to medications usually begin 24–72 hours following instillation of a topical agent. Patients are often sensitized by previous exposure to the offending drug or preservative. An acute eczema with erythema, leathery thickening, and scaling of the eyelid develops (Fig 7-2). Sequelae of chronic contact blepharoconjunctivitis include hyperpigmentation, dermal scarring, and lower eyelid ectropion. A papillary conjunctivitis and a mucoid or mucopurulent discharge may develop. Punctate epithelial erosions may be noted on the inferior cornea. Medications that are commonly associated with contact blepharoconjunctivitis include

- cycloplegics such as atropine and homatropine
- aminoglycosides such as neomycin, gentamicin, and tobramycin
- antiviral agents such as idoxuridine and trifluridine
- preservatives such as thimerosal and ethylenediaminetetraacetic acid (EDTA)

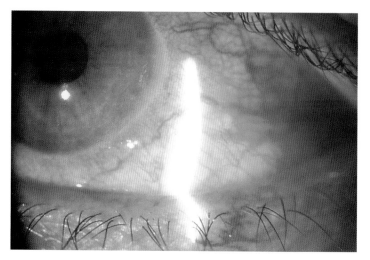

Figure 7-1 Anaphylactic allergic reaction to topical ophthalmic medication with acute conjunctival hyperemia and chemosis.

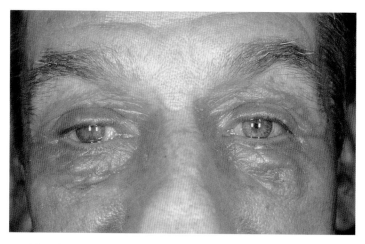

Figure 7-2 Allergic contact dermatitis secondary to topical ophthalmic medication.

MANAGEMENT Treatment of hypersensitivity reactions requires identifying and discontinuing the offending agent. Usually, the history provides the necessary clue to determine the offending agent, but sometimes a "rechallenge" is necessary to confirm a suspicion. Rechallenges should never be done in patients with a known systemic allergy to a drug.

Initial management of type I hypersensitivity reactions includes allergen avoidance or discontinuation. Adjunctive therapy may involve the use of cold compresses, artificial lubricants, topical antihistamines, mast-cell stabilizers, and nonsteroidal anti-inflammatory agents (NSAIDs) in the case of pain. Topical vasoconstrictors, either alone or in combination with antihistamines, may provide acute symptomatic relief but should not be used chronically. Delayed hypersensitivity reactions are also treated with allergen withdrawal. In severe cases, a brief (several-day) course of mild topical corticosteroids applied to the eyelids and periocular skin may speed resolution of eyelid and conjunctival inflammation.

Atopic Dermatitis

PATHOGENESIS Atopic dermatitis is a chronic condition in genetically susceptible individuals that usually begins in infancy or childhood and may or may not involve the external eye. The pathogenesis of atopic dermatitis involves increased IgE hypersensitivity, increased histamine release from mast cells and basophils, and impaired cell-mediated immunity.

CLINICAL PRESENTATION Diagnostic criteria for atopic dermatitis include pruritus, lesions on the eyelid and other sites (eg, joint flexures in adolescents and adults, face and extensor surfaces in infants and young children), and a personal or family history of other atopic disorders, such as asthma, allergic rhinitis, nasal polyps, and aspirin hypersensitivity. There is an increased incidence of ectatic corneal diseases such as keratoconus and pellucid marginal degeneration as well as an increased incidence of staphylococcal and herpes simplex infections. Other ocular findings may include periorbital darkening, exaggerated eyelid folds, ectropion, and chronic conjunctivitis. The appearance of the skin lesions varies depending on the age of the patient. Infants typically have an erythematous rash; children tend to have eczematoid dermatitis with secondary lichenification from scratching; and adults have scaly patches with thickened and wrinkled dry skin.

MANAGEMENT Allergens in the environment and in foods should be minimized whenever possible. In general, the services of an allergist should be sought. Moisturizing lotions and petrolatum gels can be useful for skin hydration. Acute lesions can be controlled with a topical corticosteroid cream or ointment (clobetasone butyrate 0.05%), but chronic use of such medications should be strongly discouraged to avoid skin thinning. Topical tacrolimus is also effective and has fewer side effects. Oral antipruritic agents such as antihistamines and mast-cell stabilizers can alleviate itching but may exacerbate dry eye with their anticholinergic activity.

Ashcroft DM, Dimmock P, Garside R, Stein K, Williams HC. Efficacy and tolerability of topical pimecrolimus and tacrolimus in the treatment of atopic dermatitis: meta-analysis of randomised controlled trials. *BMJ.* 2005;330(7490):516.

Immune-Mediated Disorders of the Conjunctiva

Hay Fever Conjunctivitis and Perennial Allergic Conjunctivitis

PATHOGENESIS Hay fever (seasonal) and perennial allergic conjunctivitis are largely IgE-mediated immediate hypersensitivity reactions. The allergen is typically airborne. It enters the tear film and comes into contact with conjunctival mast cells that bear allergen-specific IgE antibodies. Degranulation of mast cells releases histamine and a variety of other inflammatory mediators that promote vasodilation, edema, and recruitment of other inflammatory cells such as eosinophils. The activation and degranulation of mast cells in a presensitized individual can be triggered within minutes of allergen exposure.

CLINICAL PRESENTATION   Patients with hay fever conjunctivitis often suffer from other atopic conditions, such as allergic rhinitis or asthma. Symptoms develop rapidly after exposure to the allergen and consist of itching, eyelid swelling, conjunctival hyperemia, chemosis, and mucoid discharge. Intense itching is a hallmark symptom. Attacks are usually short-lived and episodic. Contributing factors, including contact lenses and dry eye, should be identified, as these can play an important role in facilitating allergen contact with the ocular surface.

LABORATORY EVALUATION   The diagnosis of hay fever conjunctivitis is generally made clinically, although conjunctival scraping can be performed in order to observe the characteristic eosinophils, which are not normally present on the ocular surface (see Chapter 6). Challenge testing with a panel of allergens can be performed.

MANAGEMENT   Efforts should first be directed at avoidance or abatement of allergen exposure. Thorough cleaning (or changing) of unclean or old carpets, linens, and bedding can be effective in removing accumulated allergens such as animal dander and house dust mites. Simple measures such as wearing glasses or goggles can also serve as physical barriers. Treatment should be based on the severity of patient symptoms and consists of one or more of the following:

Supportive
- cold compresses
- artificial tears

Topical
- topical antihistamines and mast-cell stabilizers
- topical NSAIDs
- judicious, selective use of topical corticosteroids
- topical vasoconstrictors

Systemic
- Systemic antihistamines may be effective for the short term and may be associated with increased dry eye.

Artificial tears are beneficial in diluting and flushing away allergens and other inflammatory mediators present on the ocular surface. Topical vasoconstrictors, alone or in combination with antihistamines, may provide acute symptomatic relief. However, their use for more than 5–7 consecutive days may predispose to compensatory chronic vascular dilation and rebound conjunctival hyperemia. Topical mast-cell stabilizing agents such as cromolyn sodium and lodoxamide tromethamine may be useful for treating seasonal allergic conjunctivitis, but their primary role is prophylactic. Treatment effects usually require continued use over 7 or more days, and hence these agents are generally ineffective in the acute phase of hay fever conjunctivitis. Topical cyclosporine and oral antihistamines may provide symptomatic relief in some patients. Hyposensitization injections (immunotherapy) can be beneficial if the offending allergen has been identified. Certain topical

NSAIDs have been approved by the Food and Drug Administration for use in ocular atopy, but their efficacy is highly variable. Reports of corneal perforations with the use of NSAIDs, especially the generic forms, suggest the need for careful monitoring. Refills should be limited, and follow-up appointments need to be maintained. Topical corticosteroids are very effective in ocular allergy, but they should be used with caution except in very severe cases due to their toxicity. For associated dermatitis, topical tacrolimus appears to be a useful course of treatment.

Vernal Keratoconjunctivitis

PATHOGENESIS   Usually a seasonally recurring, bilateral inflammation of the cornea and conjunctiva, *vernal* (springtime) *keratoconjunctivitis (VKC)* occurs predominantly in male children, who frequently, but not invariably, have a personal or family history of atopy. The disease may persist year-round in tropical climates. The immunopathogenesis appears to involve both types I and IV hypersensitivity reactions. The conjunctival inflammatory infiltrate in VKC consists of eosinophils, lymphocytes, plasma cells, and monocytes.

> Abu El-Asrar AM, Al-Mansouri S, Tabbara KF, Missotten L, Geboes K. Immunopathogenesis of conjunctival remodelling in vernal keratoconjunctivitis. *Eye.* 2006;20(1):71–79.
> Baudouin C, Liang H, Bremond-Gignac D, et al. CCR 4 and CCR 5 expression in conjunctival specimens as differential markers of T(H)1/ T(H)2 in ocular surface disorders. *J Allergy Clin Immunol.* 2005;116(3):614–619.
> Ono S, Abelson M. Allergic conjunctivitis: update on pathophysiology and prospects for future treatment. *J Allergy Clin Immunol.* 2005;115(1):118–122.

CLINICAL PRESENTATION   Symptoms consist of itching, blepharospasm, photophobia, blurred vision, and copious mucoid discharge. Clinically, 2 forms of VKC may be seen: palpebral and limbal.

The inflammation in *palpebral VKC* is located predominantly on the palpebral conjunctiva, where a diffuse papillary hypertrophy develops, usually more prominently on the upper rather than the lower region. Bulbar conjunctival hyperemia and chemosis may also occur. In more severe cases, giant papillae resembling cobblestones may develop on the upper tarsus (Fig 7-3).

Limbal VKC may develop alone or in association with palpebral VKC. It occurs predominantly in patients of African or Asian descent and is also more prevalent in hotter climates. The limbus has a thickened, gelatinous appearance, with scattered opalescent mounds and vascular injection. *Horner-Trantas dots,* whitish dots that represent macroaggregates of degenerated eosinophils and epithelial cells, may be observed in the hypertrophied limbus of patients with limbal VKC (Fig 7-4).

Several types of corneal changes associated with upper tarsal lesions may also develop in VKC. Punctate epithelial erosions in the superior and central cornea are frequently observed. Pannus occurs most commonly in the superior cornea, but occasionally 360° corneal vascularization may develop. Noninfectious epithelial ulcers with an oval or shieldlike shape (the so-called shield ulcer) with underlying stromal opacification may develop in the superior or central cornea (Fig 7-5). An association between VKC and keratoconus has been reported.

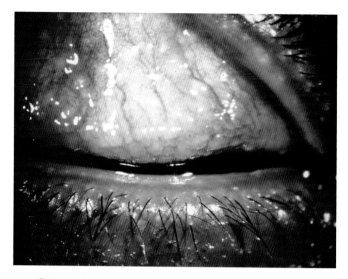

Figure 7-3 Palpebral vernal keratoconjunctivitis. *(Courtesy of James J. Reidy, MD.)*

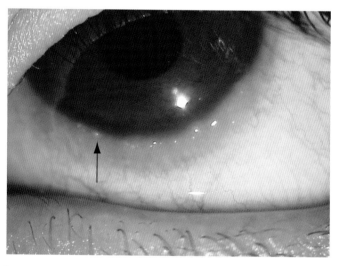

Figure 7-4 Limbal vernal keratoconjunctivitis. Note the Horner-Trantas dots *(arrow).* *(Courtesy of Charles S. Bouchard, MD.)*

MANAGEMENT Therapy should be based on the severity of the patient's symptoms and of the ocular surface disease. Mild cases may be successfully managed with topical anti-histamines. Climatotherapy, such as the use of home air-conditioning or relocation to a cooler environment, can promote improvement of the condition. Patients with mild to moderate disease may respond to topical mast-cell stabilizers. In patients with seasonal exacerbations, these drops should be started at least 2 weeks prior to the usual time of symptomatic onset. Patients with year-round disease can be maintained chronically on mast-cell stabilizer drops.

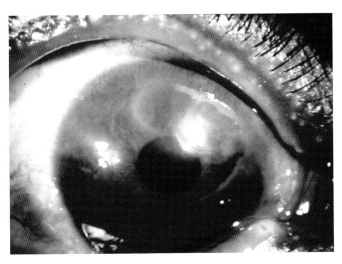

Figure 7-5 Shield ulcer in vernal keratoconjunctivitis. *(Courtesy of James J. Reidy, MD.)*

Severe cases may require the use of topical corticosteroids or topical immunomodulatory agents such as cyclosporine. Both have been shown to be effective in reducing inflammation and symptoms. Because of the likelihood that patients will develop corticosteroid-related complications from chronic administration, however, these drugs should be reserved for exacerbations with moderate to severe discomfort and/or decreased visual acuity. During these exacerbations, intermittent (pulse) therapy is very effective: topical corticosteroids are used at relatively high frequency (eg, every 2 hours) for 5–7 days and then rapidly tapered. Because of the propensity of particles of suspended corticosteroid (such as prednisolone acetate) to lodge between papillae, the use of less potent but soluble corticosteroids such as dexamethasone phosphate is preferred. Corticosteroids should be discontinued between attacks. To discourage indiscriminate use for relief of mild symptoms, the patient and family must be thoroughly informed of the potential dangers of chronic topical corticosteroid therapy. Use of systemic anti-inflammatory therapy for severe VKC has been reported, but this should be reserved for very severe cases.

Cooperative patients can be offered an alternative to topical delivery that avoids the problem of continuing self-medication: supratarsal injection of corticosteroid. The supratarsal subconjunctival space is located superior to the upper border of the superior tarsus and is most easily reached by everting the upper eyelid. This space is free of the subepithelial adhesions that bind the superior palpebral conjunctiva to the tarsal plate. After the upper eyelid is everted and the supratarsal conjunctiva has been anesthetized, supratarsal injection of 0.5–1.0 mL of either a relatively short-acting corticosteroid such as dexamethasone phosphate (4 mg/mL) or a longer-acting corticosteroid such as triamcinolone acetonide (40 mg/mL) can be performed. Monitoring of intraocular pressure is mandatory, as corticosteroid-induced pressure spikes are possible.

Topical cyclosporine applied 2–4 times daily can also be used to treat refractory cases of VKC. There are few data on exact dosing in VKC; success has been reported with 2% preparations in VKC treatment, but significantly lower concentrations (0.05%) have not been shown to be as effective. Reported side effects include punctate epithelial keratopathy and ocular surface irritation. Systemic absorption after topical instillation is minimal, but experience with this agent is limited; therefore, its use in VKC should probably be reserved for the most severe cases.

Daniell M, Constantinou M, Vu HT, Taylor HR. Randomised controlled trial of topical ciclosporin A in steroid dependent allergic conjunctivitis. *Br J Ophthalmol.* 2006;90(4): 461–464.

Heidemann DG. Atopic and vernal keratoconjunctivitis. *Focal Points: Clinical Modules for Ophthalmologists.* San Francisco: American Academy of Ophthalmology; 2001, module 1.

Tatlipinar S, Akpek EK. Topical ciclosporin in the treatment of ocular surface disorders. *Br J Ophthalmol.* 2005;89(10):1363–1367.

Atopic Keratoconjunctivitis

PATHOGENESIS   Keratoconjunctivitis may occur in patients with a history of atopic dermatitis. Approximately one third of patients with this condition develop one or more manifestations of *atopic keratoconjunctivitis (AKC).* Atopic individuals show signs of type I immediate hypersensitivity responses with seasonal variation but also have depressed systemic cell-mediated immunity. As a consequence of this altered immunity, they are susceptible to herpes simplex virus keratitis and to colonization of the eyelids with *Staphylococcus aureus.* Complications related to this predisposition to infection may contribute to, or compound, the primary immunopathogenic manifestations. AKC is primarily a type IV reaction; therefore, the use of mast-cell therapy may not be effective.

CLINICAL PRESENTATION   The ocular findings are similar to those of VKC, with the following differences:

- Patients with AKC frequently have disease year-round; seasonal exacerbation is minimal.
- Patients with AKC are older.
- The papillae are more apt to be small or medium-sized rather than giant.
- The papillae occur in the upper and lower palpebral conjunctiva.
- Milky conjunctival edema, with variable subepithelial fibrosis, is often present (Fig 7-6).
- Extensive corneal vascularization and opacification secondary to chronic epithelial disease (likely due to some degree of limbal stem cell dysfunction) can occur (Fig 7-7).
- Eosinophils seen in conjunctival cytology are less numerous and are less often degranulated.
- Conjunctival scarring often occurs and is sometimes so extensive as to produce symblepharon formation.
- Characteristic posterior subcapsular and/or multifaceted or shield-shaped anterior subcapsular lens opacities may occasionally develop.

MANAGEMENT   Treatment of AKC involves allergen avoidance and the use of pharmacotherapeutic agents similar to those used in the treatment of VKC. Cold compresses may

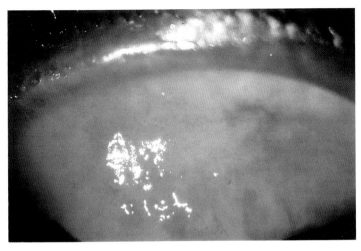

Figure 7-6 Atopic keratoconjunctivitis demonstrating small papillae, edema, and subepithelial fibrosis.

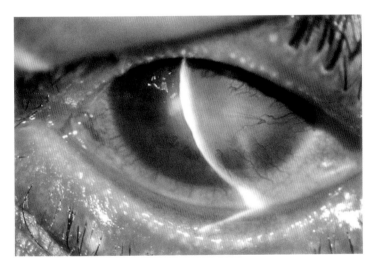

Figure 7-7 Severe corneal vascularization and scarring with atopic keratoconjunctivitis.

also be of benefit. In addition, patients should be carefully monitored for infectious disease complications that may warrant specific therapy, such as secondary staphylococcal infections. In the minority of patients in whom the disease takes a very aggressive and destructive course, local pharmacotherapies often fail to control the pathologic process. In these severe cases, the indications for systemic therapy would include chronic ocular surface inflammation unresponsive to topical treatment, discomfort, progressive cicatrization, and peripheral ulcerative keratopathy. Systemic immune suppression (eg, by oral cyclosporine 2.0–2.5 mg/kg daily) should be monitored with an internist. Systemic treatment of AKC may be beneficial in suppressing the IL-2 response, which promotes lymphocyte proliferation. Topical therapy with tacrolimus has been helpful for the dermatitis.

Ashcroft DM, Dimmock P, Garside R, Stein K, Williams HC. Efficacy and tolerability of topical pimecrolimus and tacrolimus in the treatment of atopic dermatitis: meta-analysis of randomised controlled trials. *BMJ.* 2005;330(7490):516.

Ligneous Conjunctivitis

PATHOGENESIS Ligneous conjunctivitis is a rare chronic disorder characterized by the formation of firm ("woody"), yellowish fibrinous pseudomembranes on the conjunctival surface (Fig 7-8). These membranes are composed of an admixture of fibrin, fibrin-bound tissue plasminogen activator (tPA), epithelial cells, and mixed inflammatory cells that adhere to the conjunctival surface. Latent and activated forms of matrix metalloproteinase-9 (MMP-9) have also been reported. The cause of ligneous conjunctivitis has recently been linked to severe deficiency in type 1 plasminogen, with hypofibrinolysis as the primary defect. More than 12% of patients have severe hypoplasminogenemia. The genetic defect in the plasminogen gene (PLG) is located at chromosome 6q26.

Schuster V, Hügle B, Tefs K. Plasminogen deficiency. *J Thromb Haemost.* 2007;5(12):2315–2322.

Thachil J, Reeves G, Kaye S. Ligneous conjunctivitis with plasminogen deficiency. *Br J Haematol.* 2009;145(3):269.

Watts P, Suresh P, Mezer E, et al. Effective treatment of ligneous conjunctivitis with topical plasminogen. *Am J Ophthalmol.* 2002;133(4):451–455.

CLINICAL PRESENTATION Ligneous conjunctivitis can affect all ages. Patients present with symptoms of ocular irritation and foreign-body sensation. The cardinal finding consists of yellowish, platelike masses that overlie one or more of the palpebral surfaces and are readily visible with eversion of the eyelid (see Fig 7-8). Ligneous conjunctivitis is generally bilateral and can recur after excision.

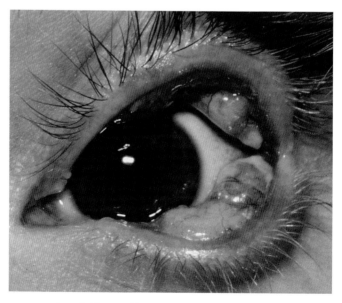

Figure 7-8 Ligneous conjunctivitis: papillary white-red lesions of firm consistency in both eyelids of the left eye. *(Reproduced with permission from Mission for Vision, 2005. Available at http://www.missionfor visionusa.org/anatomy/2006/03/what-is-ligneous-conjunctivitis.html.)*

MANAGEMENT Cultures can be taken at initial diagnosis to exclude a bacterial pseudomembranous or membranous conjunctivitis. Surgical excision with or without adjunctive cryotherapy has been advocated. However, recurrences are frequent, and patients and their families should be informed about this possibility. Medical therapy by administration of purified plasminogen, fresh frozen plasma, heparin, corticosteroids, or azathioprine has been reported. Use of amniotic membrane has also been reported. No single treatment has been shown to be consistently effective or superior. Many cases of ligneous conjunctivitis eventually resolve spontaneously after several months to a few years.

Barabino S, Rolando M. Amniotic membrane transplantation in a case of ligneous conjunctivitis. *Am J Ophthalmol.* 2004;137(4):752–753.

Heidemann DG, Williams GA, Hartzer M, Ohanian A, Citron ME. Treatment of ligneous conjunctivitis with topical plasmin and topical plasminogen. *Cornea.* 2003;22(8):760–762.

Schuster V, Seregard S. Ligneous conjunctivitis. *Surv Ophthalmol.* 2003;48(4):369–388.

Contact Lens–Induced Conjunctivitis

PATHOGENESIS The pathogenesis of contact lens–induced conjunctivitis is not fully understood and may be multifactorial (allergic, dry eye, infectious). Patients with ocular prostheses and exposed monofilament sutures have shown reactions similar to those seen in patients with contact lens–induced conjunctivitis, suggesting that an immune-related response may result from a variety of insults, including repeated mechanical trauma of the superior tarsus by the sharp or rough surface of a contact lens, prosthesis, or suture. A hypersensitivity reaction to the contact lens polymer itself (or to antigens or other foreign material adhering to it) has also been postulated but not formally demonstrated. Although most patients who develop contact lens–induced conjunctivitis do not have clinically significant dry eye, the latter condition is present in a significant minority (particularly because contact lenses diminish blinking and hence increase evaporative loss of tears) and may facilitate adhesion of antigens to the surface epithelium.

The histologic findings in contact lens–induced conjunctivitis are similar to those observed in VKC. An abnormal accumulation of mast cells, basophils, and eosinophils is noted in the epithelium and/or the substantia propria of the superior tarsus. Abnormally elevated concentrations of immunoglobulins, specifically IgE, IgG, and IgM, and complement components have been found in the tears of affected patients. These findings suggest a combined mechanical and immune-mediated pathophysiology for the condition. Surface deposits on worn contact lenses are a known risk factor for the development and persistence of contact lens–induced conjunctivitis.

CLINICAL PRESENTATION Some patients who wear contact lenses, particularly extended-wear soft contact lenses, may develop inflammatory symptoms, including redness, itching, and mucoid discharge. One or more of the following signs may be seen during biomicroscopic examination of contact lens wearers with these symptoms:

- mild papillary reaction (papillae <0.3 mm in diameter) on the superior tarsal conjunctiva
- punctate epithelial erosions
- peripheral corneal infiltrates and vascularization

At the more severe end of the spectrum of contact lens–related inflammation is the entity known as *giant papillary conjunctivitis (GPC)*. GPC tends to develop earlier and more frequently in soft contact lens wearers than in hard contact lens wearers and may be recurrent. It may also be induced by other irritants, such as loose sutures or prosthetics. Symptoms include contact lens intolerance, itching, excessive mucus discharge, blurred vision from mucus coating of the contact lens, contact lens decentration, and conjunctival redness. In rare instances, bloody tears and ptosis secondary to inflammation of the superior tarsal conjunctiva may be observed.

The signs of GPC consist of hyperemia, thickening, and abnormally large papillae (diameter >0.3 mm) on the superior tarsal conjunctiva (Fig 7-9) due to disruption of anchoring septae. The morphologic appearance of the superior tarsal papillae may be variable in GPC. In some cases, the giant papillae cover the entire central tarsus from the posterior eyelid margin to the upper border of the tarsal plate; involvement in other cases may be less extensive. Occasionally, only a few giant papillae appear, surrounded by smaller papillae. Long-standing or involuted giant papillae on the superior tarsus can resemble follicles.

The symptoms of GPC generally resolve when contact lens wear is discontinued. The tarsal conjunctival hyperemia and thickening may resolve in several weeks, but papillae or dome-shaped scars on the superior tarsus can persist for months to years.

MANAGEMENT   The goals of GPC treatment are to resolve the symptoms and enable patients to continue wearing contact lenses, if possible. Therapeutic strategies include discarding the offending contact lenses, refitting the patient, improving lens hygiene, and treating conjunctival inflammation with drugs. Simply fitting the patient with new contact lenses frequently resolves GPC. Daily-wear rather than extended-wear soft contact lenses should be encouraged, although GPC can also occur with daily-wear or even daily disposable contact lenses. Still, periodic planned replacement of soft contact lenses is often

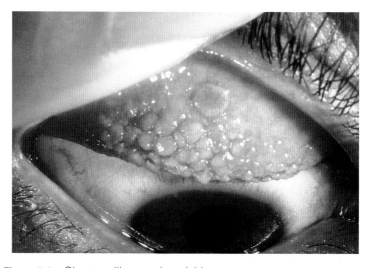

Figure 7-9   Giant papillary conjunctivitis. *(Courtesy of Kirk R. Wilhelmus, MD.)*

beneficial and can easily be done by switching the patient to disposable contact lenses that are used for daily wear and discarded every day or every 2 weeks. Reducing daily-wear time and instituting a 1-month contact lens holiday are other measures that can be helpful in many cases.

Patients should be encouraged to clean their soft contact lenses daily using agents free of preservatives, particularly thimerosal, and to rinse and store lenses in appropriate lens storage solutions. Disinfection of contact lenses with a hydrogen peroxide system appears to be the method best tolerated by the inflamed conjunctiva. Regular enzymatic treatment of contact lenses may remove inciting contact lens deposits. It is also important to store contact lenses in cases that are routinely cleaned or sterilized; periodic replacement of contact lens cases is encouraged.

If GPC persists, consideration should be given to changing the lens to a different polymer or to daily disposable lenses. Some patients do better with low-water-content lenses. Nevertheless, some patients continue to suffer from GPC as a result of soft contact lens wear despite these measures. In these cases, consideration can be given to fitting the patient with rigid gas-permeable (RGP) contact lenses, which are associated with a lower incidence of GPC. It should be noted that some patients have recurrences of GPC in spite of aggressive lens management and even RGP lens wear; these patients should be counseled about alternatives to contact lens wear.

Pharmacologic therapy can be helpful in managing patients with GPC. Many practitioners recommend discontinuing lens wear for several (2–3) weeks while treatment is initiated. Mast-cell stabilizers such as cromolyn sodium have been reported to improve early, mild GPC but have not been successful in advanced, severe cases. However, once advanced cases of GPC have been brought under control, maintenance therapy with topical mast-cell inhibitors may prevent further exacerbations. Topical corticosteroids, although effective in GPC, generally have a limited role because of their potential side effects. If used, they should be discontinued after a short period.

Elhers WH, Donshik PC. Giant papillary conjunctivitis. *Curr Opin Allergy Clin Immunol.* 2008; 8(5):445–449.

Stevens-Johnson Syndrome and Toxic Epidermal Necrolysis

PATHOGENESIS   Immune-complex deposition in the dermis and conjunctival stroma has been implicated in the pathogenesis of erythema multiforme. The most common inciting agents include drugs such as sulfonamides, anticonvulsants, salicylates, penicillin, ampicillin, and isoniazid; or infectious organisms, such as herpes simplex virus, streptococci, adenovirus, and occasionally mycoplasma.

The distinctive pathologic changes of Stevens-Johnson syndrome are subepithelial bullae and subsequent scarring. The most severe form of this condition is referred to as *toxic epidermal necrolysis (TEN).* TEN occurs more commonly in children and people with AIDS. It is characterized by keratinocyte apoptosis and epidermal necrosis with minimal inflammatory infiltrate in the dermal stroma. See Table 7-1 for a comparison of Stevens-Johnson syndrome, TEN, and other oculocutaneous immune-mediated conditions.

Table 7-1 Selected Oculocutaneous Immune-Mediated Reactions

Condition	Causes	Eye	Skin	Others
Angioedema	Drugs; foods; insect sting	Eyelid edema	Facial edema; urticaria	Cardiorespiratory distress
Cicatricial pemphigoid	Unknown	Cicatrizing conjunctivitis	Bullous eruptions	Lesions of oropharynx and genitalia
Graft-vs-host disease	Bone-marrow transplant	Dry eye; conjunctivitis	Pigmentary changes	Respiratory and gastrointestinal lesions
Stevens-Johnson syndrome	Drugs; infections	Conjunctival erosion; conjunctivitis; episcleritis	Blisters	Fever; respiratory lesions; sepsis
Toxic epidermal necrolysis	Drugs; infections	Blepharodermatitis; conjunctivitis; corneal exposure	Blisters; necrosis	Fever; respiratory and gastrointestinal lesions

Albert DM, Miller JW, Azar DT, Blodi BA. *Albert & Jakobiec's Principles and Practice of Ophthalmology.* 3rd ed. Philadelphia: Elsevier/Saunders; 2008.

CLINICAL PRESENTATION   The term *erythema multiforme* refers to an acute inflammatory vesiculobullous reaction of the skin and mucous membranes. When these hypersensitivity disorders involve only the skin, the term *erythema multiforme minor* is used; when the skin and mucous membranes are involved, the condition is known as *Stevens-Johnson syndrome,* or *erythema multiforme major,* which accounts for 20% of all patients with erythema multiforme. The incidence of Stevens-Johnson syndrome has been shown to be about 5 cases per million per year. Recent reports have suggested that patients with AIDS are at a higher risk of developing erythema multiforme, particularly patients treated for *Pneumocystis carinii* pneumonia.

Stevens-Johnson syndrome occurs most commonly in children and young adults and in females more often than males. Fever, arthralgia, malaise, and upper or lower respiratory symptoms are usually sudden in onset. Skin eruption follows within a few days with a classic "target" lesion consisting of a red center surrounded by a pale ring and then a red ring, although maculopapular or bullous lesions are also common. The mucous membranes of the eyes, mouth, and genitalia may be affected by bullous lesions with membrane or pseudomembrane formation. New lesions may appear over 4–6 weeks, with approximate 2-week cycles for each crop of lesions. The primary ocular finding is a mucopurulent conjunctivitis and episcleritis. Bullae and extensive areas of necrosis may develop (Fig 7-10). Later ocular complications are caused by cicatrization resulting in conjunctival shrinkage, keratinization, trichiasis, and tear deficiency. Patients with Stevens-Johnson syndrome are at higher risk of infection due to loss of the epithelial barrier and hence may develop severe ocular infection concurrent with the ocular surface disease. Cicatricial pemphigoid has also been reported as a rare sequela of Stevens-Johnson syndrome (see the following section).

MANAGEMENT   Management of Stevens-Johnson syndrome is mainly supportive. The mainstay of ocular therapy is lubrication with preservative-free artificial tears and ointments

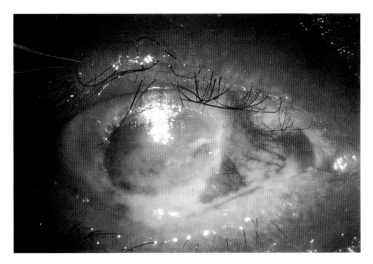

Figure 7-10 Stevens-Johnson syndrome with associated ocular disease.

and vigilant surveillance for the early manifestations of ocular infections. Topical antibiotics are occasionally used as prophylaxis. Improved supportive therapy and, in some cases, administration of systemic corticosteroids have reduced the high mortality rate previously associated with this condition. However, the role of corticosteroids remains controversial. Some authorities recommend treating severe cases (Stevens-Johnson syndrome/TEN) with oral prednisone, starting with 1 mg/kg/day. Even when used for short periods of time, however, high doses of systemic corticosteroids (primarily when administered intravenously) can be associated with serious complications: gastrointestinal hemorrhage, electrolyte imbalance, and even sudden death. Moreover, they may increase the likelihood of infection. The efficacy of topical corticosteroids for the ocular manifestations of this condition has not been established and remains controversial. On the one hand, corticosteroids may decrease surface inflammation and corneal angiogenesis; on the other hand, they may contribute to corneal thinning and infection. Hence, aggressive lubrication with drops and ointment remains the mainstay of therapy and can prevent nosocomial complications in debilitated patients.

Symblephara may form during the acute phase because the raw, necrotic palpebral and bulbar conjunctival surfaces can adhere to one another (Fig 7-11). Some authors recommend daily lysis of the symblephara and the use of symblepharon rings, but the long-term results of this therapy may be disappointing. In fact, some investigators discourage the use of these strategies, hypothesizing that repeated conjunctival lysis may exacerbate inflammation and surface morbidity.

More recently, significant long-term benefit has been demonstrated from the early transplantation of amniotic membrane over the entire ocular surface, including the eyelid margins. This is one of the few potentially beneficial therapeutic interventions for this devastating disease. A recent study also supported the use of high-dose IV corticosteroids during the acute phase, with improved ocular outcomes as well.

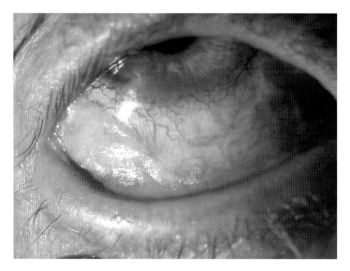

Figure 7-11 Stevens-Johnson syndrome demonstrating inferior eyelid symblepharon as well as ocular surface keratinization. *(Courtesy of Charles S. Bouchard, MD.)*

Late eyelid sequelae, such as entropion, trichiasis, and keratinization result in chronic ocular surface inflammation that is difficult to manage. Attempts to reconstruct the symblepharon and eyelid margins with mucous membrane grafting may result in further inflammation and scarring. Therapeutic contact lenses may offer temporary help. Systemic immunosuppression is often required to suppress the severe inflammatory response in these cases. Eyelid reconstruction for severe disease needs to be performed prior to any ocular surface management such as limbal stem cell transplantation or penetrating keratoplasty (PK). Because of the altered ocular surface and the corneal neovascularization that frequently develops in these patients, PK has an extremely poor prognosis and is generally reserved for progressive thinning or perforation. Rare favorable results in desperate cases have been achieved with the use of a keratoprosthesis, although the long-term stability of such devices is poor. Unfortunately, many patients suffering from this condition are young and are left with lifelong ocular morbidity.

Araki Y, Sotozono C, Inatomi T, et al. Successful treatment of Stevens-Johnson syndrome with steroid pulse therapy at disease onset. *Am J Ophthalmol.* 2009;147(6):1004–1011.

Gregory DG. The ophthalmologic management of acute Stevens-Johnson syndrome. *Ocul Surf.* 2008;6(2):87–95.

Nordlund ML, Brilakis HS, Holland EJ. Surgical techniques for ocular surface reconstruction. *Focal Points: Clinical Modules for Ophthalmologists.* San Francisco: American Academy of Ophthalmology; 2006, module 12.

Ocular Cicatricial Pemphigoid

PATHOGENESIS The exact mechanism of *ocular cicatricial pemphigoid (OCP),* or *mucous membrane pemphigoid (MMP),* remains unknown, although it may represent a cytotoxic (type II) hypersensitivity in which cell injury results from autoantibodies directed against a cell surface antigen in the basement membrane zone (BMZ). Bullous pemphigoid antigen II (BP180) and its soluble extracellular domains have been identified as possible autoantigens. Antibody activates complement with a subsequent breakdown of the conjunctival membrane. A number of proinflammatory cytokines such as IL-1 and TNF-α are overexpressed. TNF-α has been shown to induce the expression of migration inhibitory factor, a cytokine found to have elevated levels in the conjunctival tissues of patients with OCP. Macrophage colony–stimulating factor has also been shown to have an increased expression in the conjunctival tissue of patients with active OCP.

Cellular immunity may also play a role. HLA-DR4, a special genetic locus in the major histocompatibility complex (MHC), has been associated with this condition, but not all affected individuals are positive for this background; hence, HLA typing is not useful.

Pseudopemphigoid, which has a clinical picture similar to pemphigoid, has been associated with the chronic use of certain topical ophthalmic medications. Case reports have implicated pilocarpine, epinephrine, timolol, idoxuridine, echothiophate iodide, and demecarium bromide. The principal difference between pseudopemphigoid and true pemphigoid is that in the former, progression of the disease generally ceases once the offending agent is recognized and removed. The differential diagnosis of cicatrizing conjunctivitis includes 4 major categories (Table 7-2):

1. postinfectious conditions that follow severe episodes of trachoma, adenoviral conjunctivitis, or streptococcal conjunctivitis
2. autoimmune or autoreactive conditions such as sarcoidosis, scleroderma, lichen planus, Stevens-Johnson syndrome, dermatitis herpetiformis, epidermolysis bullosa, atopic blepharoconjunctivitis, and graft-vs-host disease
3. prior conjunctival trauma
4. severe blepharokeratoconjunctivitis caused by rosacea or other disorders (eg, atopic keratoconjunctivitis) that are associated with conjunctival shrinkage

The diagnosis of unilateral OCP should be made with caution, because other diseases, including many of those just listed, may masquerade as OCP. Finally, linear IgA dermatosis, a rare dermatologic condition, can result in an ocular syndrome that is clinically identical to cicatricial pemphigoid and requires similar treatment.

Oyama N, Setterfield JF, Powell AM, et al. Bullous pemphigoid antigen II (BP180) and its soluble extracellular domains are major autoantigens in mucous membrane pemphigoid: the pathogenic relevance to HLA class II alleles and disease severity. Br J Dermatol. 2006; 154(1):90–98.

Table 7-2 Differential Diagnosis of Cicatricial Conjunctivitis

Infectious	Allergic	Autoimmune	Miscellaneous
Trachoma	Atopic keratoconjunctivitis	OCP	Ocular rosacea
Adenovirus	Stevens-Johnson syndrome	Sarcoidosis	Chemical burns
Corynebacterium diphtheriae		Lupus	Trauma
		Scleroderma	Medicamentosa
		Lichen planus	Radiation
			Neoplasia

CLINICAL PRESENTATION   Cicatricial pemphigoid is a chronic cicatrizing conjunctivitis of autoimmune etiology. Although it is a chronic vesiculobullous disease primarily involving the conjunctiva, it frequently affects other mucous membranes, including the mouth and oropharynx, genitalia, and anus. The skin is involved as well in approximately 15% of the cases. Pemphigoid should not be confused with pemphigus vulgaris, a skin disease that rarely affects the eyes and with rare exceptions does not cause conjunctival scarring.

Cicatricial pemphigoid affects women more than men by a 2:1 ratio. Patients are usually older than 60 and rarely younger than 30. They frequently present with recurrent attacks of mild and nonspecific conjunctival inflammation with an occasional mucopurulent discharge. In its early phases, OCP may present with conjunctival hyperemia, edema, ulceration, and tear dysfunction.

Close examination of the conjunctiva in early stages of the disease (stage I) reveals subepithelial fibrosis (Fig 7-12). Fine gray-white linear opacities, best seen with an intense but thin slit beam, appear in the deep conjunctiva. However, in many cases insidious disease in its early stages produces nonspecific symptoms with minimal overt physical findings such as chronic red eye. Oral mucosal lesions may be a clue that can lead to early diagnosis.

Transient bullae of the conjunctivae rupture, leading to subepithelial fibrosis. Loss of goblet cells, shortening of the fornices (stage II), symblepharon formation (stage III; Fig 7-13), and, on occasion, restricted ocular motility with extensive adhesions between the lid and the globe (stage IV) can follow. Ophthalmologists should attempt to diagnose this condition in its early stages and should therefore watch for an inferior forniceal depth of less than 8 mm, which is abnormal and should prompt further evaluation. Subtle inferior symblephara can be detected when the lower eyelid is pulled down while the patient looks up.

Recurrent attacks of conjunctival inflammation can lead to destruction of goblet cells and eventually obstruction of the lacrimal gland ductules. The resultant aqueous and mucous tear deficiency leads to keratinization of the already thickened conjunctiva.

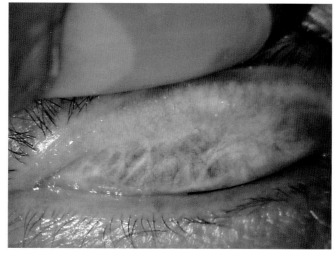

Figure 7-12   Ocular cicatricial pemphigoid showing subepithelial scarring. *(Courtesy of Charles S. Bouchard, MD.)*

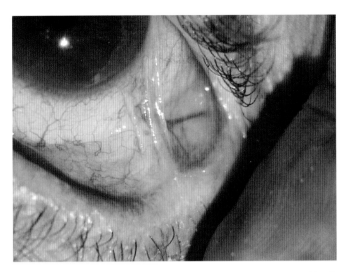

Figure 7-13 Patient with OCP demonstrating subepithelial fibrosis, symblepharon, and shortening of the inferior fornix. *(Courtesy of Charles S. Bouchard, MD.)*

Entropion and trichiasis may develop as scarring progresses, leading to abrasions, corneal vascularization, further scarring, ulceration, and epidermalization of the ocular surface. Although the clinical course is variable, progressive deterioration usually occurs in untreated cases. Remissions and exacerbations are common. Surgical intervention can incite to further scarring but may be essential in managing entropion and trichiasis.

LABORATORY EVALUATION Although OCP is a bilateral disease, 1 eye may be more severely involved than the other. Pathologic support for a diagnosis of pemphigoid can be obtained from a conjunctival biopsy sent for immunofluorescent or immunoperoxidase staining (see Table 7-2). False-negative results are not uncommon however.

Biopsy specimens should be obtained from an actively affected area of the conjunctiva or, if diffuse involvement is present, from the inferior conjunctival fornix. Oral mucosal biopsies may be useful, especially in the presence of an active lesion. Conjunctival biopsies may or may not be positive for immunoreactants in pseudopemphigoid. Immunohistochemical staining techniques can demonstrate C3, IgG, IgM, and/or IgA localized in the BMZ of the conjunctiva in pemphigoid (Fig 7-14). Circulating anti–basement membrane antibody has been identified in the sera of some patients with pemphigoid.

Mihai S, Sitaru C. Immunopathology and molecular diagnosis of autoimmune bullous diseases. *J Cell Mol Med.* 2007;11(3):462–481.

MANAGEMENT A multidisciplinary approach is often required in the management of this disease, with the involvement of ophthalmologists, dentists, dermatologists, oral surgeons, primary care physicians, gynecologists, otolaryngologists, and gastroenterologists. Classifying patients into high-risk and low-risk groups is valuable when determining appropriate therapy. Patients with OCP involving ocular, genital, nasopharyngeal, esophageal, and laryngeal mucosae, as well as patients with rapidly progressing disease, should be treated using the high-risk algorithm. This consists of initial treatment with prednisone and

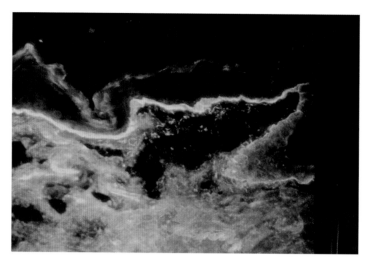

Figure 7-14 Immunofluorescent staining of basement membrane in a patient with cicatricial pemphigoid.

cyclophosphamide (Cytoxan). Cyclophosphamide remains a mainstay of therapy in severe disease. The usual therapeutic dose is 1.5–2.0 mg/kg/day in divided doses. The therapeutic target is a reduction in white blood count to the range of 2000–3000 cells/µL. Cytotoxic therapy can bring about disease remission. Consultation with an internist, dermatologist, or oncologist experienced in cytotoxic therapy is recommended when administering immunosuppressive agents such as cyclophosphamide.

Etanercept may be an effective treatment option for OCP of the oral and ocular mucous membranes. This therapy should be considered an alternative treatment option for patients who would require other aggressive systemic treatments, such as cyclophosphamide, corticosteroids, azathioprine, and intravenous immunoglobulin (IVIg).

Low-risk patients include those with disease occurring only in the oral mucosa or oral mucosa and skin. These patients have a much lower incidence of scarring; thus, they can be treated more conservatively. Because progression is often slow, careful clinical staging of the disease and photodocumentation in differing positions of gaze are generally recommended in evaluating the disease course and response to therapy. Severity of pemphigoid can be judged by measuring the shortening of the inferior fornix depth (for stage II disease) and the extent of symblepharon along the inferior fornix in quartiles (0%–25%, 25%–50%, 50%–75%, and 75%–100% for stage III–IV disease) (see Fig 7-13).

Dapsone, a drug previously used to treat Hansen disease (leprosy) and dermatitis herpetiformis, has been advocated by most authorities as the initial drug of choice in mild cases. It must be avoided in patients with glucose-6-phosphate dehydrogenase (G6PD) deficiency or sulfa allergy; therefore, testing for G6PD deficiency is recommended before initiating treatment. However, even those without this enzymatic deficiency may develop hemolytic anemia.

Topical vitamin A has been shown to reverse, to some extent, the keratinization resulting from the squamous metaplasia associated with this condition, but it is not currently commercially available as an ophthalmic preparation.

Other measures, such as surgical correction of eyelid deformities or eyelash ablation for trichiasis, are occasionally required to achieve ocular surface quiescence. Intraocular surgery is best delayed until disease activity has been under control for an extended period of time. Hard palate and buccal mucosal grafting can be useful techniques in fornix reconstruction in severe cases. Punctal occlusion, which may already have resulted from cicatrization, can be useful in managing any associated dry-eye condition. In general, patients with cicatrizing conjunctivitis have a higher rate of spontaneous extrusion of silicone punctal plugs, and thus permanent punctal occlusion with cautery is often required. Standard PK generally has a very guarded prognosis in patients who develop severe corneal disease in OCP, but keratoprosthesis surgery has been used with some success.

Kheirkhah A, Blanco G, Casas V, Hayashida Y, Raju VK, Tseng SC. Surgical strategies for fornix reconstruction based on symblepharon severity. *Am J Ophthalmol.* 2008;146(2):266–275.

Sami N, Letko E, Androudi S, Daoud Y, Foster CS, Ahmed AR. Intravenous immunoglobulin therapy in patients with ocular-cicatricial pemphigoid: a long-term follow-up. *Ophthalmology.* 2004;111(7):1380–1382.

Saw VP, Dart JK, Rauz S, et al. Immunosuppressive therapy for ocular mucous membrane pemphigoid: strategies and outcomes. *Ophthalmology.* 2008;115(2):253–261.

Tauber J. Ocular cicatricial pemphigoid. *Ophthalmology.* 2008;115(9):1639–1640.

Ocular Graft-vs-Host Disease

Graft-vs-host disease (GVHD) is a relatively common complication of allogeneic bone-marrow transplantation, performed most commonly for hematopoietic malignancies. In this condition, the grafted cells can attack the patient's tissues, including the skin, gut, lungs, liver and gastrointestinal system, and eyes. Although GVHD can be acute or chronic (developing more than 3 months after bone-marrow transplantation), most ocular complications occur as a manifestation of chronic GVHD (cGVHD). Clinical features of ocular graft-vs-host disease (keratoconjunctivitis sicca [KCS], cicatricial conjunctivitis, scleritis, and others) mirror other inflammatory ocular conditions associated with autoimmune/collagen vascular diseases. The pathogenesis of ocular surface disease in GVHD is multifactorial but has 2 main components: (1) conjunctival inflammation with or without subepithelial fibrosis, and (2) severe keratoconjunctivitis sicca from lacrimal gland infiltration by GVHD-effecting T lymphocytes. KCS occurs in 40%–60% of patients with cGVHD. Conjunctival inflammation in GVHD can be severe and even associated with limbal stem cell deficiency and secondary corneal scarring. Amniotic membrane transplantation and even autologous or allogeneic stem cell transplantation may be used for more severe cases. Fortunately, the stem cell deficiency is rare.

Aggressive lubrication and punctal occlusion are the mainstays of local therapy. A high incidence of fibrosis, which leads to extrusion of the punctual plugs, must be monitored closely. Severe filamentary keratitis can be treated further with mucolytic agents (10% acetylcysteine) or bandage soft contact lenses. Severe ocular surface disease in GVHD may be associated with active nonocular (often skin) GVHD and may require increased systemic immunosuppression by cyclosporine or tacrolimus (FK506). Topical cyclosporine may also be useful in controlling the disease. Visual disturbances are due to surface irregularity, and it is important to remember the high rate of posterior subcapsular cataracts, which

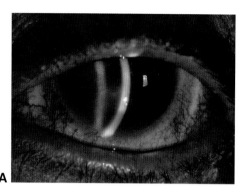
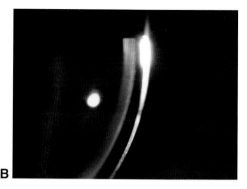

A
B

Figure 7-15   A, Patient with GVHD fitted with a therapeutic scleral contact lens. The inferior paracentral cornea demonstrates subepithelial scarring. **B,** High magnification shows the space between the contact lens and cornea. *(Courtesy of Charles S. Bouchard, MD.)*

can cause decreased vision. Gas-permeable scleral contact lenses provide an important management tool for patients with severe ocular surface disease (Fig 7-15).

Kim SK. Update on ocular graft versus host disease. *Curr Opin Ophthalmol.* 2006;17(4): 344–348.

Nakamura N, Inatomi T, Sotozono C, et al. Transplantation of autologous serum-derived cultivated corneal epithelial equivalents for the treatment of severe ocular surface disease. *Ophthalmology.* 2006;113(10):1765–1772.

Takahide K, Parker PM, Wu M, et al. Use of fluid-ventilated, gas-permeable scleral lens for management of severe keratoconjunctivitis sicca secondary to chronic graft-versus-host disease. *Biol Blood Marrow Transplant.* 2007;13(9):1016–1021.

Other Immune-Mediated Diseases of the Skin and Mucous Membranes

Other immune-mediated disorders that can, in rare cases, affect the conjunctiva include linear IgA bullous dermatosis, dermatitis herpetiformis, epidermolysis bullosa, lichen planus, paraneoplastic pemphigus, pemphigus vulgaris, and pemphigus foliaceus (Table 7-3).

Immune-Mediated Diseases of the Cornea

Thygeson Superficial Punctate Keratitis

PATHOGENESIS   The etiology of Thygeson superficial punctate keratitis (SPK) is unknown. Although many of the clinical features resemble those of a viral infection of the epithelium, attempts to confirm viral particles by electron microscopy or culture have been unsuccessful. Confocal microscopy has demonstrated clumps of markedly enlarged epithelial cells and multiple highly reflective filamentary structures in the deeper layers. Most of these lesions were linear, but some showed curled ends and others demonstrated branching lesions with "sprouts." No inflammatory cells were evident. The rapid response of the lesions to corticosteroid therapy suggests that Thygeson keratitis is largely immunopathogenically derived.

Table 7-3 Immunopathologic Features of Autoimmune Bullous Diseases

Disease	Direct Immunofluorescence	Indirect Immunofluorescence	Autoantigens
Pemphigus diseases			
Pemphigus vulgaris	Intercellular IgG and C3	Intercellular IgG (monkey esophagus)	Dsg 3, Dsg 1
Pemphigus foliaceus	Intercellular IgG and C3	Intercellular IgG (monkey esophagus)	Dsg 1
Paraneoplastic pemphigus	IgG and C3 intercellularly and at the dermal–epidermal junction	Intercellular IgG (monkey esophagus and rat bladder*)	Dsg 3, Dsg 1, plakines
IgA pemphigus	Intercellular IgA and C3	Intercellular IgA (monkey esophagus)	Dsc 1, Dsg 3
Pemphigoid diseases			
Bullous pemphigoid	Linear C3 and IgG at the dermal–epidermal junction	Epidermal IgG (SSS†)	BP180, BP230
Gestational pemphigoid	Linear C3 at the dermal–epidermal junction	Epidermal complement-fixing IgG (SSS)	BP180, BP230
Mucous membrane pemphigoid	Linear IgG, IgA, and C3 at the dermal–epidermal junction	Epidermal or dermal IgG, IgA (SSS)	BP180, Laminin 5, $\alpha_6\beta_4$ integrin
Linear IgA disease	Linear IgA (and C3) at the dermal–epidermal junction	Epidermal IgA (SSS) Dermal IgA (SSS)	LAD-1 Type VII collagen
Epidermolysis bullosa acquisita	Linear IgG, IgA, and C3 at the dermal–epidermal junction	Dermal IgG (SSS)	Type VII collagen
Dermatitis herpetiformis	Granular IgA deposits in the dermal papillae	Antiendomysium IgA (monkey esophagus)	Transglutaminase

Dsc = desmocollin, Dsg = desmoglein.
*Rat bladder is a sensitive substrate for detection of circulating autoantibodies in paraneoplastic pemphigus.
†SSS is skin incubated with 1 M NaCl, as a substrate for detecting circulating autoantibodies in subepidermal blistering diseases.

From Mihai S, Sitaru C. Immunopathology and molecular diagnosis of autoimmune bullous diseases. *J Cell Mol Med.* 2007;11(3):462–481.

Cheng LL, Young AL, Wong AK, Law RW, Lam DS. In vivo confocal microscopy of Thygeson's superficial punctate keratitis. *Clin Experiment Ophthalmol.* 2004;32(3):325–327.

CLINICAL PRESENTATION This condition, first reported by Thygeson in 1950, is characterized by recurrent episodes of tearing, foreign-body sensation, photophobia, and reduced vision. It affects children to older adults and is typically bilateral, although it may develop initially in 1 eye or may be markedly asymmetric in some cases. The hallmark finding is multiple (up to 40 but as few as 2–3) slightly elevated corneal epithelial lesions with "negative staining," which are noted during exacerbations. The epithelial lesions are round or oval conglomerates of gray, granular, or "crumblike" opacities associated with minimal conjunctival reaction, in contrast to adenoviral keratoconjunctivitis. High magnification reveals each opacity to be a cluster of multiple smaller pinpoint opacities (Fig 7-16). A characteristic feature is the waxing and waning appearance of individual epithelial opacities, which change in location and number over time. The greatest density of these lesions typically appears in the central cornea. The raised punctate epithelial lesions themselves stain faintly with fluorescein and rose bengal.

No conjunctival inflammatory reaction is noted during exacerbations, but occasionally patients will have mild bulbar conjunctival injection. In rare cases, a mild subepithelial opacity may develop underlying the epithelial lesion—more commonly in patients who have received topical antiviral therapy. The important facet of this condition is that the patient's symptoms may far exceed the apparent signs; frequently, patients complain bitterly of photophobia and foreign-body sensation in the setting of only a few central epithelial lesions.

MANAGEMENT   Supportive therapy with artificial tears is often adequate in mild cases. Treatment alternatives for persistently symptomatic cases include topical corticosteroids and bandage soft contact lenses. Antiviral therapy is not the standard of care at this time, as there are no firm data to associate this condition with an active replicative viral infection.

If a topical corticosteroid is prescribed, only a very mild preparation is needed (eg, fluorometholone 0.1%). Because the lesions are quite responsive to corticosteroids, treatment will hasten their resolution, but they frequently recur in the same or different locations on the cornea after the topical corticosteroids are stopped. Overall, the use of corticosteroids should be minimized in these cases and monitored closely. Topical cyclosporine 0.05% or tacrolimus given 2–4 times daily is also effective in causing regression of the lesions. Although there is little to suggest that this treatment is superior to corticosteroid therapy, it is the preferred treatment over corticosteroids due to the higher safety profile.

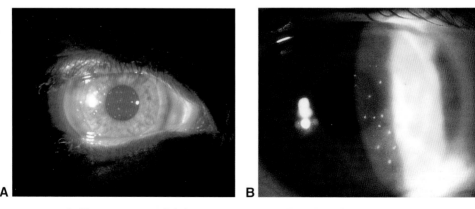

Figure 7-16   A, Thygeson superficial punctate keratitis. **B,** At higher magnification, each lesion is seen to consist of several minute dots.

Connell PP, O'Reilly J, Coughlan S, Collum LM, Power WJ. The role of common ocular viral pathogens in Thygeson's superficial punctate keratitis. *Br J Ophthalmol.* 2007;91(8):1038–1041.

Nagra PK, Rapuano CJ, Cohen EJ, Laibson PR. Thygeson's superficial punctate keratitis: ten years' experience. *Ophthalmology.* 2004;111(1):34–37.

Tatlipinar S, Akpek EK. Topical ciclosporin in the treatment of ocular surface disorders. *Br J Ophthalmol.* 2005;89(10):1363–1367.

Interstitial Keratitis Associated With Infectious Diseases

PATHOGENESIS Interstitial keratitis (IK) is a nonsuppurative inflammation of the corneal stroma that features cellular infiltration and usually vascularization without primary involvement of the epithelium or endothelium. Most cases result from a type IV hypersensitivity response to infectious microorganisms or other antigens in the corneal stroma. The topographic distribution (diffuse versus focal or multifocal) and depth of the stromal infiltration, in addition to associated systemic signs, are helpful in determining the cause of IK.

Congenital syphilis was the first infection to be linked with IK. Herpes simplex virus, which accounts for most cases of stromal keratitis, and varicella-zoster virus keratitis are discussed earlier in this volume. Many other microorganisms are much rarer causes of IK; these include

- *Mycobacterium tuberculosis*
- *M leprae*
- *Borrelia burgdorferi* (Lyme disease)
- rubeola (measles)
- Epstein-Barr virus (infectious mononucleosis)
- *Chlamydia trachomatis* (lymphogranuloma venereum)
- *Leishmania* spp
- *Onchocerca volvulus* (onchocerciasis)

Syphilitic interstitial keratitis

CLINICAL PRESENTATION Syphilitic eye disease is discussed further in BCSC Section 6, *Pediatric Ophthalmology and Strabismus,* and Section 9, *Intraocular Inflammation and Uveitis.* Systemic aspects of syphilis are discussed in BCSC Section 1, *Update on General Medicine.*

Keratitis may be caused by either congenital or acquired syphilis, although most cases are associated with congenital syphilis. Manifestations of congenital syphilis that occur early in life (within the first 2 years) are infectious. However, IK is an example of a later, immune-mediated manifestation of congenital syphilis. Affected children typically show no evidence of corneal disease in their first years; stromal keratitis lasting for several weeks develops late in the first decade of life (or even later). These patients may also have other nonocular signs of congenital syphilis:

- dental deformities: notched (Hutchinson) incisors and mulberry molars
- bone and cartilage abnormalities: saddle nose, palatal perforation, saber shins, and frontal bossing

- cranial nerve VIII (vestibulocochlear) deafness
- rhagades (circumoral radiating scars)
- mental retardation

Congenital syphilitic keratitis is usually bilateral (80%), although both eyes may not be affected simultaneously or to the same degree. Initial symptoms are pain, tearing, photophobia, and perilimbal injection. The inflammation may last for weeks if left untreated. Sectoral superior stromal inflammation and keratic precipitates are typically seen early. As the disease progresses, deep stromal neovascularization develops. Eventually, the inflammation spreads centrally, and corneal opacification and edema may develop (Fig 7-17). In some cases, the deep corneal vascularization becomes so intense that the cornea appears pink—hence the term *salmon patch*. Sequelae of stromal keratitis include corneal scarring, thinning, and ghost vessels in the deep layers of the stroma. Visual acuity may be reduced because of irregular astigmatism and stromal opacification.

Stromal keratitis develops only rarely in acquired (as opposed to congenital) syphilis and, if it does, is typically unilateral (60%). The ocular findings are similar to those seen in congenital syphilitic keratitis. In general, uveitis and retinitis are much more common manifestations of acquired syphilis than keratitis.

LABORATORY EVALUATION AND MANAGEMENT   The diagnosis can be confirmed serologically with the rapid plasmin reagin test and a treponeme-specific antibody test (FTA-ABS or MHA-TP). During the acute phase, ocular inflammation should be treated with cycloplegic agents and topical corticosteroids to limit stromal inflammation and late scarring. The corneal disease can be suppressed effectively with topical corticosteroids; however, even if left untreated, the disease typically burns out after several weeks, although it can lead to severe corneal opacification before doing so. Systemic syphilis (or neuroretinal manifestations) should be treated with penicillin or an appropriate alternative antibiotic according to the protocol appropriate for either congenital or acquired syphilis. The necessity of

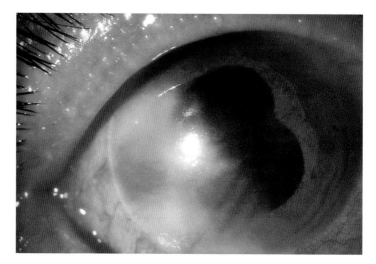

Figure 7-17   Active syphilitic interstitial keratitis with salmon patch.

lumbar puncture in syphilitic interstitial keratitis is uncertain. See BCSC Section 9, *Intraocular Inflammation and Uveitis,* for a more in-depth discussion of noncorneal syphilitic disease.

Reactive Arthritis

PATHOGENESIS   Reactive arthritis (formerly Reiter syndrome) is a systemic disorder characterized by the classic triad of ocular (conjunctivitis/episcleritis, iridocyclitis, or keratitis), urethral, and joint inflammation. The joint inflammation is often highly asymmetric and involves a few joints (oligoarticular). These manifestations can appear simultaneously or separately in any sequence. Less common manifestations include keratoderma blennorrhagicum (a scaling skin eruption), balanitis, aphthous stomatitis, fever, lymphadenopathy, pneumonitis, pericarditis, and myocarditis. Attacks are self-limited, lasting from 2 to several months, but they may recur periodically over the course of several years.

Reactive arthritis may occur after gram-negative bacterial dysentery (most frequently associated with *Salmonella, Shigella,* and *Yersinia*) or after nongonococcal urethritis caused by *Chlamydia trachomatis.* More than 75% of patients with reactive arthritis are HLA-B27 positive. See BCSC Section 9, *Intraocular Inflammation and Uveitis,* for discussion of HLA-B27–related diseases and illustrations of nonocular manifestations of reactive arthritis.

CLINICAL PRESENTATION   A bilateral papillary conjunctivitis with mucopurulent discharge is the most common ocular finding in reactive arthritis; it has been reported in 30%–60% of patients. The conjunctivitis is self-limited, lasting for days to weeks. Some patients present more with episcleritis rather than with conjunctivitis. Mild nongranulomatous iritis has been reported to occur in 3%–12% of patients. Various forms of keratitis may occur in rare cases, including diffuse punctate epithelial erosions, superficial or deep focal infiltrates, and superficial or deep vascularization. Reactive arthritis should be considered in any case of chronic, nonfollicular, mucopurulent conjunctivitis with negative cultures.

MANAGEMENT   Treatment is mainly palliative. Corneal infiltrates and vascularization often respond to topical corticosteroids. Systemic antibiotic treatment of the related infection, if any, may be beneficial. Occasionally, the intraocular (uveitic) component of the disease can be very severe and require systemic immune suppression; see BCSC Section 9, *Intraocular Inflammation and Uveitis.*

Cogan Syndrome

PATHOGENESIS   Cogan syndrome is an autoimmune disorder that produces stromal keratitis, vertigo, and hearing loss. The etiology of Cogan syndrome is obscure, but the disease shares some clinicopathologic features with polyarteritis nodosa.

CLINICAL PRESENTATION   Cogan syndrome typically occurs in young adults, the majority of whom have had an upper respiratory infection 1–2 weeks prior to the onset of ocular or vestibuloauditory symptoms (vertigo, tinnitus, and hearing loss). The earliest corneal findings are bilateral faint white subepithelial infiltrates similar to those occurring in viral keratoconjunctivitis but located in the peripheral cornea. Multifocal nodular infiltrates may develop in the posterior cornea later in the course of this condition. Some patients develop a systemic vasculitis that presents as polyarteritis nodosa.

LABORATORY EVALUATION   When the cause of stromal keratitis is not apparent, VDRL or RPR and FTA-ABS or MHA-TP are obtained (VDRL and RPR may become nonreactive in congenital syphilis). Other infectious syndromes should also be considered. Because there are no specific laboratory findings, Cogan syndrome is essentially a diagnosis of exclusion.

MANAGEMENT   The acute keratitis of Cogan syndrome is treated with frequent topical corticosteroids. It is important to treat this condition promptly because the ocular and vestibular changes can proceed rapidly, and deafness is more likely if not treated early. Oral corticosteroids are recommended for the vestibuloauditory symptoms, because this treatment enhances the long-term prognosis and recovery of normal hearing. Cytotoxic agents may also have a therapeutic role but are reserved for severe and unresponsive cases.

> Gluth MB, Baratz KH, Matteson EL, Driscoll CL. Cogan syndrome: a retrospective review of 60 patients throughout a half century. *Mayo Clin Proc.* 2006;81(4):483–488.

Marginal Corneal Infiltrates Associated With Blepharoconjunctivitis

PATHOGENESIS   The limbus plays an important role in immune-mediated corneal disorders. As reviewed in Chapter 6, the limbus has a population of antigen-presenting cells that constitutively express class II MHC antigens and are capable of efficient mobilization and induction of T-cell responses. Therefore, immune-related corneal changes often occur in a peripheral location adjacent to the limbus. In addition, because the peripheral cornea is adjacent to the vascularized (posterior) limbus, circulating immune cells, immune complexes, and complement factors tend to deposit adjacent to the terminal capillary loops of the limbal vascular arcades, thereby producing a variety of immune phenomena that manifest in the corneal periphery. Predisposing causes include

- blepharoconjunctivitis
- contact lens wear
- trauma
- endophthalmitis

CLINICAL PRESENTATION   Marginal infiltrates (also referred to as *catarrhal infiltrates*) usually occur where the eyelid margins intersect with the corneal surface: the 10, 2, 4, and 8 o'clock positions. Marginal infiltrates in staphylococcal blepharitis are typically gray-white, well circumscribed, and located approximately 1 mm inside the limbus, with a characteristic clear (intervening) zone of cornea between the infiltrate and the limbus (see Fig 5-10, in Chapter 5). In chronic disease, superficial blood vessels may cross the clear interval into the area of corneal infiltration. The epithelium overlying marginal infiltrates may be intact, show punctate epithelial erosions, or be ulcerated. Stromal opacification, peripheral corneal thinning, and/or pannus may develop following resolution of the acute marginal infiltrates.

Peripheral Ulcerative Keratitis Associated With Systemic Immune-Mediated Diseases

PATHOGENESIS Autoimmune peripheral keratitis may develop in patients who have systemic immune-mediated and rheumatic diseases. Peripheral ulcerative keratitis (PUK) occurs most often in association with rheumatoid arthritis but may also be seen in Wegener granulomatosis, systemic lupus erythematosus, polyarteritis nodosa, ulcerative colitis, relapsing polychondritis, and other inflammatory diseases such as rosacea (Table 7-4). Biopsy of conjunctival tissue adjacent to marginal corneal disease—although not a standard diagnostic procedure—typically shows evidence of immune-mediated vaso-occlusive disease.

Central corneal melting in the setting of systemic collagen vascular disease may be due to a different mechanism associated with a T-lymphocyte infiltration.

CLINICAL PRESENTATION A history of connective tissue disease is often (but not invariably) present, although in some patients the ocular finding of peripheral corneal infiltration or

---

Table 7-4 Differential Diagnosis of PUK

Ocular	
Microbial	
Bacterial	*Staphylococcus, Streptococcus, Gonococcus, Moraxella, Haemophilus*
Viral	Herpes simplex, herpes zoster
Acanthamoeba	
Fungal	
Mooren ulcer	
Traumatic or postsurgical	
Terrien marginal degeneration	
Exposure keratopathy	
Rosacea	
Systemic	
Microbial	
Bacterial	Tuberculosis, syphilis, gonorrhea, borreliosis, bacillary dysentery
Viral	Herpes zoster, AIDS, hepatitis C
Helminthiasis	
Rheumatoid arthritis	
Systemic lupus erythematosus	
Wegener granulomatosis	
Polyarteritis nodosa	
Relapsing polychondritis	
Progressive systemic sclerosis and scleroderma	
Sjögren syndrome	
Behçet syndrome	
Sarcoidosis	
Inflammatory bowel disease	
α_1-Antitrypsin deficiency	
Malignancy	

Adapted with permission from Dana MR, Qian Y, Hamrah P. Twenty-five-year panorama of corneal immunology: emerging concepts in the immunopathogenesis of microbial keratitis, peripheral ulcerative keratitis, and corneal transplant rejection. *Cornea*. 2000;19(5):625–643.

frank stromal melting may be the first sign of the underlying systemic illness. Autoimmune PUK generally correlates with exacerbations of systemic disease activity. Follow-up of these patients reveals that, if they are treated inadequately, a high proportion may suffer severe disease-related morbidity. The term *keratolysis* refers to the significant (and often rapid) stromal melting seen in some cases of immune-mediated PUK associated with systemic autoimmunity.

Although autoimmune PUK can sometimes be bilateral and extensive, it is usually unilateral and limited to 1 sector of the peripheral cornea (Fig 7-18). The initial lesions appear in a zone within 2 mm of the limbus and are accompanied by varying degrees of vaso-occlusion of the adjacent limbal vascular networks. In most cases, the epithelium is absent in the affected area and the underlying stroma thinned; however, if the disease is detected early, epithelial involvement may be patchy and the stroma still of near-normal thickness. Ulceration may or may not be associated with a significant cellular infiltrate in the corneal stroma, and the adjacent conjunctiva can be minimally or severely inflamed.

MANAGEMENT   The goal of therapy is to provide local supportive measures to decrease melting. This is achieved through maneuvers directed at (1) improving wetting, (2) promoting reepithelialization, and (3) suppressing the systemic-mediated inflammation.

Maintaining enhanced lubrication of the surface is very important: first, because many rheumatoid patients have keratoconjunctivitis sicca as a manifestation of their secondary Sjögren syndrome; and second, because lubrication may help in diluting the effect of inflammatory cytokines in the preocular tear film. Melting will stop or slow appreciably if the epithelium can be made to heal by means of lubricants, patching, or a bandage soft contact lens. A number of topical collagenase inhibitors, such as sodium citrate 10%, Mucomyst 20%, medroxyprogesterone 1%, or tetracycline and systemic collagenase inhibitors, such as tetracyclines (eg, doxycycline), are of possible value. Topical cyclosporine has been shown to be potentially effective in patients with central melting that is probably not due to occlusive vasculitis but is more likely a T-cell–mediated process.

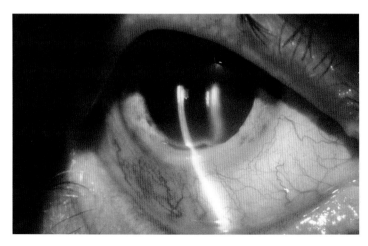

Figure 7-18   Peripheral ulcerative keratitis as a result of rheumatoid disease.

Topical corticosteroids, which also inhibit collagenase function, often have variable effects. Although they may suppress corneal inflammation when there is profound leukocyte infiltration in the cornea, they also may delay reepithelialization, predispose to superinfection, and even exacerbate melting by suppressing collagen production. In general, if the cornea has become significantly thinned, corticosteroid therapy is probably contraindicated. Excision or recession of adjacent limbal conjunctiva (as has been advocated for Mooren ulcer; see the following section) is often followed by healing of the ulcer, presumably because the procedure eliminates a source of inflammatory cells and collagenolytic enzymes.

Definitive management often cannot be achieved by local measures alone and requires institution or escalation of systemic treatment, including immunosuppressive therapy using cytotoxic agents such as cyclophosphamide or immunomodulatory agents such as methotrexate or cyclosporine. Severe, rapidly melting cases may require intravenous therapy with high-dose cyclophosphamide, with or without corticosteroid therapy. Threatened perforation should be treated with temporizing measures such as cyanoacrylate glue and bandage contact lens placement until systemic therapy has been initiated, because lamellar or penetrating grafts are also susceptible to melting. Sometimes multiple tectonic grafts are required to preserve the globe while the systemic therapy is being adjusted. Once the underlying disease process has been controlled, reconstructive keratoplasty can be performed (see Chapters 15 and 16). Although conjunctival flaps can be very helpful for controlling the stromal melting in difficult-to-manage microbial keratitis, they are probably best avoided in immune-mediated disease. The melting could potentially be accelerated by bringing the conjunctival vasculature in even closer proximity to the area of corneal disease.

Gottsch JD, Akpek EK. Topical cyclosporin stimulates neovascularization in resolving sterile rheumatoid central corneal ulcers. *Trans Am Ophthalmol Soc.* 2000;98:81–87.

Perez VL, Azar DT, Foster CS. Sterile corneal melting and necrotizing scleritis after cataract surgery in patients with rheumatoid arthritis and collagen vascular disease. *Semin Ophthalmol.* 2002;17(3-4):124–130.

Mooren Ulcer

PATHOGENESIS Although the etiology of PUK is unknown, evidence is mounting that autoimmunity plays a key role. The following have been found in patients with Mooren ulcer:

- deficiency of suppressor T cells
- increased level of IgA
- increased concentration of plasma cells and lymphocytes in the conjunctiva adjacent to the ulcerated areas
- increased $CD4^+/CD8^+$ and $B7-2^+$/antigen-presenting cell ratios as well as increased VCAM-1, VLA-4, and ICAM-1 in the vascular endothelium of conjunctival vessels
- tissue-fixed immunoglobulins and complement in the conjunctival epithelium and peripheral cornea

A significant number of resident cells in Mooren ulcer specimens express MHC class II antigens, a reflection of the degree of immune-mediated inflammation in the tissue. It has been suggested that autoreactivity to a cornea-specific antigen may play a role in the pathogenesis of this disorder, and humoral and cell-mediated immune mechanisms may be involved in the initiation and perpetuation of corneal destruction. The proximity of the ulcerative lesion to the limbus probably has pathophysiologic importance (as discussed earlier in the section on PUK), because resection or recession of the limbal conjunctiva can often have a beneficial therapeutic effect.

Although the cause of Mooren ulcer is unknown, precipitating factors include accidental trauma or surgery and exposure to parasitic infection. The latter is of considerable importance, as the incidence of Mooren ulcer is particularly high in areas where parasitic (eg, helminthic) infections are endemic. The principal hypotheses are that inflammation associated with previous injury or infection may alter the expression of corneal or conjunctival antigens (to which autoantibodies are then produced) or that cross-reactivity occurs between the immune effectors generated in response to infection and corneal autoantigens. The simultaneous presence of multiple types of inflammatory cells, adhesion, and costimulatory molecules in Mooren ulcer conjunctiva suggests that their interaction may contribute to a sustained immune activation as at least part of the pathogenic mechanism of this disorder. By definition, Mooren ulcer is of unknown cause. Cases of PUK due to known local (eg, rosacea) or systemic (eg, rheumatoid arthritis) diseases should not be called Mooren ulcer.

Gottsch JD, Stark WJ, Liu SH. Cloning and sequence analysis of human and bovine corneal antigen (CO-Ag) cDNA: identification of host-parasite protein calgranulin C. *Trans Am Ophthalmol Soc.* 1997;95:111–125.

Kafkala C, Choi J, Zafirakis P, et al. Mooren ulcer: an immunopathologic study. *Cornea.* 2006; 25(6):667–673.

Wilson SE, Lee WM, Murakami C, Weng J, Moninger GA. Mooren-type hepatitis C virus-associated corneal ulceration. *Ophthalmology.* 1994;101(4):736–745.

Zelefsky JR, Srinivasan M, Kundu A, et al. Hookworm infestation as a risk factor for Mooren's ulcer in South India. *Ophthalmology.* 2007;114(3):450–453.

CLINICAL PRESENTATION Mooren ulcer is a chronic, progressive, painful, idiopathic ulceration of the peripheral corneal stroma and epithelium. Typically, the ulcer starts in the periphery of the cornea and spreads circumferentially and then centripetally, with a leading undermined edge of deepithelized tissue (Fig 7-19). A slower movement of ulceration proceeds toward the sclera. The eye is inflamed and pain can be intense, with photophobia and tearing. Perforation may occur with minor trauma or during secondary infection. Extensive vascularization and fibrosis of the cornea may occur.

In some patients, it may be very difficult to distinguish Mooren ulcer from idiopathic PUK. An important distinguishing feature is the purely corneal involvement of Mooren; PUK has scleral involvement.

Two clinical types of Mooren ulcer have been described. Unilateral Mooren ulcer typically occurs in an older patient population. Sex distribution is equal in this form, which is slowly progressive. A second type of Mooren ulcer is more common in Africa. This form

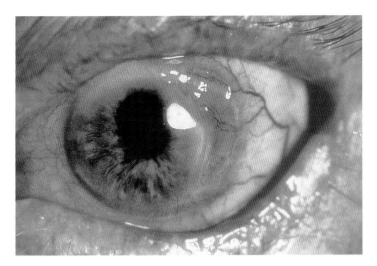

Figure 7-19 Mooren ulcer. *(Courtesy of Vincent P. deLuise, MD.)*

is usually bilateral, rapidly progressive, and poorly responsive to medical or surgical intervention (Fig 7-20). Corneal ulceration and perforation are frequent. Many of the patients with this form of Mooren ulcer also have coexisting parasitemia. It is possible that in this subgroup of West African males, Mooren ulcer may be triggered by antigen–antibody reaction to helminthic toxins or antigens deposited in the limbal cornea during the blood-borne phase of parasitic infection.

MANAGEMENT   The multitude of therapeutic strategies used against Mooren ulcer underscores the relative lack of effective treatment. Topical corticosteroids, contact lenses, acetylcysteine (Mucomyst 10%) and L-cysteine (0.2 molar), topical cyclosporine, limbal

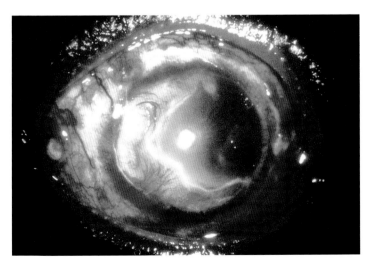

Figure 7-20   Mooren ulcer with severe superior limbal ulceration and thinning.

conjunctival excision, and lamellar keratoplasty have all been described with variable success. More recently, topical IFN-α_{2a} and topical cyclosporine 2%, as well as infliximab, have also been reported as effective alternatives. Systemic immunosuppressives such as oral corticosteroids, cyclophosphamide, methotrexate, and cyclosporine have also shown promise in these cases. Hepatitis C–associated cases of "Mooren ulcer"-type PUK have responded to interferon therapy.

Erdem U, Kerimoglu H, Gundogan F, Dagli S. Treatment of Mooren's ulcer with topical administration of interferon alfa 2a. *Ophthalmology.* 2007;114(3):446–449.

Fontana L, Parente G, Neri P, Reta M, Tassinari G. Favourable response to infliximab in a case of bilateral refractory Mooren's ulcer. *Clin Experiment Ophthalmol.* 2007;35(9):871–873.

Tandon R, Chawla B, Verma K, Sharma N, Titiyal JS. Outcome of treatment of Mooren ulcer with topical cyclosporine A 2%. *Cornea.* 2008;27(8):859–861.

Immune-Mediated Diseases of the Episclera and Sclera

Episcleritis

PATHOGENESIS   Episcleritis is a self-limited, generally benign inflammation of the episcleral tissues. The pathophysiology of this disorder remains obscure. An underlying systemic cause is found in only a minority of patients.

CLINICAL PRESENTATION   Episcleritis is typically a transient (usually days to weeks), self-limited disease of adults, usually 20–50 years of age. The chief complaint is usually ocular redness without irritation, which resolves spontaneously. Slight tenderness may be present. The disease occurs most commonly in the exposure zone of the eye, often in the area of a pinguecula, and it may recur in the same or different locations. About one third of patients have bilateral disease at one time or another.

Episcleritis is diagnosed clinically by localizing the site of inflammation to the episclera. Unlike the deeper inflammation seen in scleritis (often with associated scleral edema clearly discernible on slit-lamp examination), episcleral inflammation is superficial. The characteristic color in episcleritis is bright red or salmon pink in natural light, unlike the violaceous hue in most forms of scleritis. In addition, the redness in episcleritis (unlike that associated with scleritis) will blanch with application of 2.5% topical phenylephrine.

Episcleritis is classified as *simple* (diffuse injection) or *nodular.* In simple episcleritis, the inflammation is localized to a sector of the globe in 70% of cases, and to the entire episclera in 30% of cases. A localized mobile nodule develops in nodular episcleritis (Fig 7-21). Small peripheral corneal opacities can be observed adjacent to the area of episcleral inflammation in 10% of patients. The disease generally resolves without producing any lasting destructive effects on tissues of the eye.

MANAGEMENT   A workup for underlying causes (eg, autoimmune connective tissue disease such as Sjögren syndrome, rheumatoid arthritis, or other conditions such as gout, herpes zoster, syphilis, tuberculosis, rosacea) is rarely indicated except after multiple recurrences. Episcleritis generally clears without treatment, but topical or oral NSAIDs may

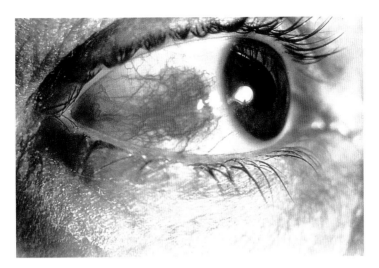

Figure 7-21 Nodular episcleritis.

be prescribed for patients bothered by pain. Most patients simply need reassurance that their condition is not sight-threatening and can be treated with lubricants alone. The use of topical corticosteroids should be kept to a minimum in this benign, self-limited condition. However, in unusual cases of severe disease that does not respond to standard therapy with lubricants and NSAIDs, a short course of corticosteroids may be necessary.

Jabs DA, Mudun A, Dunn JP, Marsh MJ. Episcleritis and scleritis: clinical features and treatment results. *Am J Ophthalmol.* 2000;130(4):469–476.

Williams CP, Browning AC, Sleep TJ, Webber SK, McGill JI. A randomised, double-blind trial of topical ketorolac vs artificial tears for the treatment of episcleritis. *Eye.* 2005;19(7):739–742.

Scleritis

PATHOGENESIS Scleritis is a much more severe ocular inflammatory condition than episcleritis. It is caused by an immune-mediated (typically immune-complex) vasculitis that frequently leads to destruction of the sclera. Scleritis is frequently associated with an underlying systemic immunologic disease; about one third of patients with diffuse or nodular scleritis and two thirds with necrotizing scleritis have a detectable connective tissue or autoimmune disease. Scleritis causes significant pain and may lead to structural alterations of the globe, with attendant visual morbidity. It is exceedingly rare in children, occurs most often in the fourth to sixth decades of life, and is more common in women. About one half of scleritis cases are bilateral at some time in their course.

Watson PG. Scleral structure, organisation and disease: a review. *Exp Eye Res.* 2004;78(3): 609–623.

CLINICAL PRESENTATION The onset of scleritis is usually gradual, extending over several days. Most patients with scleritis develop severe boring or piercing ocular pain, which may worsen at night and occasionally awaken them from sleep. The pain may be referred to other regions of the head or face on the involved side, and the globe is often tender to touch. The inflamed sclera has a violaceous hue best seen in natural sunlight. Inflamed scleral vessels have a crisscross pattern, adhere to the sclera, and cannot be moved with a cotton-tipped applicator. Scleral edema, often with overlying episcleral edema, is noted by slit-lamp examination. Scleritis can be classified clinically based on the anatomical location (anterior versus posterior scleritis) and appearance of scleral inflammation (Table 7-5).

Diffuse versus nodular anterior scleritis

Diffuse anterior scleritis is characterized by a zone of scleral edema and redness. A portion of the anterior sclera (<50%) is involved in 60% of cases, and the entire anterior segment is involved in 40% of cases (Fig 7-22). In *nodular anterior scleritis,* the scleral nodule is a deep red-purple color, immobile, and separated from the overlying episcleral tissue, which is elevated by the nodule (Fig 7-23).

Necrotizing scleritis

Necrotizing scleritis is the most destructive form of scleritis. Of the patients affected, 60% develop ocular and systemic complications, 40% suffer loss of vision, and a significant minority may die prematurely as a result of complications of vasculitis.

Table 7-5 Subtypes and Prevalence of Scleritis

Location	Subtype	Prevalence
Anterior sclera	Diffuse scleritis	40%
	Nodular scleritis	44%
	Necrotizing scleritis	14%
	with inflammation	(10%)
	without inflammation *(scleromalacia perforans)*	(4%)
Posterior sclera		2%

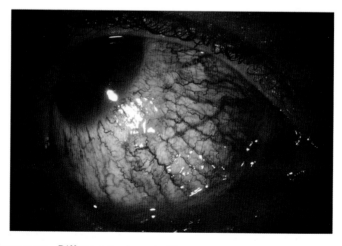

Figure 7-22   Diffuse anterior scleritis. *(Courtesy of Charles S. Bouchard, MD.)*

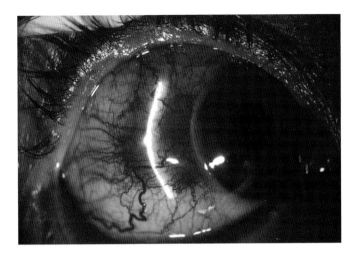

Figure 7-23 Nodular anterior scleritis. *(Courtesy of Charles S. Bouchard, MD.)*

Necrotizing scleritis with inflammation Patients with necrotizing scleritis with inflammation typically present with severe pain. Most commonly, a localized patch of inflammation is noted initially, with the edges of the lesion more inflamed than the center. In more advanced disease (25% of cases), an avascular edematous patch of sclera is seen (Fig 7-24). Untreated, necrotizing scleritis may spread posteriorly to the equator and circumferentially until the entire anterior globe is involved. Severe loss of tissue may result if treatment is not intensive and prompt. The sclera may develop a blue-gray appearance (due to thinning, which allows the underlying choroid to show) and reveal an altered deep episcleral blood vessel pattern (large anastomotic blood vessels that may circumscribe the involved area) after the inflammation subsides.

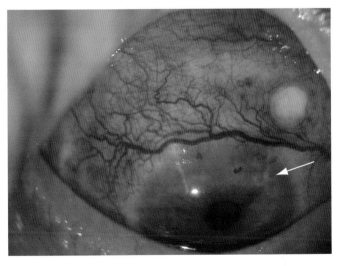

Figure 7-24 Diffuse anterior scleritis with samll area of necrotizing scleritis. Note also the partially resolved sclerokeratitis *(arrow)*. *(Courtesy of Charles S. Bouchard, MD.)*

Necrotizing scleritis without inflammation   This form of scleritis, also known as *sclero-malacia perforans*, although undoubtedly due to inflammation, is said to be "without inflammation" because its clinical presentation is distinct from those of other forms of anterior scleritis, in which typical signs (redness, edema) and symptoms (pain) of inflammation are readily apparent.

Scleromalacia perforans typically occurs in patients with long-standing rheumatoid arthritis. Signs of inflammation are minimal, and this type of scleritis is generally painless. As the disease progresses, the sclera thins and the underlying dark uveal tissue becomes visible (Fig 7-25). In many cases, the uvea is covered with only thin connective tissue and conjunctiva. Large abnormal blood vessels surround and cross the areas of scleral loss. A bulging staphyloma develops if intraocular pressure is elevated; spontaneous perforation is rare, although these eyes may rupture with minimal trauma.

Posterior scleritis

Posterior scleritis can occur in isolation or concomitantly with anterior scleritis. Some investigators include posterior scleritis as an anterior variant of inflammatory pseudotumor. Patients present with pain, tenderness, proptosis, visual loss, and, occasionally, restricted motility. Choroidal folds, exudative retinal detachment, papilledema, and angle-closure glaucoma secondary to choroidal thickening may develop. Retraction of the lower eyelid may occur in upgaze, presumably caused by infiltration of muscles in the region of the posterior scleritis. The pain may be referred to other parts of the head, and the diagnosis can be missed in the absence of associated anterior scleritis. Demonstration of thickened posterior sclera by echography, CT scan, or MRI may be helpful in establishing the diagnosis (Fig 7-26). Often, no related systemic disease can be found in patients with posterior scleritis.

Complications of scleritis

Complications of scleritis are frequent and include peripheral keratitis (37%), uveitis (30%), cataract (7%), glaucoma (18%), and scleral thinning (33%). Anterior uveitis may

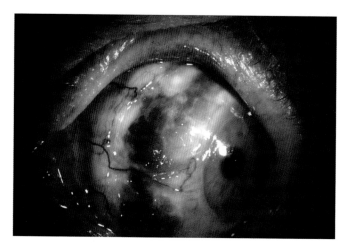

Figure 7-25   Necrotizing anterior scleritis without inflammation (scleromalacia perforans) in a patient with rheumatoid arthritis. *(Courtesy of Charles S. Bouchard, MD.)*

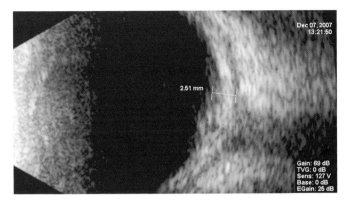

Figure 7-26 B-scan ultrasound of a patient with posterior scleritis demonstrating localized posterior scleral thickening. *(Courtesy of James J. Reidy, MD.)*

occur as a spillover phenomenon in eyes with anterior scleritis. Some degree of posterior uveitis occurs in all patients with posterior scleritis and may also occur in anterior scleritis when the overlying sclera is inflamed. Although one third of patients with scleritis have evidence of scleral translucency and/or thinning, frank scleral defects are seen only in the most severe forms of necrotizing disease and in the late stages of scleromalacia perforans.

A wide variety of corneal findings may coincide with scleritis. In rare cases, corneas may develop central stromal keratitis in conjunction with scleritis, associated with heavy vascularization and opacification in the absence of treatment. In diffuse or nodular scleritis, the corneal changes are usually localized to the area of inflammation.

In sclerokeratitis, the peripheral cornea becomes opacified by fibrosis and lipid deposition in conjunction with neighboring scleritis (which may be severe or very mild; Fig 7-27). The area of involvement may gradually move centrally, resulting in opacification

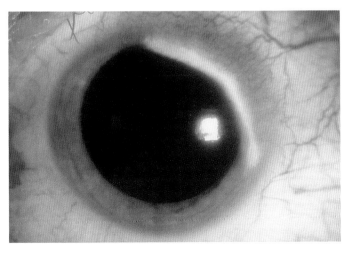

Figure 7-27 Sclerokeratitis.

of a large segment of cornea. This type of keratitis commonly accompanies herpes zoster scleritis but may also occur in rheumatic diseases.

LABORATORY EVALUATION   Scleritis can occur in association with various systemic infectious diseases, including syphilis, tuberculosis, herpes zoster, Lyme disease, cat-scratch disease, and Hansen disease. It is most frequently seen, however, in association with autoimmune connective tissue diseases such as rheumatoid arthritis, systemic lupus erythematosus, and seronegative spondyloarthropathies (eg, ankylosing spondylitis) or secondary to vasculitides such as Wegener granulomatosis, polyarteritis nodosa, or giant cell arteritis. Metabolic diseases such as gout may also, in rare instances, be associated with scleritis. More than one half of patients with scleritis have an associated identifiable systemic disease. The differential diagnosis of scleritis is similar to that of PUK (see Table 7-4).

Because patients with certain forms of scleritis, especially necrotizing scleritis, have an increased rate of extraocular morbidity, its presence should be recognized as a manifestation of a potentially serious systemic disease. The workup of scleritis should therefore include a complete physical examination, with attention to the joints, skin, and cardiovascular and respiratory systems. Usually, this is best done in conjunction with a rheumatologist or other internist with experience in diagnosing and managing these conditions. No single approach can be used in the diagnosis of these patients' possible underlying illness, and laboratory studies should always be guided by the history and physical examination. However, the following laboratory tests are generally recommended as an initial screening; other tests may then be ordered based on a more thorough rheumatologic (or infectious disease) examination:

- complete blood count (CBC) with differential
- erythrocyte sedimentation rate (ESR) or C-reactive protein (CRP)
- serum autoantibody screen (antinuclear antibodies, anti-DNA antibodies, rheumatoid factor, antineutrophil cytoplasmic antibodies)
- urinalysis
- serum uric acid
- syphilis serology
- chest x-ray
- sarcoidosis screen (serum angiotensin-converting enzyme and lysozyme), as appropriate

MANAGEMENT   Topical corticosteroids may occasionally reduce ocular inflammation in mild cases of diffuse anterior and nodular scleritis, but in general the treatment of scleritis is systemic. For nonnecrotizing disease, especially diffuse disease, oral NSAIDs may be effective. Some patients respond well to 600 mg of ibuprofen 3 times a day. Severe nodular disease and necrotizing disease almost always require more potent anti-inflammatory therapy. The use of tumor necrosis factor (TNF) inhibitors such as infliximab (Remicade) in rheumatoid arthritis–associated scleritis has shown promise in treating this difficult disease. Treatment is usually begun with oral corticosteroids. Although subconjunctival corticosteroids may be effective in reducing scleral inflammation, they have been reported to cause scleral necrosis and exacerbate epithelial defects; therefore, use of depot corticosteroid injections in these cases is generally contraindicated.

It is important to clearly define treatment goals: treatment failure may be considered as progression of disease to a more severe form (eg, nodular to necrotizing) or failure to achieve response to treatment after 2–3 weeks of therapy, in which case an alternate therapeutic strategy will need to be instituted.

Oral and/or high-dose (pulsed) IV corticosteroids may be effective for some cases of necrotizing scleritis or sclerokeratitis. If no therapeutic response is observed with corticosteroids, however, systemic immunosuppressive therapy with an antimetabolite (methotrexate), an immunomodulator (eg, cyclosporine), or a cytotoxic agent (eg, cyclophosphamide) is recommended. Although there is no consensus, most clinicians place rheumatoid arthritis patients on methotrexate and reserve more potent cytotoxic therapy for patients with active vasculitic disease such as Wegener granulomatosis. Patients receiving systemic immunosuppressive therapy for scleritis should be monitored closely for systemic complications associated with these drugs. Antituberculosis and anti-*Pneumocystis* coverage may be necessary for at-risk patients. Both the treatment and long-term management of these patients are best done as a collaborative effort between the ophthalmologist and rheumatologist.

In patients whose systemic evaluation is initially negative, it is important to repeat the workup annually.

Albert DM, Miller JW, Azar DT, Blodi BA, eds. *Albert & Jakobiec's Principles and Practice of Ophthalmology.* 3rd ed. 4 vols. Philadelphia: Elsevier/Saunders; 2008.

Jabs DA, Mudun A, Dunn JP, Marsh MJ. Episcleritis and scleritis: clinical features and treatment results. *Am J Ophthalmol.* 2000;130(4):469–476.

Clinical Approach to Neoplastic Disorders of the Conjunctiva and Cornea

In the United States, approximately 1 person in 2500 seeks ophthalmic care for a tumor of the eyelid or ocular surface each year, about 100,000 total. Benign neoplasms are at least 3 times more frequent than malignant lesions. Most of these tumors arise from the eyelid skin and are discussed in BCSC Section 4, *Ophthalmic Pathology and Intraocular Tumors,* and Section 7, *Orbit, Eyelids, and Lacrimal System.*

Neoplastic tumors of the conjunctiva and cornea are considered together because the lesions often affect both tissues in a similar fashion. These lesions are classified by cell type: epithelium, melanocytes and nevus cells, vascular endothelium, mesenchymal cells, and lymphocytes. Many are analogous to lesions affecting the eyelid. See also BCSC Section 4, *Ophthalmic Pathology and Intraocular Tumors.*

Shields JA, Shields CL. *Atlas of Eyelid and Conjunctival Tumors.* Philadelphia: Lippincott Williams & Wilkins; 1999.

Inclusion Cysts of the Epithelium

Inclusion cysts of the conjunctival epithelium are typically asymptomatic and are commonly found during routine ophthalmic examination (Fig 8-1).

PATHOGENESIS   Like epidermal cysts of the eyelids, cysts of conjunctival epithelium can be congenital or acquired. Most acquired cysts of the conjunctiva are derived from an inclusion of conjunctival epithelium into the substantia propria. As nests of epithelial cells proliferate, a central cavity forms lined by nonkeratinized conjunctival epithelium. The central cavity is filled with clear fluid. Conjunctival cysts may also form from ductal epithelium of the accessory lacrimal glands and are lined by a double layer of epithelium. Stimuli for cyst formation include chronic inflammation, trauma, and surgery.

CLINICAL FINDINGS   Conjunctival inclusion cysts typically appear clear and most commonly occur in either the bulbar conjunctiva or the conjunctival fornix. A corneal epithelial inclusion cyst is rare, but it can occur if trauma, surgery, or chronic inflammation results in conjunctival overgrowth onto the surface of the cornea. Dilated lymphatic channels may mimic an inclusion cyst of the bulbar conjunctiva.

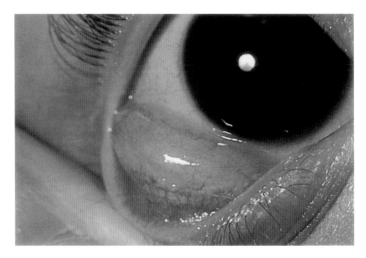

Figure 8-1 Large conjunctival epithelial inclusion cyst.

MANAGEMENT   Epithelial inclusion cysts are most commonly asymptomatic and there-fore may be simply observed. Cysts will usually re-form after simple drainage because the inner epithelial cell wall remains. Complete excision is necessary to prevent recurrence.

Tumors of Epithelial Origin

Table 8-1 lists the epithelial tumors of the conjunctiva and cornea.

Warner MA, Jakobiec FA. Squamous neoplasms of the conjunctiva. In: Krachmer JH, Mannis MJ, Holland EJ, eds. *Cornea.* 2nd ed. Vol 2. Philadelphia: Elsevier/Mosby; 2005:557–570.

Benign Epithelial Tumors

Conjunctival papilloma

The 2 forms of conjunctival papilloma, sessile and pedunculated, have etiologic, histo-logic, and clinical differences.

PATHOGENESIS   *Human papillomavirus (HPV),* subtype 6 (in children) or 16 (in adults), initiates a neoplastic growth of epithelial cells with vascular proliferation that gives rise

Table 8-1 Neoplastic Tumors of Ocular Surface Epithelium

Benign	Preinvasive	Malignant
Papilloma	Conjunctival and corneal intraepithelial neoplasia	Squamous cell carcinoma
Pseudoepitheliomatous hyperplasia		Mucoepidermoid carcinoma
Benign hereditary intra-epithelial dyskeratosis		

to a pedunculated papilloma of the conjunctiva. Although also usually benign, a sessile conjunctival lesion may represent a dysplastic or carcinomatous lesion, especially when caused by HPV-16 or HPV-18.

CLINICAL FINDINGS   A pedunculated conjunctival papilloma is a fleshy, exophytic growth with a fibrovascular core (Fig 8-2A). It often arises in the inferior fornix but can also present on the tarsal or bulbar conjunctiva or along the semilunar fold. The lesion emanates from a stalk and has a multilobulated appearance with smooth, clear epithelium and numerous underlying, small corkscrew blood vessels. Multiple lesions sometimes occur, and the lesion may be extensive in patients with compromised immunity.

A sessile papilloma is more typically found at the limbus and has a flat base (Fig 8-2B). The glistening surface and numerous red dots resemble a strawberry. The lesion may spread onto the cornea. Signs of dysplasia include keratinization (leukoplakia), symblepharon formation, inflammation, and invasion. A very rare variant is an inverted papilloma.

MANAGEMENT   Many conjunctival papillomas regress spontaneously. A pedunculated papilloma that is small, cosmetically acceptable, and nonirritating may be observed.

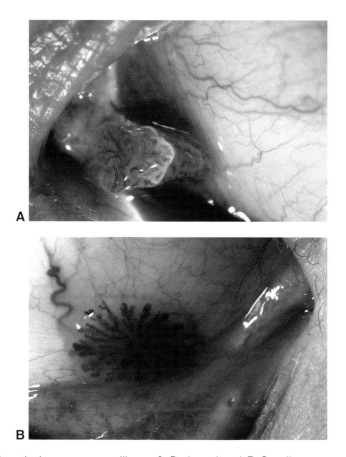

Figure 8-2   Conjunctival squamous papilloma. **A,** Pedunculated. **B,** Sessile. *(Reproduced with permission from Krachmer JH, Mannis MJ, Holland EJ, eds. Cornea. 2nd ed. Vol 1. Philadelphia: Elsevier/Mosby; 2005:559.)*

Spontaneous resolution may take months to years. An incomplete excision, however, can stimulate growth and lead to a worse cosmetic outcome. Cryotherapy alone, excision with cryotherapy to the base, or excision with adjunctive application of interferon-α_{2b} is sometimes curative, but recurrences are frequent. Surgical manipulation should be minimized to reduce the risk of virus dissemination to uninvolved healthy conjunctiva. Oral cimetidine (Tagamet) may be a systemic adjunct acting as an immunomodulator.

A sessile limbal papilloma must be observed closely or excised. If the lesion enlarges or shows clinical features suggesting dysplastic or carcinomatous growth, then excisional biopsy with adjunctive cryotherapy is indicated.

Preinvasive Epithelial Lesions

Conjunctival intraepithelial neoplasia

Conjunctival intraepithelial neoplasia (CIN), or *dysplasia,* is analogous to actinic keratosis of the eyelid skin. In CIN, the dysplastic process does not invade the underlying basement membrane and is referred to as mild (CIN I), moderate (CIN II), or severe (CIN III), depending on the extent of involvement of the epithelium with atypical cells. Related terms include *squamous dysplasia,* if atypical cells involve only part of the epithelium, and *carcinoma in situ,* when cellular atypia involves the entire thickness of the epithelial layer. See also BCSC Section 4, *Ophthalmic Pathology and Intraocular Tumors.*

PATHOGENESIS   The relative contributions to this condition of HPV infection, sunlight exposure, and host factors have not been determined. The lesion most commonly develops on exposed areas of the bulbar conjunctiva, at or near the limbus, in older male smokers with light complexions who may have been exposed to petroleum products or to the sun over long periods of time. Rapid growth may occur when the lesion is present in a person with AIDS. Systemic immunosuppression appears to potentiate squamous neoplasia. In a young adult, CIN should instigate a serologic test for HIV infection.

Macarez R, Bossis S, Robinet A, Le Collonnec A, Charlin JF, Colin J. Conjunctival epithelial neoplasias in organ transplant patients receiving cyclosporine therapy. *Cornea.* 1999;18(4): 495–497.

CLINICAL FINDINGS   CIN is usually found at the limbus in the interpalpebral zone. There are 3 principal clinical variants (Fig 8-3):

1. papilliform, in which a sessile papilloma harbors dysplastic cells
2. gelatinous, as a result of acanthosis and dysplasia
3. leukoplakic, caused by hyperkeratosis, parakeratosis, and dyskeratosis

Mild inflammation and various degrees of abnormal vascularization may accompany CIN lesions, but large feeder blood vessels indicate a higher probability of invasion beneath the epithelial basement membrane. CIN lesions are slow-growing tumors nearly always centered at the limbus but with the potential to spread to other areas of the ocular surface, including the cornea.

MANAGEMENT   The surgical management of CIN is the same as for squamous cell carcinoma of the conjunctiva and cornea. Excision should include 3–4 mm of surrounding,

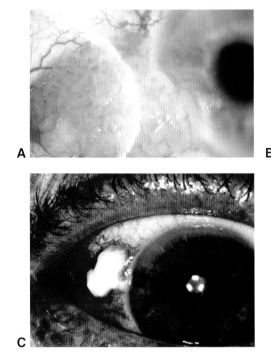
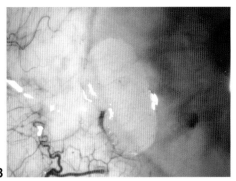

Figure 8-3 Conjunctival intraepithelial neoplasia: **A,** Papilliform. **B,** Gelatinous. **C,** Leukoplakic. *(Part A courtesy of James Chodosh, MD; parts B and C courtesy of James J. Reidy, MD.)*

clinically uninvolved, tissue. Rose bengal or lissamine green staining is useful to help delineate tumor margins. CIN has been reported to recur in approximately one third of eyes with negative surgical margins within 10 years and in one half of eyes with positive surgical margins. Lesions with dysplastic cells at the excision edge recur sooner than lesions that have been completely excised. Therefore, although excisional biopsy with adjunctive cryotherapy is still recommended, recent reports have focused on topical chemotherapeutic agents with the potential to treat the entire ocular surface without regard to surgical margins. Interferon-α_{2b}, mitomycin C, and 5-fluorouracil applied topically as eyedrops appear in some cases to completely eradicate CIN lesions. Long-term studies of newer therapies are still pending. Figure 8-4 summarizes the various treatment options for CIN and invasive squamous cell carcinoma.

Hardten DR, Samuelson TW. Ocular toxicity of mitomycin-C. *Int Ophthalmol Clin.* 1999;39(2): 79–90.

Koreishi AF, Karp CL. Ocular surface neoplasia. *Focal Points: Clinical Modules for Ophthalmologists.* San Francisco: American Academy of Ophthalmology; 2007, module 1.

Corneal intraepithelial neoplasia

The cornea adjacent to intraepithelial neoplasia of the conjunctiva can also be affected. Sometimes, the conjunctival or limbal component is not clinically apparent, and only a sheet or individual islands of well-demarcated, geographic, epithelial granularity are seen.

PATHOGENESIS Corneal intraepithelial neoplasia is associated with the same risk factors as CIN and presumably shares the same pathogenesis.

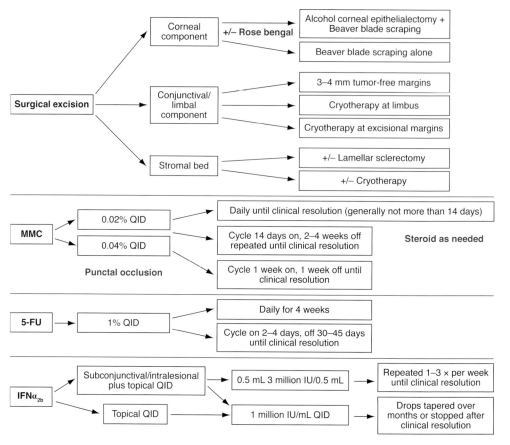

Figure 8-4 Treatment options for conjunctival intraepithelial neoplasia and invasive squamous cell carcinoma. *(Reproduced from Koreishi AF, Karp CL. Ocular surface neoplasia. Focal Points: Clinical Modules for Ophthalmologists. San Francisco: American Academy of Ophthalmology; 2007, module1.)*

CLINICAL FINDINGS　A granular, translucent, gray epithelial sheet broadly based at the limbus extends onto the cornea. Occasionally, free islands of punctate granular epithelium are present on the cornea. The edges of corneal lesions have characteristic fimbriated margins and pseudopodia-like extensions (Fig 8-5). Rose bengal and lissamine green staining help define the edges of the lesion. Corneal neovascularization does not typically occur, which helps to differentiate CIN lesions from limbal stem cell failure.

MANAGEMENT　Corneal involvement may be treated by applying absolute alcohol for 30–40 seconds to the affected part of the cornea and extending 1–2 mm into the normal cornea, followed by copious irrigation with balanced salt solution. The devitalized epithelium is then gently removed from the underlying Bowman layer with a surgical sponge, a blunt spatula, or a No. 64 Beaver blade. Care should be taken not to penetrate the Bowman layer. Excision of the grossly normal but often histologically abnormal adjacent limbal tissue is important, even if the lesion appears to be primarily corneal. Cryotherapy of the excisional margins of the conjunctiva, using a double rapid-freeze-slow-thaw technique,

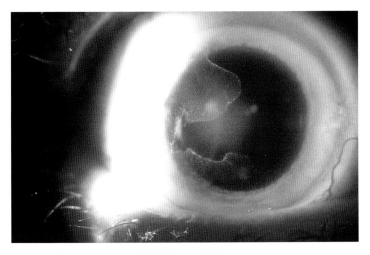

Figure 8-5   Corneal intraepithelial neoplasia. *(Courtesy of James Chodosh, MD.)*

can destroy any residual abnormal cells and possibly reduce the likelihood of recurrence. In cases where extensive surgical excision may lead to future ocular surface disease, or in cases of recurrent tumor, topical chemotherapy using mitomycin C, 5-fluorouracil, or interferon-α_{2b} has successfully eradicated ocular surface neoplasia. See the references in "Conjunctival intraepithelial neoplasia."

Malignant Epithelial Lesions

Squamous cell carcinoma

Squamous cell carcinoma, a plaquelike, gelatinous, or papilliform growth, occurs in limbal and bulbar conjunctiva in the interpalpebral fissure zone of older individuals.

PATHOGENESIS   Ultraviolet radiation is an important influence on the development of squamous cell carcinoma, but viral and genetic factors probably also play a role. Squamous cell carcinoma is more common and more aggressive in patients with compromised immunity and in those with xeroderma pigmentosum.

CLINICAL FINDINGS   A broad base is usually present along the limbus. The lesion tends to grow outward with sharp borders and may appear leukoplakic (Fig 8-6). Although histologic invasion beneath the epithelial basement membrane is present, growth usually remains superficial, infrequently penetrating the sclera or Bowman layer. Pigmentation can occur in dark-skinned patients. Engorged conjunctival vessels feed the tumor.

MANAGEMENT   When possible, complete local excision of the tumor, accompanied by adjunctive cryotherapy, is suggested. The treatment of choice includes excision of conjunctiva 4 mm beyond the clinically apparent margins of the tumor, along with a thin lamellar scleral flap beneath the tumor; treatment of the remaining sclera with absolute alcohol; and cryotherapy applied to the conjunctival margins. As with CIN, the risk of recurrence depends on the status of the surgical margins. If neglected, squamous cell carcinoma can

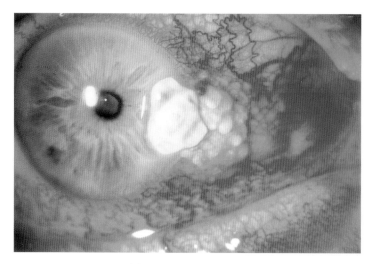

Figure 8-6 Limbal squamous cell carcinoma.

eventually invade the interior of the eye, where the tumor can exhibit vigorous growth. Invasion of the iris or trabecular meshwork provides the tumor with access to the systemic circulation and may be the route by which metastases occur. Orbital invasion may necessitate orbital exenteration. Radiation therapy may be indicated as adjunctive therapy in select cases.

The area of surgical resection may be closed primarily or left open to heal if the area of resection is small in size. An amniotic membrane graft may be used to cover larger defects. Amniotic membrane facilitates reepithelialization and minimizes postoperative inflammation. The graft should be cut slightly larger than the defect and may be fixated with either absorbable (9-0 or 10-0 polyglactin) or nonabsorbable suture (10-0 nylon). Tissue adhesive (eg, Tisseel; Baxter Healthcare, Dearfield, IL) may also be used to fixate the graft, thereby avoiding the need for suture removal and possible complications related to the presence of the sutures. If greater than two thirds of the limbus is removed, stem cell transplantation may be required.

Nordlund ML, Brilakis HS, Holland EJ. Surgical techniques for ocular surface reconstruction. *Focal Points: Clinical Modules for Ophthalmologists.* San Francisco: American Academy of Ophthalmology; 2006, module 12.

Shields CL, Shields JA. Tumors of the conjunctiva and cornea. *Surv Ophthalmol.* 2004;49: 3–24.

Tseng SCG, Tsubota K. Amniotic membrane transplantation for ocular surface reconstruction. In: Holland EJ, Mannis MJ, eds. *Ocular Surface Disease: Medical and Surgical Management.* New York: Springer-Verlag; 2002:226–231.

Warner MA, Jakobiec FA. Squamous neoplasia of the conjunctiva. In: Krachmer JH, Mannis MJ, Holland EJ, eds. *Cornea.* 2nd ed. Vol 1. Philadelphia: Elsevier/Mosby; 2005:557–570.

Mucoepidermoid carcinoma

Mucoepidermoid carcinoma, a very rare carcinoma of the limbal conjunctiva, fornix, or caruncle, clinically resembles an aggressive variant of squamous cell carcinoma. In addition to neoplastic epithelial cells, malignant goblet cells can be shown with mucin stains. Compared to squamous cell carcinoma, mucoepidermoid carcinoma is more likely to invade the globe or orbit. Treatment is wide surgical excision; adjuvant therapy can include cryotherapy and radiotherapy.

Spindle cell carcinoma

Spindle cell carcinoma is a rare, highly malignant tumor of the bulbar or limbal conjunctiva in which the anaplastic cells appear spindle-shaped like fibroblasts.

Glandular Tumors of the Conjunctiva

Oncocytoma

A slow-growing cystadenoma, an oncocytoma arises from ductal and acinar cells of main and accessory lacrimal glands. In older individuals, an oncocytoma may present as a reddish brown nodule on the surface of the caruncle.

Sebaceous Gland Carcinoma

Sebaceous gland carcinomas account for approximately 1% of all eyelid tumors and 5% of eyelid malignancies. They affect older individuals but may be seen in younger individuals after radiation therapy. They may masquerade as chalazia or as chronic unilateral blepharoconjunctivitis (Fig 8-7). See also BCSC Section 7, *Orbit, Eyelids, and Lacrimal System.*

Tumors of Neuroectodermal Origin

Table 8-2 lists the ocular surface tumors that arise from melanocytes, nevus cells, and other neuroectodermal cells. Some pigmented lesions of the globe are normal. For example, a *pigment spot of the sclera* is a collection of melanocytes associated with an intrascleral nerve loop or perforating anterior ciliary vessel. The term *melanosis* refers to excessive pigmentation without an elevated mass that may be congenital (whether epithelial or subepithelial) or acquired (whether primary or secondary). Conjunctival pigmentation can also occur from chronic exposure to epinephrine, silver, or mascara.

McLean IW. Melanocytic neoplasms of the conjunctiva. In: Krachmer JH, Mannis MJ, Holland EJ, eds. *Cornea.* 2nd ed. Vol 1. Philadelphia: Elsevier/Mosby; 2005:571–578.

Shields CL, Demirci H, Karatza E, Shields JA. Clinical survey of 1643 melanocytic and nonmelanocytic conjunctival tumors. *Ophthalmology.* 2004;111(9):1747–1754.

Benign Pigmented Lesions

Congenital epithelial melanosis

A conjunctival freckle, or *ephelis,* is a flat brown patch, usually of the bulbar conjunctiva near the limbus. It is more common in darkly pigmented individuals and is present at an early age.

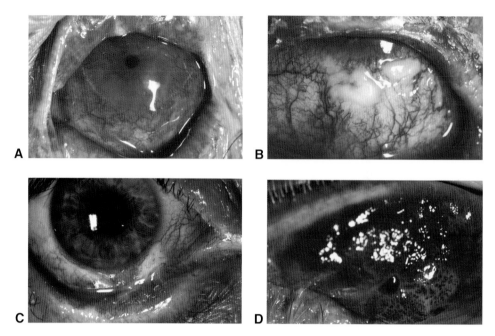

Figure 8-7 Sebaceous gland carcinoma: various presentations. **A,** Presents as a unilateral blepharoconjunctivitis with injection, pannus, thickened lid margin, and eyelash loss. **B,** White nodules composed of neoplastic sebaceous cells may be present near the limbus. **C,** Neoplastic symblepharon is present nasally. **D,** Upper palpebral conjunctival thickening. Papillary fronding may be present. *(Reproduced with permission from Krachmer JH, Mannis MJ, Holland EJ, eds. Cornea. 2nd ed. Vol 1. Philadelphia: Elsevier/Mosby; 2005:568.)*

Table 8-2 Neoplastic Tumors and Related Conditions of Neuroectodermal Cells of the Ocular Surface

Cell of Origin	Benign	Preinvasive/Malignant
Epithelial melanocytes	Freckle Benign acquired melanosis	Primary acquired melanosis Melanoma
Subepithelial melanocytes	Ocular melanocytosis Blue nevus Melanocytoma	Melanoma
Nevus cells	Intraepithelial nevus Compound nevus Subepithelial nevus	Melanoma
Neural and other cells	Neurofibroma	Leiomyosarcoma

Benign melanosis

Increasing pigmentation of the conjunctiva of both eyes is a common occurrence in middle-aged individuals with dark skin. This pigmentation is often most apparent in the bulbar conjunctiva. The stimulus to melanocytic hyperplasia is unknown but may be related to sunlight exposure. Benign melanosis is characterized by light brown pigmentation of the perilimbal (Fig 8-8) and interpalpebral bulbar conjunctiva. Streaks and whorls called *striate melanokeratosis* sometimes extend into the peripheral corneal epithelium.

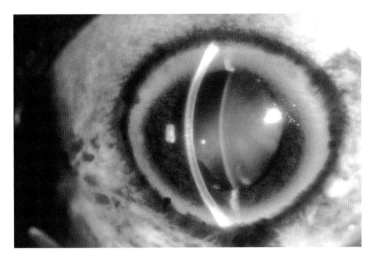

Figure 8-8 Benign acquired melanosis in a patient with corneal arcus. *(Courtesy of James Chodosh, MD.)*

Ocular melanocytosis

Congenital melanosis of the episclera occurs in about 1 in every 2500 individuals and is more common in the black, Hispanic, and Asian populations.

PATHOGENESIS Ocular melanocytosis consists of focal proliferation of subepithelial melanocytes (blue nevus).

CLINICAL FINDINGS Patches of episcleral pigmentation appear slate gray through the normal conjunctiva (Fig 8-9) and are immobile and usually unilateral. Affected patients may have a diffuse nevus of the uvea evident as increased pigmentation of the iris and choroid. About one half of patients with ocular melanocytosis have ipsilateral dermal melanocytosis (nevus of Ota) and a proliferation of dermal melanocytes in the periocular skin of

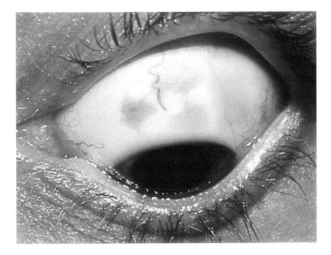

Figure 8-9 Episcleral pigmentation in a patient with congenital ocular melanocytosis.

the first and second dermatomes of cranial nerve V. The combined ocular and cutaneous pigmentations are referred to as *oculodermal melanocytosis.* Approximately 5% of cases are bilateral.

MANAGEMENT   Secondary glaucoma occurs in the affected eye in 10% of patients. Malignant transformation is possible but rare and seems to occur only in patients with a fair complexion. Malignant melanoma can develop in the skin, conjunctiva, uvea, or orbit. The lifetime risk of uveal melanoma in a patient with ocular melanocytosis is about 1 in 400, significantly greater than the approximate 6 per million risk of the general population.

Nevus

Nevocellular nevi of the conjunctiva are hamartias that arise during childhood and adolescence. A nevus can be junctional, compound, or subepithelial.

PATHOGENESIS   Pure intraepithelial nevi are rare except in children, and these junctional nevi may be difficult to distinguish histopathologically from primary acquired melanosis. The subepithelial nevus of the conjunctiva is the equivalent of the intradermal nevus of the skin.

CLINICAL FINDINGS   A nevus near the limbus is usually almost flat. Those appearing elsewhere on the bulbar conjunctiva, semilunar fold, caruncle, or eyelid margin tend to be elevated. Pigmentation of conjunctival nevi is variable; they may be light tan in color or amelanotic (Fig 8-10). A subepithelial nevus often has a cobblestone appearance.

Small epithelial inclusion cysts occur within about half of all conjunctival nevi, particularly the compound or subepithelial varieties. Secretion of mucin by goblet cells in the inclusion cysts can cause a nevus to enlarge, producing a false impression of malignant change. Cellular proliferation may induce secondary lymphocytic inflammation. Rapid enlargement can occur at puberty, giving rise to a clinical impression of conjunctival melanoma. When inflamed, an amelanotic, vascularized nevus may resemble an angioma.

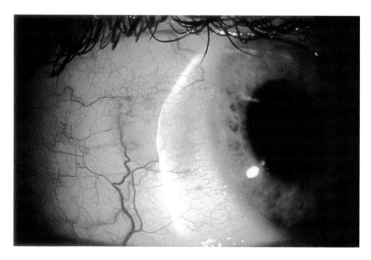

Figure 8-10   Amelanotic conjunctival nevus.

MANAGEMENT   Conjunctival nevi rarely become malignant and can be followed every 6–12 months with serial photography or detailed slit-lamp drawings that include dimensional measurements. Excisional biopsy should be performed on lesions that change. Because nevi are rare on the palpebral conjunctiva, pigmented lesions on the tarsal conjunctiva, the caruncle, or plica semilunaris, or in the fornix should be biopsied rather than observed.

Shields CL, Fasiudden A, Mashayekhi A, Shields JA. Conjunctival nevi: clinical features and natural course in 410 consecutive patients. *Arch Ophthalmol.* 2004;122(2):167–175.

Preinvasive Pigmented Lesions

Primary acquired melanosis

Primary acquired melanosis (PAM), an acquired pigmentation of the conjunctival epithelium, may be analogous to lentigo maligna of the skin (Hutchinson freckle), a preinvasive intraepidermal lesion of sun-exposed skin. It is usually unilateral and most often seen in light-skinned individuals. The term *primary acquired melanosis* refers to flat, brown lesions of the conjunctival epithelium (Fig 8-11). By definition, the condition differs from congenital pigmented lesions and from secondary acquired melanosis, such as that caused by Addison disease, radiation, or pregnancy. Table 8-3 compares the various pigmentary lesions of the conjunctiva. Most types of acquired melanosis remain benign, but in one study, PAM associated with cellular atypia progressed to conjunctival melanoma in 46% of cases. See BCSC Section 4, *Ophthalmic Pathology and Intraocular Tumors.*

Folberg R, McLean IW, Zimmerman LE. Primary acquired melanosis of the conjunctiva. *Hum Pathol.* 1985;16(2):129–135.

PATHOGENESIS   Abnormal melanocytes proliferate in the basal conjunctival epithelium of middle-aged, light-skinned individuals for reasons that are unknown. Pigmentation in an individual with dark skin is called *benign acquired melanosis* rather than PAM, but the 2 conditions may be related.

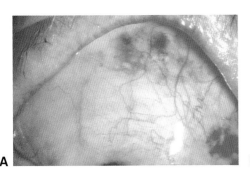
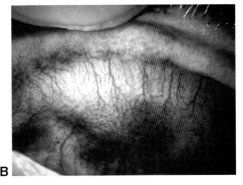

Figure 8-11   A, Primary acquired melanosis of the bulbar conjunctiva. **B,** Primary acquired melanosis of the palpebral conjunctiva. *(Part A courtesy of James Chodosh, MD; part B courtesy of James J. Reidy, MD.)*

Table 8-3 Clinical Comparison of Conjunctival Pigmentary Lesions

Lesion	Onset	Appearance	Location	Malignant Potential
Nevus	1st or 2nd decade	Discrete, brown or amelanotic, cysts	Conjunctival epithelium/ stroma	<1%
Ocular (racial) melanosis	Adulthood, dark-skinned, bilateral	Flat, patchy, brown	Conjunctival epithelium	Very rare
Ocular and oculodermal melanocytosis	Congenital	Flat, gray-brown	Episcleral	<1%, uveal melanoma
Primary acquired melanosis	Middle age, most often in Caucasians, unilateral	Flat, patchy, or diffuse	Conjunctival epithelium	50% with atypia
Malignant melanoma	Middle- to older-aged	Conjunctival stroma	Brown or amelanotic, nodular, vascular, growth	Overall mortality 25%

CLINICAL FINDINGS   Multiple flat, brown patches of noncystic pigmentation appear within the superficial conjunctiva of 1 eye. Changes in size may be associated with inflammation or may be the result of hormonal influences. Presence or absence of cellular atypia within these lesions can be definitively established only by biopsy. Malignant transformation should be suspected when a lesion shows nodularity, enlargement, or increased vascularity. Pigmented lesions located on the palpebral conjunctiva, conjunctival fornix, plica, or caruncle should increase clinical suspicion and lead to a biopsy.

MANAGEMENT   All suspicious pigmentary lesions of the ocular surface should be biopsied. If the lesions are multifocal, then multiple biopsies should be performed in order to establish the presence of atypia and its location. If the diagnosis of PAM without atypia is made, then the lesion(s) may be followed every 6–12 months. If atypia is present, then an excisional biopsy using the same techniques as for squamous neoplasia of the conjunctiva should be performed. For lesions that show atypia or malignancy, topical mitomycin C or interferon-α_{2b} may also be useful. Regional lymph nodes should be checked regularly.

McLean IW. Melanocytic neoplasms of the conjunctiva. In: Krachmer JH, Mannis MJ, Holland EJ, eds. *Cornea.* 2nd ed. Vol 2. Philadelphia: Elsevier/Mosby; 2005:571–578.

Malignant Pigmented Lesions

Melanoma

With a prevalence of approximately 1 per 2 million in the population of European ancestry, conjunctival melanomas make up less than 1% of ocular malignancies. Conjunctival melanomas are rare in black and Asian populations. Although malignant melanoma of the conjunctiva has a better prognosis than cutaneous melanoma, the overall mortality rate is 25%.

PATHOGENESIS   Conjunctival melanomas may arise from PAM (70%) or nevi (2%), or be de novo (10%). Intralymphatic spread increases the risk of metastasis. In rare cases, an underlying ciliary body melanoma can extend through the sclera.

CLINICAL FINDINGS   Although conjunctival melanomas can arise in palpebral conjunctiva, they are most commonly found in bulbar conjunctiva or at the limbus (Fig 8-12). The degree of pigmentation is variable; approximately 25% of conjunctival melanomas are amelanotic. Because heavy vascularization is common, these tumors may bleed easily. They grow in a nodular fashion and can invade the globe or orbit. Poor prognostic indicators include location in the palpebral conjunctiva, caruncle, or fornix; invasion into deeper tissues; thickness >1.8 mm; involvement of the eyelid margin; pagetoid or full-thickness intraepithelial spread; lymphatic invasion; or mixed cell type. Conjunctival melanomas may metastasize to regional lymph nodes, the brain, lungs, liver, and bone.

MANAGEMENT   An excisional biopsy should be considered for any suspicious pigmented epibulbar lesions; biopsy seems not to increase the risk of metastasis. The recommended treatment comprises excision of conjunctiva 4 mm beyond the clinically apparent margins of the tumor, along with a thin lamellar scleral flap beneath the tumor; treatment of the remaining sclera with absolute alcohol; and cryotherapy applied to the conjunctival margins. Primary closure is performed when feasible, but conjunctival or amniotic membrane grafts are necessary for large excisions. Sentinel lymph node biopsy performed prior to

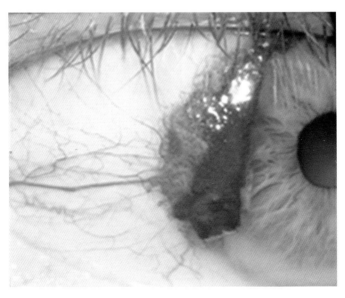

Figure 8-12   Malignant melanoma of the limbal conjunctiva. *(Reproduced with permission from Helm CJ. Melanoma and other pigmented lesions of the ocular surface. Focal Points: Clinical Modules for Ophthalmologists. San Francisco: American Academy of Ophthalmology; 1996, module 11. Photograph courtesy of Thomas Pettit, MD.)*

surgical excision may be helpful in establishing prognosis. Topical mitomycin C has been used after excision and cryotherapy to treat residual disease. Orbital exenteration is performed for advanced disease when local excision or enucleation would be insufficient to completely excise the tumor (when metastases have been excluded) or as palliative treatment for advanced, aggressive tumors.

Conjunctival malignant melanomas are potentially deadly tumors. In one study, metastasis was detected in 26% of patients, and death occurred in 13% of patients 10 years after surgical excision. Melanomas arising de novo (not in preexisting nevi or from PAM), tumors not involving the limbus, and residual involvement at the surgical margins were especially poor prognostic factors. The role of adjunctive radiotherapy has not been determined. Gene expression profiling is currently being evaluated to determine prognosis and might be beneficial in the future to determine response to targeted chemotherapies that are under development.

Esmaeli B. Regional lymph node assessment for conjunctival melanoma: sentinel lymph node biopsy and positron emission tomography. *Br J Ophthalmol.* 2008;92(4):443–445.

Finger PT, Sedeek RW, Chin KJ. Topical interferon alfa in the treatment of conjunctival melanoma and primary acquired melanosis complex. *Am J Ophthalmol.* 2008;145(1):124–129.

Seregard S. Conjunctival melanoma. *Surv Ophthalmol.* 1998;42(4):321–350.

Shields CL, Shields JA. Tumors of the conjunctiva and cornea. *Surv Ophthalmol.* 2004;49(1): 3–24.

Shields CL, Shields JA, Gündüz K, et al. Conjunctival melanoma: risk factors for recurrence, exenteration, metastasis, and death in 150 consecutive patients. *Arch Ophthalmol.* 2000; 118(11):1497–1507.

Neurogenic and Smooth Muscle Tumors

Subconjunctival peripheral nerve sheath tumors such as *neurofibromas, schwannomas,* and *neuromas* have been reported, especially in multiple endocrine neoplasia (MEN). A neurofibroma of the conjunctiva or eyelid is almost always a manifestation of neurofibromatosis, an autosomal dominant phakomatosis (see BCSC Section 6, *Pediatric Ophthalmology and Strabismus*). A *neurilemoma* is a very rare tumor of the conjunctiva that originates from Schwann cells of a peripheral nerve sheath. A *leiomyosarcoma* is a very rare limbal lesion with the potential for orbital invasion.

Vascular and Mesenchymal Tumors

Vascular lesions of the eyelid margin or conjunctiva generally are benign hamartomas or secondary reactions to infection or other stimuli (Table 8-4).

Benign Tumors

Hemangioma

Isolated capillary and cavernous hemangiomas of the bulbar conjunctiva are rare and are more likely to represent extension from adjacent structures. The palpebral conjunctiva is frequently involved with an eyelid capillary hemangioma. The presence of diffuse hemangiomatosis of the palpebral conjunctiva or conjunctival fornix indicates an orbital

Table 8-4 Neoplastic Tumors of Blood Vessels of the Eyelid and Conjunctiva*

Hamartoma	Reactive	Malignant
Nevus flammeus	Pyogenic granuloma	Kaposi sarcoma
Capillary hemangioma	Glomus tumor	Angiosarcoma
Cavernous hemangioma	Intravascular papillary endothelial hyperplasia	

*Tumors are not listed in a particular order, and lesions in 1 column do not necessarily correspond to those in parallel columns.

capillary hemangioma. A cavernous hemangioma of the orbit may present initially under the conjunctiva.

Nevus flammeus, a congenital lesion described as a port-wine stain, may occur alone or as part of Sturge-Weber syndrome, associated with vascular hamartomas, secondary glaucoma, and/or leptomeningeal angiomatosis. Some cases result from a genetic mutation coding for the vascular endothelial protein receptor for angiopoietin 1, which controls the assembly of perivascular smooth muscle. *Ataxia-telangiectasia* is a syndrome of epibulbar telangiectasis, cerebellar abnormalities, and immune alterations.

Inflammatory vascular tumors

Inflammatory conjunctival lesions often show vascular proliferation. *Pyogenic granuloma,* a common type of reactive hemangioma, is misnamed because it is not suppurative and does not contain giant cells. The lesion may occur over a chalazion or when minor trauma or surgery stimulates exuberant healing tissue with fibroblasts (granulation tissue) and proliferating capillaries that grow in a radiating pattern. This rapidly growing lesion is red, pedunculated, and smooth (Fig 8-13), bleeds easily, and stains with fluorescein dye.

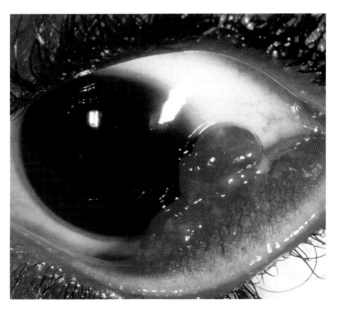

Figure 8-13 Pyogenic granuloma (in association with a chronically inflamed chalazion). *(Reproduced with permission from Krachmer JH, Mannis MJ, Holland EJ, eds. Cornea. 2nd ed. Vol 1. Philadelphia: Elsevier/ Mosby; 2005:452.)*

Topical or intralesional corticosteroids may be curative. Excision with cauterization to the base, primary closure of the wound, and generous postoperative topical corticosteroids may minimize recurrences.

Subconjunctival granulomas may form around parasitic and mycotic infectious foci. They have also occurred with connective tissue diseases such as rheumatoid arthritis. Sarcoid nodules appear as tan-yellow elevations that can resemble follicles. *Juvenile xanthogranuloma* is a histiocytic disorder that can present as a conjunctival mass. A *fibrous histiocytoma,* composed of fibroblasts and histiocytes with lipid vacuoles, arises on rare occasions on the conjunctiva or limbus. *Nodular fasciitis* is a very rare benign tumor of fibrovascular tissue in the eyelid or under the conjunctiva; it may originate at the insertion site of a rectus muscle. *Necrobiotic xanthogranuloma* is a very rare tumor that may affect the anterior orbit and eyelids. These lesions can present as subconjunctival or subdermal nodular fibrovascular tissue. Biopsy is essential to establish the diagnosis because it is often associated with paraproteinemias, multiple myeloma, or lymphoma.

Malignant Tumors

Kaposi sarcoma

Kaposi sarcoma, a malignant neoplasm of vascular endothelium, involves the skin and mucous membranes. Internal organs are occasionally involved as well.

PATHOGENESIS   Infection with Kaposi sarcoma–associated herpesvirus/human herpesvirus 8 (KSHV) is responsible for this disease. In young patients, it occurs most often in the setting of AIDS.

CLINICAL FINDINGS   On the eyelid skin, Kaposi sarcoma presents as a purplish nodule. Orbital involvement may produce eyelid and conjunctival edema. In the conjunctiva, Kaposi sarcoma presents as a reddish, highly vascular subconjunctival lesion that may simulate a subconjunctival hemorrhage. Lesions are most often found in the inferior fornix and may be nodular or diffuse (Fig 8-14). Nodular lesions may be relatively less responsive to therapy.

MANAGEMENT   Treatment may not be curative. Options for controlling symptoms include surgical debulking, cryotherapy, and radiotherapy. Local or systemic chemotherapy may be required. Intralesional interferon-α_{2a} has been reported to be effective.

Other malignant tumors

Malignant mesenchymal lesions that rarely involve the conjunctiva include malignant fibrous histiocytoma, liposarcoma, leiomyosarcoma, and rhabdomyosarcoma.

Lymphatic and Lymphocytic Tumors

Lymphoid tumors of the conjunctiva may be benign, malignant, or indeterminate. Many of these lesions have overlapping clinical and pathologic features. About 20% of patients with a conjunctival lymphoid tumor have detectable extraocular lymphoma.

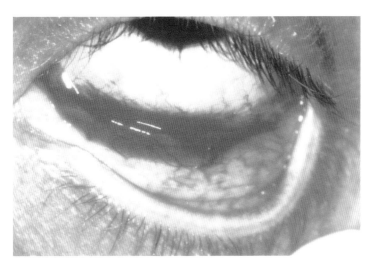

Figure 8-14 Kaposi sarcoma of the conjunctiva. *(Reproduced with permission from Holland GN, Pepose JS, Pettit TH, Gottlieb MS, Yee RD, Foos RY. Acquired immune deficiency syndrome. Ocular manifestations.* Ophthalmology. *1983;90(8):859–873. Photograph courtesy of Gary N. Holland, MD.)*

Lymphangiectasia and Lymphangioma

Lymphangiectasia appears on the eye as irregularly dilated lymphatic channels in the bulbar conjunctiva. It may be a developmental anomaly or can follow trauma or inflammation. Anomalous communication with a venule can lead to spontaneous filling of the lymphatic vessels with blood. *Lymphangiomas* are proliferations of lymphatic channel elements. Like a capillary hemangioma, lymphangiomas are usually present at birth and may enlarge slowly. The lesion appears as a patch of vesicles with edema. Intralesional hemorrhage, producing a "chocolate cyst," makes differentiation from a hemangioma difficult.

Lymphoid Hyperplasia

PATHOGENESIS Formerly called *reactive hyperplasia,* this benign-appearing accumulation of lymphocytes and other leukocytes may represent a low-grade B-cell lymphoma. Most patients are older than 40 years, although, in rare instances, extranodal lymphoid hyperplasia has occurred in children.

CLINICAL FINDINGS This mass presents as a minimally elevated, salmon-colored subepithelial tumor with a pebbly appearance corresponding to follicle formation (Fig 8-15); it is clinically indistinguishable from conjunctival lymphoma. It is often moderately or highly vascularized. Primary localized amyloidosis can have a similar appearance.

MANAGEMENT Lymphoid hyperplasia may resolve spontaneously, but these lesions have been treated with local excision, topical corticosteroids, or radiation. Biopsy specimens require special handling to complete many of the histochemical and immunologic studies. Fresh tissue is required for immunohistochemistry, flow cytometry, and gene rearrangement studies. Because a patient with an apparently benign polyclonal lymphoid lesion has the potential to develop a systemic lymphoma, general medical consultation is advisable.

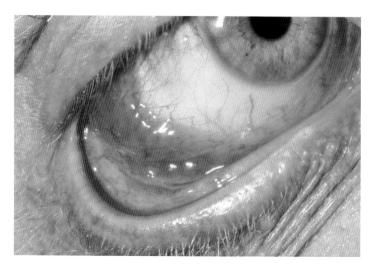

Figure 8-15 Conjunctival lymphoid hyperplasia.

Lymphoma

A neoplastic lymphoid lesion of the conjunctiva is generally a monoclonal proliferation of B lymphocytes.

PATHOGENESIS A lymphoma can arise in conjunctival lymphoid follicles. Some lymphomas are limited to the conjunctiva; others occur in conjunction with systemic malignant lymphoma. Some are polyclonal, but most conjunctival lymphomas are monoclonal B-cell lymphomas. Conjunctival plasmacytoma, Hodgkin lymphoma, and T-cell lymphomas are less common.

CLINICAL FINDINGS Non–Hodgkin B-cell lymphoma has essentially the same clinical appearance as benign lymphoid hyperplasia. It appears as a salmon pink, mobile mass on the conjunctiva (Fig 8-16). The lesions are usually unilateral; however, 20% are bilateral. A diffuse lesion may masquerade as chronic conjunctivitis. An epibulbar mass fixed to the underlying sclera may be a sign of extrascleral extension of uveal lymphoid neoplasia. Most patients with conjunctival lymphoma are either over 50 years of age or immunosuppressed.

LABORATORY EVALUATION AND MANAGEMENT Patients should be referred to an oncologist for systemic evaluation. Unless a tumor is small enough to be removed completely, incisional biopsy is indicated for histopathologic diagnosis. Local external beam radiation therapy is usually curative for lesions confined to the conjunctiva, but systemic chemotherapy is required for the treatment of systemic lymphoma. Cryotherapy and chemotherapy with interferon-α_{2b} have also been described.

Warner MA, Jakobiec FA. Subepithelial neoplasms of the conjunctiva. In: Krachmer JH, Mannis MJ, Holland EJ, eds. *Cornea*. 2nd ed. Vol 1. Philadelphia: Elsevier/Mosby; 2005:579–600.

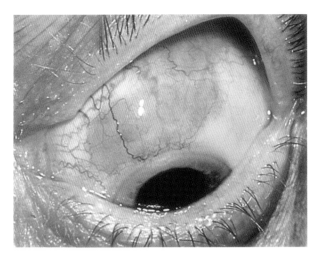

Figure 8-16 Conjunctival lymphoma.

Metastatic Tumors

Metastatic tumors to the conjunctiva are much less common than those to the uveal tract and orbit, but such tumors have arisen from cancer of the breast, lung, kidney, and elsewhere, including cutaneous melanoma. Metastatic lesions to the uveal tract, orbit, or paranasal sinuses can extend into the conjunctiva. Metastases or leukemic infiltrates to the limbus or cornea also occur.

Epibulbar Choristoma

Epibulbar Dermoid

The congenital *epibulbar dermoid* typically occurs on the inferotemporal globe or temporal limbus as a smooth, elevated, solid mass embedded in the superficial sclera and/or cornea (Fig 8-17). About 1 in 10,000 individuals is affected.

PATHOGENESIS An epibulbar dermoid results from faulty development of the eyelid folds and consists of displaced embryonic tissue that was destined to become skin. Dermoids are composed of fibrous tissue and occasionally hair with sebaceous glands; they are covered by conjunctival epithelium. Epibulbar dermoids are solid rather than cystic and are not fully entrapped beneath the surface, unlike dermoid cysts.

CLINICAL FINDINGS Dermoids are well circumscribed, porcelain white, round to oval lesions that occur most often at the inferotemporal limbus, but they can also be found on the central cornea, in the subconjunctival space, or in the orbit. Fine hairs may protrude from some dermoids. A limbal dermoid often has an arcuslike deposition of lipid along its anterior corneal border. Corneal astigmatism caused by a dermoid can lead to

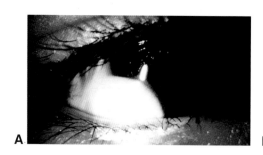 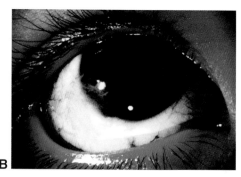

Figure 8-17 **A,** Limbal dermoid; note the fine hairs. **B,** Lamellar keratoplasty following resection of a limbal dermoid. *(Courtesy of James J. Reidy, MD.)*

anisometropic amblyopia. The flattest meridian of the cornea is adjacent to the limbal dermoid.

Dermoids are often associated with a congenital malformation known as *Goldenhar syndrome* (oculoauriculovertebral dysplasia), a sporadic or autosomal dominant syndrome of the first branchial arch, characterized by the presence of epibulbar dermoid, coloboma of the upper eyelid, preauricular skin tags, aural fistulae, and vertebral anomalies. BCSC Section 6, *Pediatric Ophthalmology and Strabismus*, discusses and illustrates Goldenhar syndrome in greater detail.

MANAGEMENT Dermoids grow along with the child and the eye and have virtually no malignant potential. The elevated portion of a dermoid may be excised, but the lesion often extends deep into underlying tissues. Some corneal astigmatism often remains after a shaving dissection of a limbal dermoid. Often, however, excision or shaving allows the fitting of a rigid contact lens. A relaxing incision or other corrective measure may also be considered. Lamellar keratoplasty can improve the cosmetic appearance and may reduce postoperative astigmatism.

Dermolipoma

A dermolipoma is a pale yellow dermoid containing adipose tissue that should be distinguished from herniation of orbital fat. It typically occurs superotemporally and may extend posteriorly.

Ectopic Lacrimal Gland

Lacrimal gland tissue occurring outside of the lacrimal fossa may be associated with a complex choristoma (see the following section), or it may occur alone as a round, pink, vascularized mass at the limbus.

Other Choristomas

A *complex choristoma,* usually on the superotemporal globe, consists of multiple tissues, including cartilage, bone, lacrimal gland lobules, hair follicles, hair, sebaceous glands, and

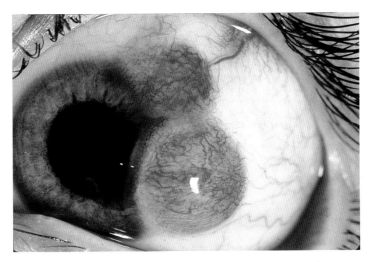

Figure 8-18   Complex choristoma showing rose coloring caused by the presence of richly vascularized ectopic lacrimal gland tissue. *(Reproduced with permission from Margo CE. Nonpigmented lesions of the ocular surface.* Focal Points: Clinical Modules for Ophthalmologists. *San Francisco: American Academy of Ophthalmology; 1996, module 9.)*

adipose tissue (Fig 8-18). An *osseous choristoma* is a solitary nodule of bone surrounded by fibrous tissue that is also located superotemporally. A *neuroglial choristoma* is more diffuse. A *phakomatous choristoma* is a subcutaneous nodule in the inferomedial eyelid composed of disorganized lens cells.

CHAPTER 9

Basic and Clinical Concepts of Congenital Anomalies of the Cornea and Sclera

Congenital anomalies are also discussed in depth in BCSC Section 6, *Pediatric Ophthalmology and Strabismus*. Chapter 18 of that volume covers diseases of the cornea and anterior segment. See also BCSC Section 2, *Fundamentals and Principles of Ophthalmology*.

Developmental Anomalies of the Globe and Sclera

Cryptophthalmos

Cryptophthalmos, or "hidden eye," is a very rare condition, with fewer than 150 reported cases. It is usually bilateral. The eyelids and associated structures of the brows and lashes fail to form *(ablepharon)*. The cornea is merged with the epidermis, and the anterior chamber, iris, and lens are variably formed or are absent (Fig 9-1). The conjunctiva is typically absent. *Pseudocryptophthalmos* occurs when the eyelids and associated structures form but fail to separate *(ankyloblepharon)*.

PATHOGENESIS Cryptophthalmos occurs in both isolated and syndromic form. The principal syndromic form is Fraser syndrome, a recessive disorder with a combination of acrofacial and urogenital malformations with or without cryptophthalmos. The disorder

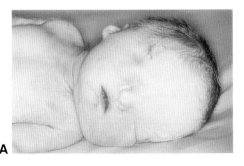
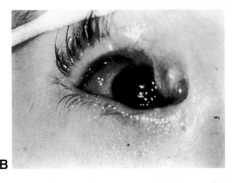

A   **B**

Figure 9-1   A, Complete cryptophthalmos, both eyes. **B,** Incomplete cryptophthalmos of the right eye, with eyelid fused to cornea superonasally.

results from mutations in the *FRAS1* gene located at 4q21, which encodes a putative extracellular matrix (ECM) protein.

CLINICAL FINDINGS Cryptophthalmos demonstrates equal sex distribution and equal occurrence in male and female siblings, consanguinity in families with more than 1 affected child, and lack of vertical transmission—strongly suggesting autosomal recessive inheritance. Associated ocular findings include corneal and conjunctival dermoid, absence of the lacrimal glands and canaliculi, and anterior segment dysgenesis.

MANAGEMENT Cryptophthalmos requires surgical intervention only for cosmesis or relief of pain from absolute glaucoma. Pseudocryptophthalmos may benefit from fornix reconstruction using buccal mucosal and amniotic membrane grafts, but ongoing management of the reconstructed eyelids to prevent secondary complications is necessary. See also BCSC Section 6, *Pediatric Ophthalmology and Strabismus*.

McGregor L, Makela V, Darling SM, et al. Fraser syndrome and mouse blebbed phenotype caused by mutations in FRAS1/Fras1 encoding a putative extracellular matrix protein. *Nat Genet*. 2003;34(2):203–208.

Stewart JM, David S, Seiff SR. Amniotic membrane graft in the surgical management of cryptophthalmos. *Ophthal Plast Reconstr Surg*. 2002;18(5):378–380.

Thomas IT, Frias JL, Felix V, Sanchez de Leon L, Hernandez RA, Jones MC. Isolated and syndromic cryptophthalmos. *Am J Med Genet*. 1986;25(1):85–98.

Microphthalmos

Microphthalmos is a small disorganized globe (Fig 9-2). There is often an associated cystic outpouching of the posteroinferior sclera. This condition has been associated with failure of the fetal fissure to close properly, and colobomatous defects of the iris, ciliary body, uvea, and optic nerve are often present.

PATHOGENESIS Normal embryonic development proceeds through at least the formation of the optic vesicle. Multiple associations have been made with microphthalmos,

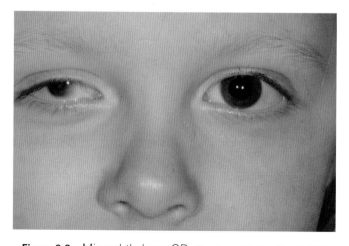

Figure 9-2 Microphthalmos OD *(Courtesy of Jeffrey Nerad, MD.)*

including trisomies of almost every chromosome (typically, trisomy 13), maternal infections, and exposure to toxins and radiation. Most cases of nonsyndromic microphthalmos are sporadic, although autosomal dominant, autosomal recessive, and X-linked forms have been reported. Isolated, nonsyndromic microphthalmos has been reported to map to the 14q23-q24.3 and 2q11-14 gene loci. Syndromic microphthalmos has been reported to map to the following gene loci: Xp22, 15q24.1, and 14q-22-q23. Mutations in the autosomal *CHX10, MAF, PAX6, PAX2, RAX, SHH, SIX3,* and *SOX2* genes have all been shown to be involved in the development of various forms of microphthalmos.

CLINICAL FINDINGS Associated ocular abnormalities may include leukomas, anterior segment disorders, retinal dysplasia, colobomas, cysts, marked internal dysgenesis, persistent fetal vasculature (PFV), small orbit, ptosis, and blepharophimosis. Systemic associations are numerous, including mental retardation and dwarfism among many others.

MANAGEMENT Associated conditions should be sought and managed appropriately, and genetic counseling should be considered. A cosmetic shell or contact lens may be indicated in selected patients.

Ferda Percin E, Ploder LA, Yu JJ, et al. Human microphthalmia associated with mutations in the retinal homeobox gene CHX10. *Nat Genet.* 2000;25(4):397–401.

Li H, Wang JX, Wang CY, et al. Localization of a novel gene for congenital nonsyndromic simple microphthalmia to chromosome 2q11-14. *Hum Genet.* 2008;122(6):589–593.

Verma AS, FitzPatrick DR. Anophthalmia and microphthalmia. *Orphanet J Rare Dis.* 2007;2:47.

Nanophthalmos

Nanophthalmos is characterized by a small, functional eye with relatively normal internal organization and proportions. Patients have a high degree of hyperopia (7–15 diopters [D]) due to a short axial length (15–20 mm). Patients also have a high lens-to-eye volume ratio that can lead to crowding of the anterior segment and angle-closure glaucoma.

PATHOGENESIS Nanophthalmos may be sporadic or hereditary, and both autosomal dominant (nanophthalmos 1) and autosomal recessive (nanophthalmos 2) inheritance patterns have been reported. One gene locus for the autosomal dominant form has been mapped to chromosome arm 11p. The recessive form of the disease is caused by a mutation in the gene encoding membrane-type frizzled protein (MFRP).

CLINICAL FINDINGS Patients have high hyperopia due to short axial length, high lens–eye volume ratio, thickened sclera, steep corneal curvature, narrow palpebral fissures, and crowded anterior segments associated with angle-closure glaucoma. Many patients have strabismus.

Histopathologic examination of the sclera from nanophthalmos patients has revealed frayed collagen fibrils and glycogen-like deposits. These findings might contribute to scleral inelasticity, which in turn leads to reduced intraocular volume, choroidal congestion, choroidal detachment, and/or exudative retinal detachment. Peripheral choroidal effusion can occur spontaneously. Large choroidal effusions or hemorrhage has been frequently encountered during anterior segment surgery.

MANAGEMENT Hyperopia and glaucoma are managed medically. Peripheral laser iridotomy, sometimes combined with peripheral laser iridoplasty, may be effective treatment of the angle-closure component. Cataract surgery may be complicated by uveal effusion or hemorrhage and exudative retinal detachment, although advances in small-incision surgery have reduced the frequency of these complications. Extremely high intraocular lens powers are required to achieve emmetropia.

Faucher A, Hasanee K, Rootman DS. Phacoemulsification and intraocular lens implantation in nanophthalmic eyes: report of a medium-size series. *J Cataract Refract Surg.* 2002;28(5): 837–842.

Othman MI, Sullivan SA, Skuta GL, et al. Autosomal dominant nanophthalmos (NNO1) with high hyperopia and angle-closure glaucoma maps to chromosome 11. *Am J Hum Genet.* 1998;63(5):1411–1418.

Yamani A, Wood I, Sugino I, Wanner M, Zarbin MA. Abnormal collagen fibrils in nanophthalmos: a clinical and histologic study. *Am J Ophthalmol.* 1999;127(1):106–108.

Blue Sclera

The striking clinical picture of blue sclera is related to generalized scleral thinning, with increased visibility of underlying uvea. This anomaly must be distinguished from the slate-gray appearance of ocular melanosis bulbi and from acquired causes of scleral thinning such as rheumatoid arthritis or staining from minocycline treatment.

PATHOGENESIS Genetic mutations and altered proteins have been identified for 2 syndromes associated with blue sclera:

1. *Osteogenesis imperfecta type I* is a somewhat common, dominantly inherited, generalized connective tissue disorder characterized mainly by bone fragility and blue sclerae. "Functional null" alleles of *COL1A1* on chromosome 17q21.31 or *COL1A2* on chromosome 7q22.1 lead to reduced amounts of normal type I collagen in most cases.

2. *Ehlers-Danlos syndrome type VI (EDS VI)* is a somewhat rare syndrome with autosomal recessive inheritance characterized by joint hyperextensibility, moderate to severe kyphoscoliosis, cardiac anomalies, and skin abnormalities of easy bruisability, abnormal scarring, and soft distensibility. EDS VI is associated with molecular defects in the gene for lysyl hydroxylase located on 1p36.3-p36.2 in some patients.

A third syndrome of brittle cornea, blue sclera, keratoglobus, and joint hyperextensibility may be the same as EDS VI but with a normal level of lysyl hydroxylase.

CLINICAL FINDINGS All 3 syndromes may share similar manifestations of fractures from minor trauma in childhood, kyphoscoliosis, joint extensibility, and elastic skin. Decreased hearing and tinnitus may also occur.

MANAGEMENT Regular hearing evaluations after adolescence are recommended. Oral bisphosphonate therapy may be specifically indicated for these patients. Postmenopausal women should engage in a long-term physical therapy program to strengthen the paraspinal muscles. Estrogen and progesterone replacement and adequate calcium and vitamin D intake are indicated. Fractures are treated with standard methods. Future therapies may include stem cell transplantation and gene therapy. See also Chapter 15.

Developmental Anomalies of the Anterior Segment

Anomalies of Size and Shape of the Cornea

Microcornea

Microcornea is a somewhat common condition that refers to a clear cornea of normal thickness whose diameter is less than 10 mm (or 9 mm in a newborn). If the whole anterior segment is small, the term *anterior microphthalmos* applies. If the entire eye is small and malformed, the term *microphthalmos* is used in contrast to *nanophthalmos,* in which the eye is small but otherwise normal.

PATHOGENESIS   The cause is unknown and may be related to fetal arrest of growth of the cornea in the fifth month. Alternatively, it may be related to overgrowth of the anterior tips of the optic cup, which leaves less space for the cornea to develop.

CLINICAL FINDINGS   Microcornea may be transmitted as an autosomal dominant or recessive trait with equal sex predilection. Dominant transmission is more common. Because their corneas are relatively flat, patients with microcornea are usually hyperopic and have a higher incidence of angle-closure glaucoma. Of patients who avoid angle-closure glaucoma, 20% develop open-angle glaucoma later in life. Important ocular anomalies often associated with microcornea include PFV, congenital cataracts, anterior segment dysgenesis, and optic nerve hypoplasia. Significant systemic associations include myotonic dystrophy, fetal alcohol syndrome, achondroplasia, and Ehlers-Danlos syndrome.

MANAGEMENT   If microcornea occurs as an isolated finding, the patient has an excellent visual prognosis with spectacles to treat the hyperopia resulting from the flat cornea. Concurrent ocular pathology such as cataract, PFV, and glaucoma may require treatment following the usual procedures for those conditions.

Megalocornea

Megalocornea is a bilateral, nonprogressive corneal enlargement with an X-linked recessive inheritance pattern. Rare cases of autosomal recessive inheritance have been reported. Affected subjects have histologically normal corneas measuring 13.0–16.5 mm in diameter (Fig 9-3). Males are more typically affected, but heterozygous women may demonstrate a slight increase in corneal diameter.

PATHOGENESIS   The etiology may be related to failure of the optic cup to grow and of its anterior tips to close, leaving a larger space for the cornea to fill. Alternatively, megalocornea may represent arrested buphthalmos and exaggerated growth of the cornea in relation to the rest of the eye. An abnormality in collagen production is suggested by the association

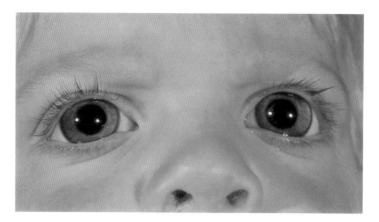

Figure 9-3 Megalocornea.

of megalocornea with systemic disorders of collagen synthesis (Marfan syndrome). The gene locus has been identified at Xq21.3-q22.

CLINICAL FINDINGS Megalocornea may be associated with iris translucency (diaphany), miosis, goniodysgenesis, cataract, ectopia lentis, arcus juvenilis, mosaic corneal dystrophy (central cloudy dystrophy of François), and glaucoma (but not congenital glaucoma). Systemic associations include craniosynostosis, frontal bossing, hypertelorism, facial anomalies, dwarfism, facial hemiatrophy, mental retardation, hypotonia, Down syndrome, Marfan syndrome, Alport syndrome, osteogenesis imperfecta, mucolipidosis type II, or occasionally other genetic syndromes.

MANAGEMENT Congenital glaucoma must be ruled out by IOP testing and careful biomicroscopy. Ultrasonography may be of value in determining the short vitreous length, deep lens and iris position, and normal axial length that distinguish megalocornea from buphthalmos caused by congenital glaucoma. Myopia and with-the-rule astigmatism are managed as in unaffected patients. Care must be taken during cataract surgery to implant the intraocular lens into the lens capsular bag. Standard-sized posterior chamber lenses are typically too short to be fixated in the ciliary sulcus, and anterior chamber lenses are similarly problematic in the enlarged anterior chamber.

Mackey DA, Buttery RG, Wise GM, Denton MJ. Description of X-linked megalocornea with identification of the gene locus. *Arch Ophthalmol.* 1991;109(6):829–833.

Cornea plana

Cornea plana is a rare condition that refers to a flat cornea, where the radius of curvature is less than 43 D, and readings of 30–35 D are common. Corneal curvature that is the same as that of the adjacent sclera is pathognomonic. Sclerocornea also features flat corneas, but it is distinguished by the loss of transparency as well (see Fig 9-8).

PATHOGENESIS Both autosomal recessive and dominant forms of cornea plana have been associated with mutations of the *KERA* gene (12q22), which codes for keratan sulfate proteoglycans (keratocan, lumican, and mimecan). These proteins are thought to play an important role in the regular spacing of corneal collagen fibrils. Investigators have speculated that mutations in the *KERA* gene cause an alteration of the tertiary structure of the keratan sulfate proteoglycans that leads to the cornea plana phenotype.

CLINICAL FINDINGS   Cornea plana is often seen in association with sclerocornea or microcornea. Other associated ocular or systemic abnormalities include cataracts, anterior and posterior colobomas, and Ehlers-Danlos syndrome. Cornea plana usually produces hyperopia, but any type of refractive error may be present because of variations in globe size. Angle-closure glaucoma occurs because of a morphologically shallow anterior chamber, and open-angle glaucoma occurs because of angle abnormalities. The majority of isolated cases appear in patients of Finnish ancestry.

MANAGEMENT   Refractive errors are corrected and glaucoma must be controlled either medically or surgically. Loss of central clarity may indicate penetrating keratoplasty (PK), but cornea plana increases the risk of graft rejection and postkeratoplasty glaucoma.

Lehmann OJ, El-Ashry MF, Ebenezer ND, et al. A novel keratocan mutation causing autosomal recessive cornea plana. *Invest Ophthalmol Vis Sci.* 2001;42(13):3118–3122.

Tahvanainen E, Villanueva AS, Forsius H, Salo P, and de la Chapelle A. Dominantly and recessively inherited cornea plana congenita map to same small region of chromosome 12. *Genome Res.* 1996;6(4):249–254.

Abnormalities of Corneal Structure and/or Clarity

The following group of conditions is associated with various congenital and/or developmental anomalies of the cornea and anterior segment. Reese and Ellsworth were among the first to link many of these conditions together, based on proposed anomalies during embryologic development, under the designation of *anterior chamber cleavage syndrome.* Other terms used in the past include *mesodermal dysgenesis, mesenchymal dysgenesis, iridogoniodysgenesis,* and *neurocristopathy.* Because of advances in our understanding of genetic control of embryonic development, these classification systems have become less useful.

Mihelec M, St Heaps L, Flaherty M, et al. Chromosomal rearrangements and novel genes in disorders of eye development, cataract and glaucoma. *Twin Res Hum Genet.* 2008;11(4):412–421.

Reese AB, Ellsworth RM. The anterior chamber cleavage syndrome. *Arch Ophthalmol.* 1966; 75(3):307–318.

Posterior embryotoxon

Posterior embryotoxon involves a thickened and centrally displaced anterior border ring of Schwalbe. The Schwalbe ring represents the junction of the trabecular meshwork with the termination of Descemet's membrane, and it is visible in 8%–30% of normal eyes as an irregular, opaque ridge 0.5–2.0 mm central to the limbus. The term *posterior embryotoxon* is used when the Schwalbe ring is visible by external examination (Fig 9-4). Posterior embryotoxon is usually inherited as a dominant trait. The eye is usually normal but can manifest a number of other anterior segment anomalies that are part of ocular or systemic syndromes, such as Alagille syndrome (arteriohepatic dysplasia), X-linked ichthyosis, and familial aniridia.

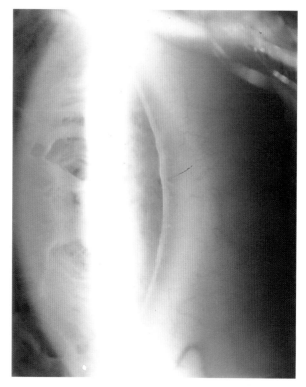

Figure 9-4   Posterior embryotoxon displaying a prominent and anteriorly displaced Schwalbe ring.

Axenfeld-Rieger syndrome

The conditions previously referred to as *Axenfeld anomaly* and *syndrome* and *Rieger anomaly* and *syndrome* have overlapping findings and have now been grouped into a single entity known as *Axenfeld-Rieger syndrome*. This syndrome represents a spectrum of disorders characterized by an anteriorly displaced Schwalbe ring (posterior embryotoxon) with attached iris strands, iris hypoplasia, and glaucoma in 50% of the cases occurring in late childhood or in adulthood (Fig 9-5). Associated skeletal, cranial, facial, and dental abnormalities are often present.

Transmission is usually dominant (75%) for the Axenfeld-Rieger group, but it can be sporadic. Evidence suggests that a spectrum of mutations of transcription factors located in chromosome region 6p25, known as *forkhead genes,* are responsible for many developmental defects of the anterior chamber of the eye.

> Nishimura DY, Searby CC, Alward WL, et al. A spectrum of FOXC1 mutations suggests gene dosage as a mechanism for developmental defects of the anterior chamber of the eye. *Am J Hum Genet.* 2001;68(2):364–372.

Peters anomaly

Peters anomaly is a central corneal opacity present at birth that may be associated with variable degrees of iridocorneal adhesion extending from the region of the iris collarette

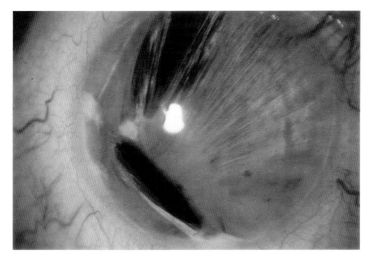

Figure 9-5 Axenfeld-Rieger syndrome exhibiting iris atrophy, corectopia, and pseudopolycoria. *(Courtesy of Vincent P. deLuise, MD.)*

to the border of the opacity (Fig 9-6). Approximately 60% of cases are bilateral. Associated ocular abnormalities are present in approximately 50% of cases. Ocular abnormalities include keratolenticular touch, cataract, congenital glaucoma, microcornea, aniridia, and PFV. Characteristic histopathologic findings in Peters anomaly include a localized absence of the corneal endothelium and Descemet's membrane beneath the area of opacity.

Peters anomaly has been associated with systemic malformations in up to 60% of patients. These abnormalities include developmental delay, heart defects, external ear abnormalities, hearing loss, CNS deficits, spinal defects, gastrointestinal and genitourinary defects, facial clefts, and skeletal anomalies. Although systemic malformations may

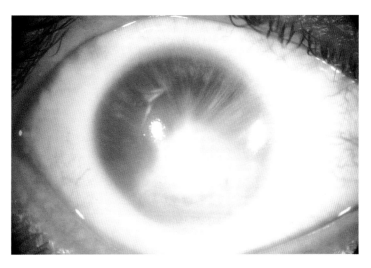

Figure 9-6 Peters anomaly.

be associated with genetically transmitted syndromes (trisomy 13–15, Peters-plus syndrome, Kivlin syndrome, Pfeiffer syndrome), these associations are the exception rather than the rule.

Most cases of Peters anomaly occur sporadically; however, both autosomal recessive and dominant modes of inheritance have been reported. Peters anomaly can be caused by mutations in the *PAX6* gene (11p13), the *PITX2* gene (4q25-26), the *CYP1B1* gene (2p22-21), and the *FOXC1* gene (6p25).

> Kivlin JD, Apple DJ, Olson RJ, Manthey R. Dominantly inherited keratitis. *Arch Ophthalmol.* 1986;104(11):1621–1623.
>
> Traboulsi EI, Maumenee IH. Peters' anomaly and associated congenital malformations. *Arch Ophthalmol.* 1992;110(12):1739–1742.

Circumscribed posterior keratoconus

The presence of a localized central or paracentral indentation of the posterior cornea without any protrusion of the anterior surface, as is seen in typical keratoconus, characterizes circumscribed posterior keratoconus. A variable amount of overlying stromal haze is also usually present. Loss of stromal substance can lead to corneal thinning approaching one third of normal (Fig 9-7A, B). Descemet's membrane and endothelium are usually present in the area of defect. Focal deposits of pigmentation and guttae are often present at the margins of the opacity. Most cases are unilateral, nonprogressive, and sporadic. Irregular astigmatism and/or amblyopia may occur. An autosomal recessive form of disease is associated with bilateral corneal changes, short stature, mental retardation, cleft lip and palate, and vertebral anomalies.

> Young ID, Macrae WG, Hughes HE, Crawford JS. Keratoconus posticus circumscriptus, cleft lip and palate, genitourinary abnormalities, short stature, and mental retardation in sibs. *J Med Genet.* 1982;19(5):332–336.

Sclerocornea

Sclerocornea, a nonprogressive, noninflammatory scleralization of the cornea, may be limited to the corneal periphery, or the entire cornea may be involved. The limbus is usually ill-defined, and superficial vessels that are extensions of normal scleral, episcleral, and conjunctival vessels cross the cornea (Fig 9-8). The most common associated ocular finding is cornea plana, which occurs in 80% of cases. Angle structures are also commonly malformed. No sex predilection is evident, and 90% of cases are bilateral. Multiple systemic anomalies have been reported in association with sclerocornea.

Sclerocornea is usually sporadic, but both autosomal dominant and recessive patterns of inheritance have been reported.

Keratectasia and congenital anterior staphyloma

Keratectasia and congenital anterior staphyloma are very rare unilateral conditions that are both characterized by protrusion of the opaque cornea between the eyelids at birth. They differ only in the presence of a uveal lining of the cornea in congenital anterior staphyloma. See Table 9-1 for a summary of developmental anomalies of the anterior segment.

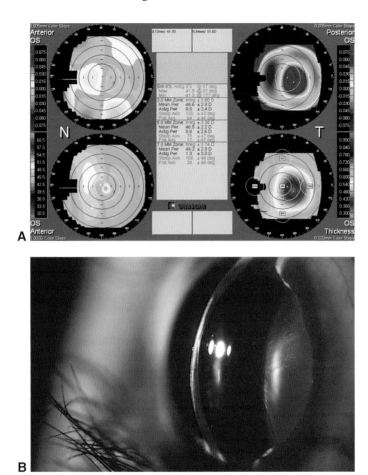

Figure 9-7 Circumscribed posterior keratoconus. **A,** Scanning-slit corneal topography shows a nasally displaced anterior corneal apex *(top left),* temporal paracentral posterior corneal vaulting *(top right),* normal anterior keratometry *(bottom left),* and significant loss of stromal thickness *(bottom right).* **B,** A slit-lamp photograph shows loss of stromal thickness, stromal haze, and posterior corneal crater. *(Courtesy of Kenneth M. Goins, MD.)*

PATHOGENESIS   Intrauterine perforation from an infection or from thinning following secondary failure of neural crest cell migration results in dermoid transformation of the cornea to stratified squamous epithelium, sparing the eyelids and conjunctiva. Keratectasia is probably not the result of abnormal development but rather of intrauterine keratitis or vitamin deficiency and subsequent corneal perforation. Histopathologically, Descemet's membrane and endothelium are absent, and a uveal lining is present (except in keratectasia). The cornea is variably thinned and scarred and the anterior segment disorganized, with the lens occasionally adherent to the posterior cornea, resembling unilateral Peters anomaly.

CLINICAL FINDINGS   An opaque, bulging cornea (Fig 9-9) is accompanied by a deep anterior segment. These cases are typically unilateral, and all are sporadic, with no familial or systemic association.

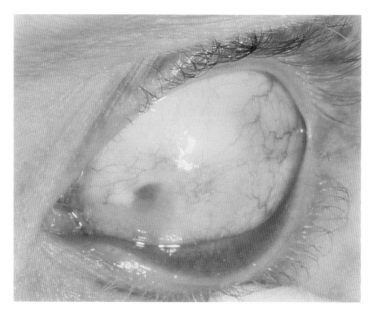

Figure 9-8 Sclerocornea.

MANAGEMENT   Except in very mild cases, visual prognosis is poor because of associated severe damage to the anterior segment. Penetrating keratoplasty and sclerokeratoplasty techniques may be useful to preserve the globe and improve cosmesis; however, enucleation may be required for a blind, glaucomatous, painful eye.

Other congenital corneal opacities

Congenital hereditary stromal dystrophy (CHSD)   This extremely rare dominant stationary dystrophy presents at birth with bilateral central superficial corneal clouding. The anterior corneal stroma exhibits an ill-defined flaky or feathery appearance. The cornea is clear peripherally. No edema, photophobia, or tearing occurs, but the opacities can be sufficiently dense to cause a reduction in vision.

Congenital hereditary endothelial dystrophy (CHED)   CHED is a cause of bilateral congenital corneal edema, but more common causes, such as birth trauma, posterior polymorphous corneal dystrophy (PPMD), and congenital glaucoma, must be ruled out. Two forms of CHED are recognized. The dominant form (CHED 1) presents in the first or second year of life, although expressivity is variable. It is slowly progressive and accompanied by pain, photophobia, and tearing, but nystagmus is not present. The cornea exhibits a diffuse, blue-gray, ground-glass appearance. The primary abnormality is thought to be a degeneration of endothelial cells during or after the fifth month of gestation.

The more common autosomal recessive type (CHED 2) presents at birth, remains stationary, and is accompanied by nystagmus. The bluish white cornea may be 2–3 times normal thickness and have a ground-glass appearance, but this finding is not associated with tearing or photophobia. There may be diffuse nonbullous epithelial edema. A uniform

Table 9-1 Developmental Anomalies of the Anterior Segment

Anomaly	Unilateral/ Bilateral	Clinical Findings	Associated Ocular Anomalies	Associated Systemic Anomalies	Inheritance	Gene Loci
Microcornea	Unilateral or bilateral	Corneal diam <10 mm or <9 mm in newborn; flat corneas with narrow AC; hyperopia	Persistent fetal vasculature; congenital cataracts; AC dysgenesis; optic nerve hypoplasia; cornea plana	Myotonic dystrophy; fetal alcohol syndrome; achondroplasia; Ehlers-Danlos syndrome	Dominant > recessive	
Megalocornea	Bilateral	Corneal diam. 13 mm or greater; typically seen in males	Iris hypoplasia; miosis; goniodysgenesis; cataract; ectopia lentis; arcus juvenilis; central cloudy dystrophy; glaucoma	Craniosynostosis; frontal bossing; hypertelorism; facial anomalies; dwarfism; facial hemiatrophy; mental retardation; hypotonia; Down syndrome; Marfan syndrome; Alport syndrome; osteogenesis imperfecta; mucolipidosis type II	X-linked recessive	Xq21.3–q22
Cornea plana	Unilateral or bilateral	Corneal curvature <43 D, typically 30–35 D. Cornea is clear; hyperopia is typical	Cataracts; anterior and posterior colobomas; narrow angle; angle closure; microcornea	Ehlers-Danlos syndrome	Dominant and recessive Finnish ancestry	12q22 KERA gene
Posterior embryotoxon	Usually bilateral	Thickened, centrally displaced Schwalbe line; seen in 8%–30% of normal eyes	Usually none	Alagille syndrome; X-linked ichthyosis; familial aniridia	Usually dominant	
Axenfeld-Rieger syndrome	Unilateral or bilateral	Anterior displaced Schwalbe line with attached iris strands	Iris hypoplasia and atrophy; corectopia; pseudopolycoria; glaucoma	Skeletal; cranial, facial, and dental anomalies	Dominant or sporadic	6p25 forkhead genes
Peters anomaly	60% bilateral	Central corneal edema present at birth; variable degrees of iridocorneal adhesion	Keratolenticular touch; cataract; congenital glaucoma; microcornea; aniridia; persistent fetal vasculature	Developmental delay; heart defects; external ear anomalies; hearing loss; CNS deficits; spinal defects; GI and GU anomalies; facial clefts; skeletal anomalies	Most cases are sporadic; however, both dominant and recessive inheritance have been reported	11p13: PAX6 gene 4q25-26: PITX2 gene 2p22-21: CYP1B1 gene 6p25: FOXC1 gene

(Continued)

Table 9-1 *(continued)*

Anomaly	Unilateral/Bilateral	Clinical Findings	Associated Ocular Anomalies	Associated Systemic Anomalies	Inheritance	Gene Loci
Posterior keratoconus	Typically unilateral	Localized central or pericentral indentation of the posterior cornea with normal anterior topography; overlying stromal haze; focal pigment deposits and guttae often present at the margins of the opacity	Astigmatism and amblyopia often present	Usually none	Sporadic	
Sclerocornea	90% bilateral	Nonprogressive, noninflammatory scleralization of the cornea. May be partial or complete. Limbus is ill-defined; vascularized	Cornea plana; angle anomalies	Multiple systemic anomalies have been reported	Most cases are sporadic; however, both dominant and recessive inheritance have been reported	
Congenital anterior staphyloma	Typically unilateral	Large, ectatic cornea protruding forward between the eyelids at birth lined by uveal tissue	Anterior segment anomalies; glaucoma; cataract	None	Sporadic	
Keratectasia	Typically unilateral	Large, ectatic cornea protruding forward between the eyelids at birth	Anterior segment anomalies; glaucoma; cataract	None	Sporadic	

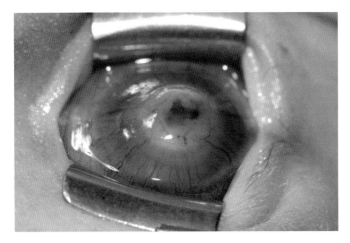

Figure 9-9 Congenital anterior staphyloma in Peters anomaly. *(Courtesy of Wallace LM Alward, MD.)*

thickening of Descemet's membrane may be seen, but no guttate changes are present. For further discussion, see Chapter 10.

Ehlers N, Módis L, Moller-Pedersen T. A morphological and functional study of congenital hereditary endothelial dystrophy. *Acta Ophthalmol Scand.* 1998;76(3):314–318.

Congenital Corneal Opacities in Hereditary Syndromes and Chromosomal Aberrations

Mucopolysaccharidoses (MPS) and *mucolipidoses* are disorders caused by abnormal carbohydrate metabolism. Corneal clouding and haziness may be present in early life in varying degrees in many of these entities, including Scheie syndrome (MPS I S) and Hurler syndrome (MPS I H). A more detailed discussion of these conditions appears in Chapter 11.

Secondary Abnormalities Affecting the Fetal Cornea

Intrauterine Keratitis: Bacterial and Syphilitic

Maternally transmitted congenital infections can cause ocular damage in several different ways:

- through direct action of the infecting agent, which damages tissue
- through a teratogenic effect resulting in malformation
- through a delayed reactivation of the agent after birth, with inflammation that damages developed tissue

A posterior corneal defect called *von Hippel internal corneal ulcer* may follow intrauterine inflammation. Often, signs of inflammation may still be present after birth, including corneal infiltrates and vascularization, keratic precipitates, and uveitis. Iris adhesions are extensive and may arise from areas apart from the collarette; the lens is usually involved.

Corneal ulcers and endophthalmitis were common complications of gonococcal ophthalmia neonatorum before the widespread use of silver nitrate prophylaxis and antibiotics. Neonatal conjunctivitis is discussed in Chapter 5.

Congenitally acquired syphilis infections caused by the *Treponema pallidum* spirochete can lead to fetal death or premature delivery. A variety of systemic manifestations have been described. Interstitial keratitis can develop in the first decade of life in children with untreated congenital syphilis. It presents as a rapidly progressive corneal edema followed by abnormal vascularization in the deep stroma adjacent to Descemet's membrane. The cornea may assume a salmon pink color because of intense vascularization, giving rise to the term *salmon patch*. Over several weeks to months, blood flow through these vessels gradually ceases, leaving empty "ghost" vessels in the corneal stroma. (See Chapter 7 for a more complete discussion of interstitial keratitis.)

Congenital Corneal Keloid

Corneal keloids are relatively rare lesions, most commonly described following corneal perforation or trauma. Congenital corneal keloids, often bilateral, have been described in Lowe disease (oculocerebrorenal syndrome) and the ACL syndrome (acromegaly, cutis gyrata, cornea leukoma syndrome). They can be seen in association with cataracts, aniridia, and glaucoma and may represent a developmental anomaly with failure of normal differentiation of corneal tissue. Histopathologic examination reveals thick collagenase bundles haphazardly arranged, with focal areas of myofibroblastic proliferation. Autosomal dominant inheritance has been observed in the ACL syndrome. Acquired corneal keloid is discussed in Chapter 12.

Congenital Corneal Anesthesia

Congenital corneal anesthesia is a rare condition that is often misdiagnosed as herpes simplex virus keratitis, recurrent corneal erosion, and dry eye. Most cases are bilateral and present with painless corneal opacities and sterile epithelial ulcerations during infancy and childhood. Rosenberg classified the disorder into 3 distinct groups: group I is associated with isolated trigeminal anesthesia, probably due to primary hypoplasia of the hindbrain; group II is associated with mesenchymal anomalies, which include Goldenhar syndrome, Möbius syndrome, and Riley-Day syndrome or familial dysautonomia (FD); group III is associated with focal brainstem signs without evidence of mesenchymal dysplasia.

A thorough systemic examination, including neuroradiologic studies, should be performed to rule out associated systemic conditions. In family linkage studies, FD, also referred to as *hereditary sensory and autonomic neuropathy type III,* is an autosomal recessive disorder that maps to chromosome 9q31-q33.

Treatment should include frequent topical lubrication, punctal occlusion, nighttime lid splinting, lateral tarsorrhaphy, amniotic membrane transplantation, scleral contact lenses and, in recalcitrant cases, conjunctival flap to stabilize the ocular surface.

Mathen MM, Vishnu S, Prajna NV, Vijayalakshmi P, Srinivasan M. Congenital corneal anesthesia: a series of four case reports. *Cornea.* 2001;20(2):194–196.

Rosenberg ML. Congenital trigeminal anaesthesia: a review and classification. *Brain.* 1984; 107(Pt 4):1073–1082.

Verpoorten N, De Jonghe P, Timmerman V. Disease mechanisms in hereditary sensory and autonomic neuropathies. *Neurobiol Dis.* 2006;21(2):247–255.

Congenital Glaucoma

Primary congenital glaucoma is evident either at birth or within the first few years of life. It is believed to be caused by dysplasia of the anterior chamber angle without other ocular or systemic abnormalities. Characteristic findings in the newborn include the triad of epiphora, photophobia, and blepharospasm. External eye examination may reveal buphthalmos, with corneal enlargement greater than 12 mm in diameter during the first year of life. (The normal horizontal corneal diameter is 9.5–10.5 in full-term infants.) Corneal edema is present in 25% of affected infants at birth and in more than 60% by the sixth month. It may range from mild haze to dense opacification in the corneal stroma because of elevated IOP. Tears in Descemet's membrane called *Haab striae* may occur acutely as a result of corneal stretching. They are typically oriented horizontally or concentric to the limbus. BCSC Section 6, *Pediatric Ophthalmology and Strabismus,* also discusses pediatric glaucoma.

Birth Trauma

Progressive corneal edema developing during the first few postnatal days, accompanied by vertical or oblique posterior striae, may be caused by birth trauma (Fig 9-10). Ruptures occur in Descemet's membrane and the endothelium. Healing usually takes place but leaves a hypertrophic ridge of Descemet's membrane. The edema may or may not clear; if it does clear, the cornea can again become edematous at any time later in life. High

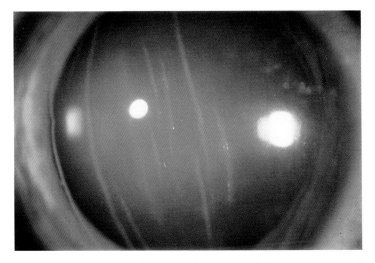

Figure 9-10 Birth trauma demonstrating vertical ruptures of Descemet's membrane secondary to traumatic delivery. *(Courtesy of Vincent P. deLuise, MD.)*

astigmatism and amblyopia may be associated. Congenital glaucoma can present with similar findings and should be considered in the differential diagnosis.

Arcus Juvenilis

Arcus juvenilis, a deposition of lipid in the peripheral corneal stroma, occasionally occurs as a congenital anomaly. Usually the condition involves only a sector of the peripheral cornea and is not associated with abnormalities of serum lipid.

CHAPTER 10

Corneal Dystrophies and Ectasias

Historically, *corneal dystrophies* are defined as bilateral, symmetric, inherited conditions that appear to have little or no relationship to environmental or systemic factors. Dystrophies begin early in life but may not become clinically apparent until later. They tend to be slowly progressive and more pronounced with age. Corneal dystrophies can be classified according to genetic pattern, severity, histopathologic features, biochemical characteristics, or anatomical location. The anatomical scheme that classifies the dystrophies according to the levels of the cornea that are involved is the one that has been used most often.

However, there are exceptions to each part of the dystrophy definition, as some dystrophies are unilateral and/or asymmetric, have no obvious heredity, and have associated systemic findings. In addition, dystrophies that appear the same phenotypically may map to different chromosomes, and dystrophies that map to the same gene (eg, *TGFBI*) may have different phenotypes. In order to more accurately reflect the genetic, clinical, and histopathologic characteristics of the dystrophies, the International Committee for the Classification of Corneal Dystrophies has revised the dystrophy nomenclature. The system is upgradable and can be retrieved at www.corneasociety.org.

According to the new system, each dystrophy is still organized according to the anatomical level affected, with a template summarizing genetic, clinical, and pathologic information. Furthermore, each dystrophy is assigned a category number reflecting the level of evidence supporting its existence:

Category 1: A well-defined corneal dystrophy in which the gene has been mapped and identified and specific mutations are known.

Category 2: A well-defined corneal dystrophy that has been mapped to one or more specific chromosomal loci, but the gene(s) remains to be identified.

Category 3: A well-defined corneal dystrophy in which the disorder has not yet been mapped to a chromosomal locus.

Category 4: Reserved for a suspected new, or previously documented, corneal dystrophy, although the evidence for its being a distinct entity is not yet convincing.

The category assigned to a corneal dystrophy may change with time as more information about it is obtained. Eventually, all valid corneal dystrophies should attain category 1 status. The new IC3D classification is summarized in Table 10-1. The genetics of corneal dystrophies is summarized in Table 10-2.

Weiss JS, Møller H, Lisch W, et al. The IC3D classification of the corneal dystrophies. *Cornea.* 2008;27(10:Suppl 2):S1–S42.

Corneal Dystrophies

Table 10-3 lists the MIM (Mendelian Inheritance in Man) numbers and abbreviations and the IC3D abbreviations.

Table 10-1 **The IC3D Classification of Corneal Dystrophies**

Epithelial and Subepithelial Dystrophies
1. Epithelial basement membrane dystrophy (EBMD): majority degenerative, some C1
2. Mutation in keratin genes: Meesmann corneal dystrophy (MECD): C1
3. Lisch epithelial corneal dystrophy (LECD): C2
4. Gelatinous droplike corneal dystrophy (GDLD): C1

Bowman Layer Dystrophies
1. Reis-Bücklers corneal dystrophy (RBCD), granular corneal dystrophy type 3: C1
2. Thiel-Behnke corneal dystrophy (TBCD): C1; potential variant: C2

Stromal Dystrophies
1. *TGFBI* corneal dystrophies
   A. Lattice corneal dystrophy
      a. Lattice corneal dystrophy, *TGFBI* type (LCD): classic lattice corneal dystrophy (LCD1): C1; variants (III, IIIA, I/IIIA, and IV): C1
      b. Lattice corneal dystrophy, gelsolin type (LCD2): C1 (this is not a true corneal dystrophy but is included here for ease of differential diagnosis)
   B. Granular corneal dystrophy: C1
      a. Granular corneal dystrophy type 1 (classic) (GCD1): C1
      b. Granular corneal dystrophy type 2 (granular-lattice) (GCD2): C1
      c. Granular corneal dystrophy type 3 (Reis-Bücklers, RBCD): C1
2. Non-*TGFBI* corneal dystrophies
   A. Macular corneal dystrophy (MCD): C1
   B. Schnyder corneal dystrophy (SCD): C1
   C. Congenital stromal corneal dystrophy (CSCD): C1
   D. Fleck corneal dystrophy (FCD): C1
   E. Posterior amorphous corneal dystrophy (PACD): C3
   F. Central cloudy dystrophy of François (CCDF): C4
   G. Pre-Descemet corneal dystrophy (PDCD): C4

Descemet Membrane and Endothelial Dystrophies
1. Fuchs endothelial corneal dystrophy (FECD): C1, C2, or C3
2. Posterior polymorphous corneal dystrophy (PPCD): C1 or C2
3. Congenital hereditary endothelial dystrophy (CHED1): C2
4. Congenital hereditary endothelial dystrophy (CHED2): C1

C = category.

Modified from Weiss JS, Møller H, Lisch W, et al. The IC3D classification of the corneal dystrophies. *Cornea.* 2008;27(10:Suppl 2):S1–S42.

Table 10-2 Genetics of Corneal Dystrophies

Dystrophy	Gene Locus	Gene	Category
Epithelial basement membrane	5q31	*TGFBI* in the minority of cases	C1 (in a minority of cases); most are sporadic
Meesmann	12q13 17q12	Keratin K3 (*KRT3*) Keratin K12 (*KRT12*)	C1
Lisch	Xp22.3	Unknown	C2
Gelatinous droplike	1p32	TACSTD2	C1
Reis-Bücklers	5q31	TGFBI	C1
Thiel-Behnke	5q31	TGFBI	C1
	10q24	Unknown	C2
Lattice type 1	5q31	TGFBI	C1
Lattice type 2	9q34	Gelsolin (*GSN*)	C1 (not a true dystrophy)
Granular type 2	5q31	TGFBI	C1
Macular	16q22	Carbohydrate sulfotransferase 6 (*CHST6*)	C1
Schnyder	1p36	UbiA prenyltransferase domain-containing protein 1 (*UBIAD1*)	C1
Congenital stromal	12q21.33	Decorin (*DCN*)	C1
Fleck	2q35	Phosphatidylinositol-3-phosphate/phosphatidylinositol 5-kinase type III (PIP5K3)	C1
Posterior amorphous	Unknown	Unknown	C3
Central cloudy dystrophy of François	None	None	C4
Pre-Descemet	Unknown	Unknown	C4
Fuchs	None (most commonly)	None	C3 (Fuchs in patients with no known inheritance)
	13pTel-13q12.13,15q,18q21.2-q21.32	Unknown	C2 (Fuchs with known genetic loci but gene not yet localized)
	Early-onset variant: 1p34.3-p32	COL8A2	C1 (early-onset Fuchs)
Posterior polymorphous	PPCD1: 20p11.2-q11.2	Unknown	C2
	PPCD2: 1p34.3-p32.3	COL8A2	C1
	PPCD3: 10p11.2	ZEB1	C1
Congenital hereditary 1	20p11.2-q11.2	Unknown	C2
Congenital hereditary 2	20p13	SLC4A11	C1

C = category.

From Weiss JS, Møller H, Lisch W, et al. The IC3D classification of the corneal dystrophies. *Cornea.* 2008;27(10:Suppl 2).

Table 10-3 The IC3D Classification—Abbreviations and MIM Number

	MIM Abbreviation	IC3D Abbreviation	MIM #
Epithelial basement membrane dystrophy	EBMD	EBMD	121820
Meesmann CD	None	MECD	122100
Lisch epithelial CD	None	LECD	None
Gelatinous droplike CD	GDLD, CDGDL	GDLD	204870
Reis-Bücklers CD	CDB1, CDRB, RBCD	RBCD	608470
Thiel-Behnke CD	CDB2, CDTB	TBCD	602082
Classic lattice CD	CDL1	LCD1	122200
Lattice CD, gelsolin type	None	LCD2	105120
Granular CD, type 1	CGDD1	GCD1	121900
Granular CD, type 2 (granular–lattice)	CDA, ACD	GCD2	607541
Macular CD	MCDC1	MCD	217800
Schnyder CD	None	SCD	121800
Congenital stromal CD	CSCD	CSCD	610048
Fleck CD	None	FCD	121850
Posterior amorphous CD	None	PACD	None
Central cloudy dystrophy of François	None	CCDF	217600
Pre-Descemet CD	None	PDCD	None
Fuchs endothelial CD	FECD1	FECD	136800
Posterior polymorphous CD	PPCD1	PPCD	122000
Congenital hereditary endothelial dystrophy 1	CHED1	CHED1	121700
Congenital hereditary endothelial dystrophy 2	CHED2	CHED2	217700

CD = corneal dystrophy, MIM = Mendelian Inheritance in Man.

From OMIM (http://www.ncbi.nlm.nih.gov/omim) and from Weiss JS, Møller H, Lisch W, et al. The IC3D classification of the corneal dystrophies. *Cornea*. 2008;27(10:Suppl 2):S6.

Epithelial and Subepithelial Dystrophies

Epithelial basement membrane dystrophy (EBMD)

Alternative names Map-dot-fingerprint dystrophy, Cogan microcystic epithelial dystrophy, anterior basement membrane dystrophy

Inheritance May have dominant inheritance (often with incomplete penetrance) but is more often sporadic (ie, no documented inheritance)

Genetics Locus 5q31; gene *TGFBI* (previously referred to as *Big-H3*) in a minority of cases

Category Most cases are sporadic; some are category 1.

PATHOLOGY EBMD is an abnormality of epithelial turnover, maturation, and production of basement membrane. Histopathologic findings include the following:

- a thickened basement membrane with extension into the epithelium
- abnormal epithelial cells with microcysts (often with absent or abnormal hemidesmosomes)
- fibrillar material between the basement membrane and Bowman layer

CLINICAL FINDINGS EBMD occurs in 6%–18% of the population, more commonly in women, with increasing frequency over the age of 50 years. Gray patches, microcysts, and/or fine lines in the corneal epithelium are seen on examination. These are usually best seen with sclerotic scatter, retroillumination, or a broad tangential beam. Four kinds of lesions are seen in the epithelium and its immediately subjacent basement membrane:

1. fingerprint lines
2. map lines
3. dots or microcysts
4. bleb or cobblestone-like pattern

These abnormalities occur in varying combinations and change in number and distribution from time to time. *Fingerprint lines* are thin, relucent, hairlike lines; several of them are often arranged in a concentric pattern so they resemble fingerprints. *Map lines* are the same as fingerprint lines except thicker, more irregular, and surrounded by a faint haze; they resemble irregular coastlines or geographic borders on maps (Fig 10-1). Maps and fingerprints consist of thickened or multilaminar strips of epithelial basement membrane. Dots (in Cogan microcystic epithelial dystrophy) are intraepithelial spaces containing the debris of epithelial cells that have collapsed and degenerated before having reached the epithelial surface (Fig 10-2). The gray-white dots have discrete edges.

Symptoms that are related to recurrent epithelial erosions and to transient blurred vision are more common in patients older than 30 but can be seen at any age. It is estimated that 10% of patients with EBMD will have corneal erosions and that 50% of patients with recurrent epithelial erosions have evidence of this anterior dystrophy. Both eyes must be examined because evidence of the dystrophy may be found in the uninvolved

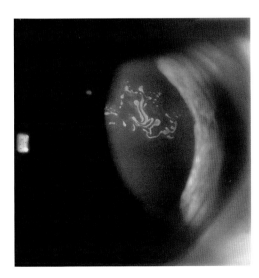

Figure 10-1 Epithelial basement membrane dystrophy, showing thick geographic map lines, or "putty marks."

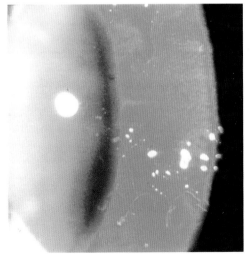

Figure 10-2 Epithelial basement membrane dystrophy, showing microcysts and geographic map line areas. *(Courtesy of Vincent P. deLuise, MD.)*

eye. Unilateral epithelial basement membrane changes may be related to localized trauma rather than a dystrophy. In some circumstances, clinical findings may mimic corneal intraepithelial dysplasia, and removed material should be submitted for histopathology.

MANAGEMENT   Treatment may need to be extended for months. It consists of varying combinations of the following (see also the discussion of recurrent corneal erosions in Chapter 3):

- 5% sodium chloride drops or ointment vs. lubricating drops or ointment
- epithelial debridement
- patching
- fitting of a thin, loose bandage (soft contact) lens

Recalcitrant cases of recurrent corneal erosion may benefit from anterior stromal puncture of the epithelium using a bent 20- to 25-gauge needle (0.1 mm is sufficient depth). The visual axis should be avoided. Multiple small punctures disturb the Bowman layer, thereby promoting a tighter adhesion and stimulating the cornea to produce functional basement membrane complexes. The Nd:YAG laser and 5-mm diamond burr have also been reported to be effective in creating anterior stromal disturbance as treatment of recurrent erosion. Removal of damaged epithelium alone may be very effective. *Phototherapeutic keratectomy (PTK)* with excimer laser into the anterior 2–4 μm of Bowman membrane after removal of the epithelium may be used for central or recurrent erosions. Recurrence of erosive symptoms after PTK occurs in 13%–44% of patients and may require repetition of PTK.

Boutboul S, Black GC, Moore JE, et al. A subset of patients with epithelial basement membrane corneal dystrophy have mutations in TGFBI/BIGH3. *Hum Mutat.* 2006;27(6):553–557.

Mutation in keratin genes: Meesmann corneal dystrophy (MECD)

Alternative names   Juvenile hereditary epithelial dystrophy; variant: Stocker-Holt

Inheritance   Autosomal dominant

Genetics   Locus 12q13; gene: keratin K3 *(KRT3)*; Stocker-Holt variant: locus 17q12, gene: keratin K12 *(KRT12)*

Category   1 (including the Stocker-Holt variant)

PATHOLOGY   In MECD, epithelial microcysts are seen that consist of degenerated epithelial cell products (PAS-positive cellular debris that fluoresces). The epithelial cells contain an electron-dense accumulation of granular and filamentary material ("peculiar substance"). There are frequent mitoses and a thickened basement membrane with projections into the basal epithelium; the basal epithelial cells have increased glycogen. On confocal microscopy, hyporeflective areas are seen in the basal epithelium ranging from 40 to 150 μm in diameter, with potential reflective spots inside.

CLINICAL FINDINGS   MECD appears very early in life. Tiny epithelial vesicles are seen—most easily with retroillumination—extending out to the limbus. These appear as tiny,

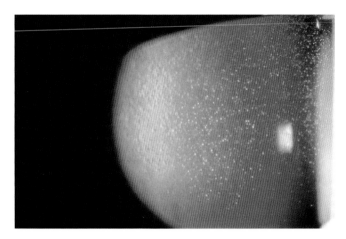

Figure 10-3 Meesmann dystrophy, appearing as tiny, bubblelike blebs against the red reflex. *(Courtesy of Vincent P. deLuise, MD.)*

bubblelike blebs and are most numerous in the interpalpebral area (Fig 10-3). The surrounding epithelium is clear. Whorled and wedge-shaped epithelial patterns may be seen. The cornea may be slightly thinned and corneal sensation may be reduced. Symptoms are usually limited to mild irritation and a slight decrease in visual acuity. Some patients complain of glare and light sensitivity. Painful recurrent erosions may occur.

MANAGEMENT   Most patients require no treatment, but soft contact lens wear may be helpful if patients show frequent symptoms. In rare instances, superficial PTK may be useful for reducing symptoms.

> Tuft S, Bron AJ. Imaging the microstructural abnormalities of Meesmann corneal dystrophy by in vivo confocal microscopy. *Cornea.* 2006;25(7):868–870.

Lisch epithelial corneal dystrophy (LECD)

Alternative names   Band-shaped and whorled microcystic dystrophy of the corneal epithelium

Inheritance   X-chromosomal dominant

Genetics   Locus Xp22.3; gene unknown

Category   2

PATHOLOGY   Diffuse cytoplasmic vacuolization of affected cells is seen in light and transmission electron microscopy. On immunohistochemistry, there is scattered staining on Ki67 without evidence of increased mitotic activity. Confocal microscopy shows many solitary dark round and oval lesions (50–100 μm). Some lesions show central reflective points (probably cell nuclei).

CLINICAL FINDINGS   On direct slit-lamp examination, gray, band-shaped, and feathery lesions appear in whorled patterns. Retroillumination reveals intraepithelial, densely

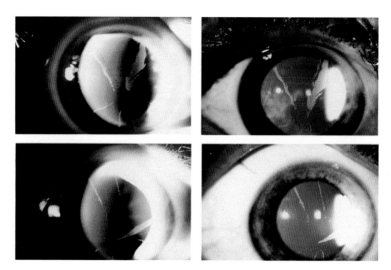

Figure 10-4 Lisch corneal dystrophy characterized by bands of gray, feathery opacities. Retroillumination shows clear, densely crowded microcysts. *(Reproduced with permission from Lisch W, Büttner A, Oeffner F, et al. Lisch corneal dystrophy is genetically distinct from Meesmann corneal dystrophy and maps to xp22.3. Am J Ophthalmol. 2000;130(4):461–468.)*

crowded clear microcysts. The surrounding epithelium is clear (Fig 10-4). In Meesmann dystrophy, such band-shaped, feathery lesions in whorled patterns do not exist. Also, the intraepithelial cysts of Meesmann are not as densely crowded as in Lisch dystrophy but are isolated, with clear spaces between the cysts.

MANAGEMENT   Patients with Lisch dystrophy are pain-free. There may be an associated decrease in acuity. Corneal debridement may be attempted but often results in recurrence. Contact lenses may be helpful for more severe cases.

Alvarez-Fischer M, de Toledo JA, Barraquer RI. Lisch corneal dystrophy. *Cornea.* 2005;24(4): 494–495.

Lisch W, Büttner A, Oeffner F, et al. Lisch corneal dystrophy is genetically distinct from Meesmann corneal dystrophy and maps to xp22.3. *Am J Ophthalmol.* 2000;130(4):461–468.

Gelatinous droplike corneal dystrophy (GDLD)

Alternative names   Subepithelial amyloidosis, primary familial amyloidosis

Inheritance   Autosomal recessive

Genetics   Locus 1p32; gene: tumor-associated calcium signal transducer 2 *(TACSTD2)*

Category   1

PATHOLOGY   Light microscopy demonstrates subepithelial and stromal amyloid deposits. Disruption of epithelial tight junctions leads to abnormally high epithelial permeability. Amyloid deposition is noted in the basal epithelial layer on transmission electron microscopy.

CLINICAL FINDINGS   Onset occurs in the first to second decade of life with subepithelial lesions that may appear similar to band keratopathy or with groups of small multiple nodules (mulberry configuration). The lesions show on fluorescein staining. There is a significant decrease in vision, with photophobia, irritation, and tearing, and a progression of protruding subepthelial lesions. Superficial vascularization is often seen. Stromal opacification or larger nodular lesions (kumquat-like lesions) may develop (Fig 10-5).

MANAGEMENT   Recurrence within a few years occurs in all patients following superficial keratectomy, lamellar keratoplasty (LK), or penetrating keratoplasty (PK). Soft contact lenses are effective in managing the abnormal epithelial permeability to decrease recurrences.

Ide T, Nishida K, Maeda N, et al. A spectrum of clinical manifestations of gelatinous drop-like corneal dystrophy in Japan. *Am J Ophthalmol.* 2004;137(6):1081–1084.

Kinoshita S, Nishida K, Dota A, et al. Epithelial barrier function and ultrastructure of gelatinous drop-like corneal dystrophy. *Cornea.* 2000;19(4):551–555.

Bowman Layer Corneal Dystrophies

Reis-Bücklers corneal dystrophy (RBCD)

Alternative names   Corneal dystrophy of Bowman layer type 1 (CDB1), geographic corneal dystrophy, superficial granular corneal dystrophy, atypical granular corneal dystrophy, granular corneal dystrophy type 3, anterior limiting membrane dystrophy type 1 (ALMD1)

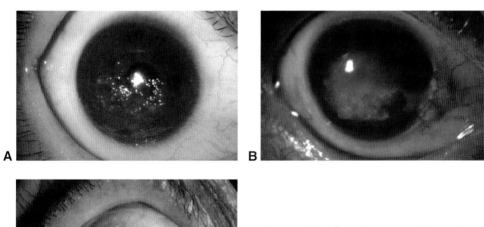

Figure 10-5 Gelatinous droplike corneal dystrophy. **A,** Mulberry type. **B,** Band keratopathy type. **C,** Kumquat-like type. *(Reproduced with permission from Weiss JS, Møller H, Lisch W, et al. The IC3D classification of the corneal dystrophies. Cornea. 2008;27(10:Suppl 2):S11.)*

Inheritance   Autosomal dominant

Genetics   Locus 5q31; gene *TGFBI*

Category   1

PATHOLOGY   On light microscopy, Bowman layer is disrupted or absent and replaced by a sheetlike connective tissue layer with granular Masson trichrome-red deposits. Transmission electron microscopy shows electron-dense, rod-shaped bodies. The rod-shaped bodies are immunopositive for the TGFBI (transforming growth factor β–induced) protein keratoepithelin. Electron microscopy is needed to histologically distinguish RBCD from TBCD (which has curly fibers; see the next section). On confocal microscopy, distinct deposits are found in the epithelium and Bowman layer. The basal epithelial cell layer shows high reflectivity from small granular material without any shadows. Bowman layer is replaced by highly reflective irregular material. Fine deposits may be noted in the anterior stroma.

CLINICAL FINDINGS   RBCD appears in the first few years of life and mainly affects Bowman layer. Confluent, irregular, and coarse geographic opacities with varying densities develop at the level of Bowman layer and superficial stroma, mostly centrally. With time, the opacities may extend to the limbus and deeper stroma (Fig 10-6).

The posterior cornea appears normal. In advanced cases, anterior scarring can lead to surface irregularity. Symptoms often begin in the first or second decade with painful

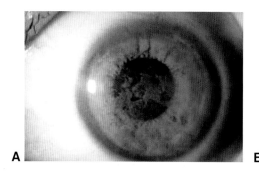

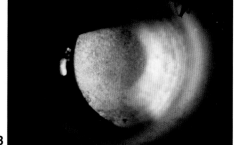

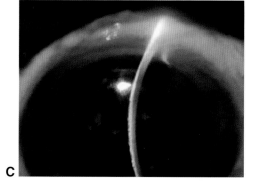

Figure 10-6 Reis-Bücklers corneal dystrophy. **A,** Coarse geographic opacity of the superficial cornea. **B,** Broad, oblique illumination showing dense, reticular, superficial opacity. **C,** Slit-lamp view showing irregularities in Bowman layer. *(Reproduced with permission from Weiss JS, Møller H, Lisch W, et al. The IC3D classification of the corneal dystrophies. Cornea. 2008;27(10:Suppl 2):S12.)*

recurrent epithelial erosions. Erosions are usually more severe and frequent than with TBCD. The recurrent erosions may resolve with time. Vision is reduced by both anterior scarring with surface irregularity and anterior stromal edema.

MANAGEMENT Initial treatment is aimed at the recurrent erosions. Superficial keratectomy, LK, PTK, or, in rare instances, PK may be performed. Recurrence in the graft is common.

> Kobayashi A, Sugiyama K. In vivo laser confocal microscopy findings for Bowman's layer dystrophies (Thiel-Behnke and Reis-Bücklers corneal dystrophies). *Ophthalmology.* 2007;114(1): 69–75.
>
> Laibson PR. Anterior corneal dystrophies. In: Krachmer JH, Mannis MJ, Holland EJ, eds. *Cornea.* 2nd ed. Vol 1. Philadelphia: Elsevier/Mosby; 2005:897–906.

Thiel-Behnke corneal dystrophy (TBCD)

Alternative names Corneal dystrophy of Bowman layer type 2 (CDB2), honeycomb-shaped corneal dystrophy, anterior limiting membrane dystrophy type 2 (ALMD2), curly fibers corneal dystrophy, Waardenburg-Jonkers corneal dystrophy

Inheritance Autosomal dominant

Genetics Loci 5q31, 10q24; gene *TGFBI* (5q31), unknown (10q24)

Category 1 (*TGFBI* variant), 2 (10q24 variant)

PATHOLOGY Light microscopy shows thickening of the epithelial layer, which allows for ridges and furrows in the underlying stroma and focal absences of the epithelial basement membrane. Bowman layer is replaced by fibrocellular material in a pathognomonic wavy "saw-toothed" pattern. On electron microscopy, curly fibers (9–15 nm) distinguish this dystrophy from RBCD. These curly fibers are immunopositive for the TGFBI protein keratoepithelin associated with the 5q31 genetic locus. On confocal microscopy, distinct deposits are found in the epithelium and Bowman layer. The deposits in the basal epithelial cell layer show reflectivity, with round edges and dark shadows. Bowman layer is replaced with irregular reflective material that is less reflective than in RBCD.

CLINICAL FINDINGS Onset is in the first or second decade, with symmetric subepithelial reticular (honeycomb) opacities, sparing the peripheral cornea (Fig 10-7). Opacities may progress to deep stromal layers and corneal periphery. Clinically distinguishing TBCD from RBCD is difficult. Recurrent erosions cause ocular discomfort and pain, with worsening of vision from corneal opacification. Erosions are less frequent and severe than with RBCD and may resolve with time. Vision decreases secondary to increased corneal opacification.

MANAGEMENT Management is similar to that used in RBCD.

> Kobayashi A, Sugiyama K. In vivo laser confocal microscopy findings for Bowman's layer dystrophies (Thiel-Behnke and Reis-Bücklers corneal dystrophies). *Ophthalmology.* 2007;114(1): 69–75.

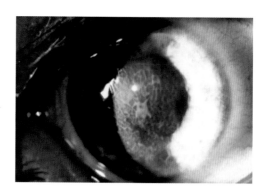

Figure 10-7 Thiel-Behnke corneal dystrophy. *(Reproduced with permission from Weiss JS, Møller H, Lisch W, et al. The IC3D classification of the corneal dystrophies. Cornea. 2008;27(10:Suppl 2):S13.)*

Küchle M, Green WR, Völcker HE, Barraquer J. Reevaluation of corneal dystrophies of Bowman's layer and the anterior stroma (Reis-Bücklers and Thiel-Behnke types): a light and electron microscopic study of eight corneas and a review of the literature. *Cornea.* 1995;14(4):333–354.

Stromal Corneal Dystrophies: *TGFBI* Dystrophies

Table 10-4 provides information on the histopathologic identification of the classic stromal corneal dystrophies.

Lattice corneal dystrophy (LCD): classic lattice corneal dystrophy (LCD1) and variants (the variants are multiple subtypes of lattice, which are not described here)

Alternative names   Classic LCD, LCD type 1, Biber-Haab-Dimmer

Inheritance   Autosomal dominant

Genetics   Locus 5q31; gene *TGFBI*

Category   1

PATHOLOGY   Light microscopy of lattice dystrophy shows amyloid deposits concentrated most heavily in the anterior stroma. Amyloid may also accumulate in the subepithelial area, giving rise to poor epithelial–stromal adhesions. Epithelial atrophy and disruption, with degeneration of basal epithelial cells, and focal thinning or absence of Bowman layer increases

Table 10-4 Histopathologic Differentiation of Granular, Macular, and Lattice Dystrophies

Dystrophy	Deposited Material	Masson	Alcian Blue	PAS	Amyloid*	Birefringence
Granular	Hyaline	+	−	−	−	−
Macular	Mucopolysaccharide	−	+	−	−	−
Lattice	Amyloid	+	−	+	+	+
Avellino	Hyaline amyloid	+	−	+	+	+

*Stains for amyloid: Congo red, crystal violet, and thioflavine T.

progressively with age. An eosinophilic layer between the epithelial basement membrane and Bowman layer develops, with stromal deposition of the amyloid substance distorting the corneal lamellar architecture. Amyloid stains rose to orange-red with Congo red dye and metachromatically with crystal violet dye, and it exhibits dichroism and birefringence. Electron microscopy reveals extracellular masses of fine 8–10-μm fibrils that are electron-dense and randomly aligned. In vivo confocal microscopy reveals characteristic linear images that should be differentiated from those seen in infection with fungal hyphae.

CLINICAL FINDINGS Lattice dystrophy is relatively common and is characterized by typical glasslike branching lines in the stroma. The spectrum of corneal changes is broad, and the classic branching lattice figures may not be present in all cases. Refractile lines, central and subepithelial ovoid white dots, and diffuse anterior stromal haze appear early in life. The refractile lines, so-called *lattice lines,* are best seen against a red reflex or with retroillumination (Fig 10-8). These lines start centrally and superficially and spread centrifugally and deeper. The stroma can take on a ground-glass appearance, but the peripheral cornea remains clear. Recurrent epithelial erosions occur often. Stromal haze and epithelial surface irregularity may decrease vision.

MANAGEMENT Recurrent erosions are managed with therapeutic contact lenses, superficial keratectomy, or PTK. Severe cases of lattice dystrophy with visual loss are treated with lamellar keratoplasty (DALK) or PK. Recurrence of this dystrophy may occur in the corneal graft. It is thought that lattice dystrophy recurs more frequently after grafting than does granular or macular dystrophy. One recent study suggested that granular dystrophy recurred more often than lattice; the study, however, had a 5-year follow-up; the mean time of recurrence for lattice is 9 years (range 3–26 years).

Marcon AS, Cohen EJ, Rapuano CJ, Laibson PR. Recurrence of corneal stromal dystrophies after penetrating keratoplasty. *Cornea.* 2003;22(1):19–21.

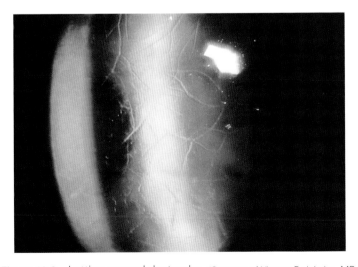

Figure 10-8 Lattice corneal dystrophy. *(Courtesy of Vincent P. deLuise, MD.)*

Lattice corneal dystrophy (LCD): gelsolin type (LCD2)

Alternative names   Familial amyloidosis, Finnish type (FAF); Meretoja syndrome; amyloidosis V; familial amyloidotic polyneuropathy type IV (FAP-IV)

Inheritance   Autosomal dominant

Genetics   Locus 9q34; gene: gelsolin *(GSN)*

Category   1 (Due to systemic involvement, this is not a true corneal dystrophy.)

PATHOLOGY   Light microscopy shows amyloid in the lattice lines as a discontinuous band under Bowman layer and within the sclera. The amyloid in this condition is related to gelsolin and does not stain for type AA or AP. The mutated gelsolin is seen deposited in the conjunctiva, sclera, and ciliary body, along the choriocapillaris, in the ciliary nerves and vessels, and in the optic nerve. Extraocularly, amyloid is detected in arterial walls, peripheral nerves, and glomeruli. On confocal microscopy, deposits are seen along the basal epithelial cells and stromal nerves.

CLINICAL FINDINGS   This form of LCD combines lattice corneal changes with coexisting systemic amyloidosis and presents in the third to fourth decade. Patients have a characteristic facial mask; dermatochalasis; lagophthalmous, pendulous ears; cranial and peripheral nerve palsies; and dry, lax skin with amyloid deposition (Fig 10-9). The risk of open-angle glaucoma may be increased. The classic corneal lattice lines are less numerous and more peripheral, and they spread centripetally from the limbus. The central cornea is relatively spared; corneal sensation is reduced. Dry eye and recurrent erosions may occur late in life.

Granular corneal dystrophy type 1 (GCD1)

Alternative names   Groenouw corneal dystrophy type I

Inheritance   Autosomal dominant

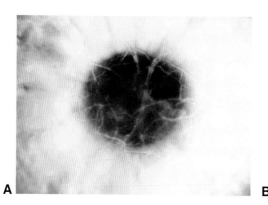
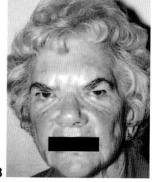

Figure 10-9   A, Diffuse lattice lines in lattice corneal dystrophy, gelsolin type (Meretoja). **B,** Typical facies of the Meretoja syndrome. *(Reproduced with permission from Weiss JS, Møller H, Lisch W, et al. The IC3D classification of the corneal dystrophies. Cornea. 2008;27(10:Suppl 2):S16.)*

Genetics   Locus 5q31; gene *TGFBI*

Category   1

PATHOLOGY   Microscopically, the granular material is hyaline and stains bright red with Masson trichrome stain. An electron-dense material made up of rod-shaped bodies immersed in an amorphous matrix is seen on electron microscopy. Histochemically, the deposits are noncollagenous protein that may derive from the corneal epithelium and/or keratocytes. Hyper-reflective opacities are seen on confocal microscopy. Although the exact cause is unknown, a mutation different from that of RBCD, LCD1, and GCD2 has been identified in the *TGFBI* gene on chromosome 5q31, which is responsible for the formation of keratoepithelin.

CLINICAL FINDINGS   Onset occurs early in life with crumblike opacities that may broaden into a disklike appearance as the patient reaches the teens. On direct illumination, the opacities appear white, but on indirect illumination, they are seen to be composed of small translucent dots with vacuoles and a glassy splinter or crushed breadcrumb appearance. The lesions do not extend to the limbus but can extend anteriorly through focal breaks in Bowman layer (Fig 10-10). The dystrophy is slowly progressive, with vision only rarely dropping to 20/200 after age 40. Patients complain of glare and photophobia. Recurrent erosions occur and vision decreases as the opacities become more confluent.

MANAGEMENT   Early in the disease process, no treatment is needed. Recurrent erosions may be treated with therapeutic contact lenses, superficial keratectomy, or PTK. When visual acuity is affected, DALK or PK has a good prognosis. Recurrence in the graft (anteriorly and peripherally) may occur after many years as fine subepithelial opacities varying from the original presentation.

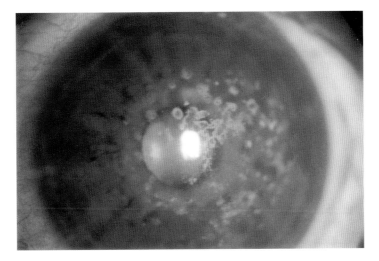

Figure 10-10   Granular dystrophy type 1.

Granular corneal dystrophy type 2 (granular-lattice) (GCD2)

Alternative names Combined granular-lattice corneal dystrophy, Avellino corneal dystrophy

Inheritance Autosomal dominant

Genetics Locus 5q31; gene *TGFBI*

Category 1

PATHOLOGY Pathologically, both the hyaline deposits typical of granular dystrophy and the amyloid deposits typical of lattice dystrophy are seen. These extend from the basal epithelium to the deep stroma. Individual opacities stain with either the Masson trichrome or Congo red stain. Rod-shaped bodies are seen on electron microscopy, as are randomly aligned fibrils of amyloid. Findings on confocal microscopy are a combination of GCD1 and LCD.

CLINICAL FINDINGS Affected patients have a granular dystrophy both histologically and clinically, with lattice lesions in addition to the granular lesions. Clinical findings differ from those of GCD1. Stellate-shaped, snowflake-like, and icicle-like opacities appear between the superficial and mid stroma. Lattice lines are also seen deeper than the snowflake opacities. Older patients have anterior stromal haze between deposits, which reduces visual acuity. Pain may occur with mild corneal erosions (Fig 10-11).

MANAGEMENT PTK, LK, or PK may be useful, depending on the depth of the deposits. LASIK and LASEK may result in increased opacification and are contraindicated.

Holland EJ, Daya SM, Stone EM, et al. Avellino corneal dystrophy. Clinical manifestations and natural history. *Ophthalmology.* 1992;99(10):1564–1568.

Kim TI, Hong JP, Ha BJ, Stulting RD, Kim EK. Determination of treatment strategies for granular corneal dystrophy type 2 using Fourier-domain optical coherence tomography. *Br J Ophthalmol.* 2010;94(3):341–345.

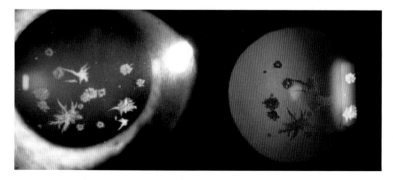

Figure 10-11 Granular dystrophy type 2. *(Reproduced with permission from Weiss JS, Møller H, Lisch W, et al. The IC3D classification of the corneal dystrophies. Cornea. 2008;27(10:Suppl 2):S18.)*

Stromal Dystrophies: Non–*TGFBI* Dystrophies

Macular corneal dystrophy (MCD)

Alternative names   Groenouw corneal dystrophy type II, Fehr spotted dystrophy

Inheritance   Autosomal recessive

Genetics   Locus 16q22; gene: carbohydrate sulfotransferase 6 *(CHST6)*

Category   1

PATHOLOGY   The deposits in macular dystrophy are glycosaminoglycans (GAGs; acid mucopolysaccharide), and they stain with colloidal iron and Alcian blue. They accumulate in the endoplasmic reticulum and not in lysosomal vacuoles, as seen in systemic mucopolysaccharidoses. Electron microscopy reveals keratocytes and endothelial cells that stain positive for GAGs, as well as extracellular clumps of fibrogranular material that also stains for GAGs. On confocal microscopy, blurred accumulations of light-reflective material are seen in the anterior corneal stroma.

CLINICAL FINDINGS   Macular dystrophy is the least common of the 3 classic stromal dystrophies (lattice, granular, and macular). Unlike most corneal dystrophies, it has an autosomal recessive inheritance, involves the entire corneal stroma and periphery, and may involve the corneal endothelium. The corneas are clear at birth and begin to cloud at ages 3–9 years. The age of presentation of clinical findings is youngest in macular dystrophy, followed by lattice dystrophy and then granular dystrophy.

Patients with macular dystrophy show focal, gray-white, superficial stromal opacities that progress to involve full stromal thickness and extend to the corneal periphery. Macular spots have indefinite edges, and the stroma between the opacities is diffusely cloudy (Fig 10-12). Involvement of Descemet's membrane and the endothelium is indicated by the presence of cornea guttae. Epithelial erosions are possible, but symptoms usually involve a decrease in vision, between the ages of 10 and 30. Central corneal thinning and hypoesthesia have been noted. The 3 types of macular dystrophy are distinguished based on biochemical differences.

Patients with *type I macular dystrophy,* the most prevalent form of macular dystrophy, lack antigenic keratan sulfate (AgKS) in their cornea, serum, and cartilage. These patients have a normal synthesis of dermatan sulfate-proteoglycan. Errors occur in the synthesis of keratan sulfate and in the activity of specific sulfotransferases involved in the sulfation of the keratan sulfate lactose aminoglycan side chain.

In *type IA macular dystrophy,* keratocytes manifest AgKS reactivity, but the extracellular material does not. There is no AgKS in the serum.

Patients with *type II macular dystrophy* synthesize a normal ratio of keratan sulfate and dermatan sulfate-proteoglycans, but total synthesis is 30% below normal. Moreover, the dermatan sulfate-proteoglycan chains are 40% shorter than normal.

An enzyme-linked immunosorbent assay (ELISA) measures sulfated keratan sulfate. This test can help in the diagnosis of macular dystrophy, even in preclinical forms and carriers.

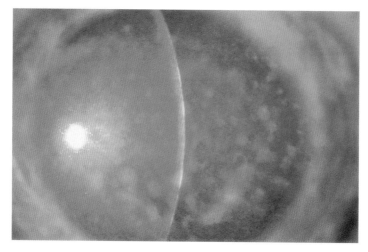

Figure 10-12 Macular dystrophy, showing involvement to the limbus with diffuse haze.

MANAGEMENT Recurrent erosions are treated as for other stromal dystrophies, and photophobia may be reduced with tinted contact lenses. PTK may be used for symptomatic anterior macular dystrophy. Definitive treatment requires penetrating corneal transplantation, although recurrences may be seen.

Schnyder corneal dystrophy (SCD)

Alternative names Schnyder crystalline corneal dystrophy (SCCD), Schnyder crystalline dystrophy sine crystals, hereditary crystalline stromal dystrophy of Schnyder, crystalline stromal dystrophy, central stromal crystalline corneal dystrophy, corneal crystalline dystrophy of Schnyder, Schnyder corneal crystalline of dystrophy

Inheritance Autosomal dominant

Genetics Locus 1p36; gene: UbiA prenyltransferase domain-containing protein 1 (*UBIAD1*)

Category 1

PATHOLOGY This condition is thought to be a local disorder of corneal lipid metabolism. Pathologically, the opacities are accumulations of unesterified and esterified cholesterol and phospholipids. Oil red O stains the phospholipids red. In the normal process of embedding tissue in paraffin, cholesterol and other fatty substances are dissolved; therefore, the pathologist must be made aware of the requirements for special stains. Electron microscopy shows abnormal accumulation of lipid and dissolved cholesterol in the epithelium, in Bowman layer, and throughout the stroma. Confocal microscopy reveals disruption of the basal epithelial/subepithelial nerve plexus, with highly reflective intracellular and extracellular deposits.

CLINICAL FINDINGS Schnyder corneal dystrophy is a rare, slowly progressive stromal dystrophy that may become apparent as early as the first year of life. However, diagnosis is usually made by the second or third decade, although it may be further delayed in patients who have the acrystalline form of the disease. Central subepithelial crystals are seen in only 50% of patients and do not involve the epithelium. Vision and corneal sensation decrease with age. Glare complaints increase due to progressive corneal haze.

Affected patients show predictable progressive changes on the basis of age, beginning with central corneal opacification (Fig 10-13):

1. central corneal opacification (can affect the entire corneal stromal thickness) ± subepithelial crystals (in individuals younger than 23 years)
2. dense corneal arcus lipoides (third decade)
3. midperipheral corneal opacification (fourth decade; affects entire corneal stromal thickness)
4. decreased corneal sensation

MANAGEMENT Schnyder corneal dystrophy disproportionately reduces photopic vision (despite maintenance of excellent scotopic vision), leading to corneal transplantation in most patients over 50. The dystrophy can recur after PK. PTK has been used to treat decreased vision from subepithelial crystals, but it does not treat panstromal haze. Abnormal serum lipids are managed by diet and/or medication but do not affect the progression of the corneal dystrophy. A fasting lipid profile should be done for possible hyperlipoproteinemia (type IIa, III, or IV) or hyperlipidemia. Most patients have elevated serum cholesterol that often responds to diet or medication. Unaffected family members may also have an abnormal lipid profile.

Weiss JS. Visual morbidity in thirty-four families with Schnyder crystalline corneal dystrophy (an American Ophthalmological Society thesis). *Trans Am Ophthalmol Soc.* 2007;105: 616–648.

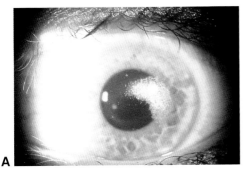 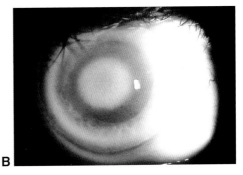

Figure 10-13 Schnyder crystalline dystrophy with **(A)** central subepithelial crystalline deposition and **(B)** central panstromal corneal opacity and arcus lipoides. No crystals are present. *(Courtesy of Jayne S. Weiss, MD.)*

Congenital stromal corneal dystrophy (CSCD)

Alternative names   Congenital hereditary stromal dystrophy, congenital stromal dystrophy of the cornea

Inheritance   Autosomal dominant

Genetics   Locus 12q21.33; gene: decorin *(DCN)*

Category   1

PATHOLOGY   The stromal lamellae are separated from each other in a regular manner, sometimes with areas of amorphous deposition. On electron microscopy, the collagen fibril diameter is about half the normal size in all lamellae. Abnormal lamellar layers consisting of thin filaments arranged in an electron-lucent ground substance separates the lamellae of normal appearance. The keratocytes and endothelium are normal. The absence of the anterior banded zone of Descemet's membrane has been reported. The epithelial cells are normal on confocal microscopy. Stromal evaluation is not possible due to increased reflectivity.

CLINICAL FINDINGS   Congenital diffuse, bilateral corneal clouding with flakelike whitish opacities is found throughout the stroma. The corneas are thickened. The course is nonprogressive or slowly progressive, with moderate to severe visual loss (Fig 10-14).

MANAGEMENT   PK is used in advanced cases.

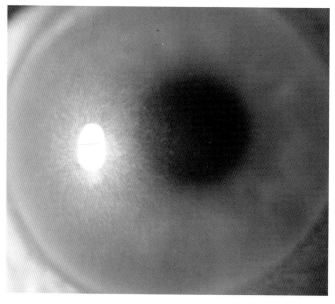

Figure 10-14   Congenital stromal corneal dystrophy: diffuse bilateral clouding with flakelike opacities throughout the stroma. *(Reproduced with permission from Weiss JS, Møller H, Lisch W, et al. The IC3D classification of the corneal dystrophies. Cornea. 2008;27(10:Suppl 2):S22.)*

Bredrup C, Knappskog PM, Majewski J, Rødahl E, Boman H. Congenital stromal dystrophy of the cornea caused by a mutation in the decorin gene. *Invest Ophthalmol Vis Sci.* 2005;46(2):420–426.

Fleck corneal dystrophy (FCD)

Alternative names   François-Neetens speckled corneal dystrophy

Inheritance   Autosomal dominant

Genetics   Locus 2q35; gene: phosphatidylinositol-3-phosphate/phosphatidylinositol 5-kinase type III *(PIP5K3)*

Category   1

PATHOLOGY   Affected keratocytes are vacuolated and contain 2 abnormal substances: excess glycosaminoglycan, which stains with Alcian blue and colloidal iron; and lipids, demonstrated by Sudan black B and oil red O. Transmission electron microscopy shows membrane-based inclusions with delicate granular material. Confocal microscopy shows an accumulation of pathologic material in stromal cells and inclusions in the basal nerves.

CLINICAL FINDINGS   Discrete, flat, gray-white, dandruff-like (sometimes ring-shaped) opacities appear throughout the stroma to its periphery. The epithelium, Bowman layer, Descemet's membrane, and endothelium are not involved. Symptoms are minimal, and vision is usually not reduced. The condition is nonprogressive and may be asymmetric or unilateral. Fleck dystrophy may be associated with decreased corneal sensation, limbal dermoid, keratoconus, central cloudy dystrophy, punctate cortical lens changes, pseudoxanthoma elasticum, or atopy (Fig 10-15).

MANAGEMENT   None is indicated

Purcell JJ Jr, Krachmer JH, Weingeist TA. Fleck corneal dystrophy. *Arch Ophthalmol.* 1977; 95(3):440–444.

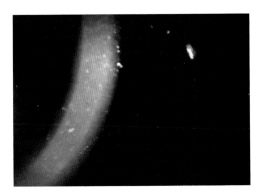

Figure 10-15 Dandruff-like opacities seen in Fleck corneal dystrophy. *(Reproduced with permission from Weiss JS, Møller H, Lisch W, et al. The IC3D classification of the corneal dystrophies. Cornea. 2008;27(10:Suppl 2):S23.)*

Posterior amorphous corneal dystrophy (PACD)

Alternative names   Posterior amorphous stromal dystrophy

Inheritance   Autosomal dominant

Genetics   No identified gene locus

Category   3 (PACD may be a mesodermal dysgenesis rather than a corneal dystrophy.)

PATHOLOGY   Focal attenuation of endothelial cells and irregular stromal architecture anterior to Descemet's membrane are seen on light microscopy. On electron microscopy, there is disorganization of the posterior stromal lamellae. A fibrillar layer interrupts Descemet's membrane. On confocal microscopy, there are microfolds and a hyperreflective layer in the posterior stroma.

CLINICAL FINDINGS   PACD presents in the first decade of life with a diffuse, gray-white, sheetlike opacity of the cornea, usually posteriorly. The condition is slowly progressive or nonprogressive. The cornea is flat (<41 D) and thin (as low as 380 μm) and there is associated hyperopia. Descemet's membrane and the endothelium may be indented by opacities. Focal endothelial abnormalities have been observed, as have a prominent Schwalbe line, fine iris processes, pupillary remnant, iridocorneal adhesions, corectopia, pseudopolycoria, and anterior stromal tags. There is no associated glaucoma. Visual acuity is only mildly affected (Fig 10-16).

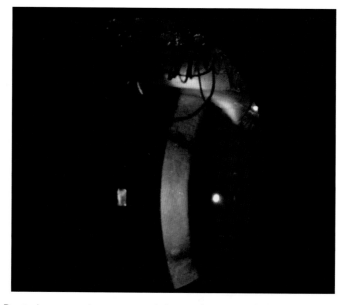

Figure 10-16   Posterior amorphous corneal dystrophy: central deep stromal, pre-Descemet opacity. *(Reproduced with permission from Weiss JS, Møller H, Lisch W, et al. The IC3D classification of the corneal dystrophies. Cornea. 2008;27(10:Suppl 2):S24.)*

MANAGEMENT   Although usually no treatment is required, PK is sometimes performed.

Johnson AT, Folberg R, Vrabec MP, Florakis GJ, Stone EM, Krachmer JH. The pathology of posterior amorphous corneal dystrophy. *Ophthalmology.* 1990;97(9):104–109.

Central cloudy dystrophy of François (CCDF)

Alternative names   None

Inheritance   Unknown (Autosomal dominant inheritance has been reported, but the condition may be a degeneration.)

Genetics   No identified gene locus

Category   4 (most consistent with posterior crocodile shagreen, a degeneration)

PATHOLOGY   In one case without known heredity, histopathologic examination showed folds of the deep stroma, with extracellular deposition of mucopolysaccharide and lipid-like material. Extracellular vacuoles, some with fibrogranular material and electron-dense deposition, are seen on electron microscopy. Endothelial vacuoles may have fibrogranular material. On confocal microscopy, small, highly refractile granules and deposits are seen in the anterior stroma.

CLINICAL FINDINGS   Opacities consist of multiple nebulous, polygonal, gray areas separated by cracklike intervening clear zones. Theses opacities are densest centrally and posteriorly and fade both anteriorly and peripherally (Fig 10-17). The epithelium, Bowman layer, stromal thickness, Descemet's membrane, and endothelium are normal. Vision is usually

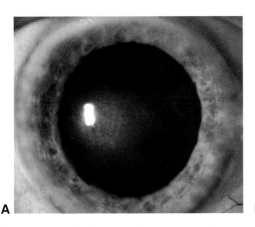
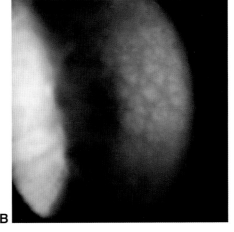

Figure 10-17   A, Central cloudy dystrophy of François. **B,** Broad, oblique illumination demonstrating nebulous, polygonal gray areas with cracklike intervening clear zones. *(Reproduced with permission from Krachmer JH, Mannis MJ, Holland EJ, eds. Cornea. 2nd ed. Vol 1. Philadelphia: Elsevier/Mosby; 2005:920.)*

not reduced. CCDF is phenotypically indistinguishable from posterior crocodile shagreen, which is a corneal degeneration.

MANAGEMENT   None indicated

De Sousa LB, Mannis MJ. The stromal dystrophies. In: Krachmer JH, Mannis MJ, Holland EJ, eds. *Cornea*. 2nd ed. Vol 1. Philadelphia: Elsevier/Mosby; 2005:907–927.

Pre-Descemet corneal dystrophy (PDCD)

Alternative names   None

Inheritance   No definite pattern of inheritance, although it has been described in families over 2–4 generations

Genetics   No identified gene locus

Category   4 (may be a degeneration or associated with systemic diseases)

PATHOLOGY   Large keratocytes are seen in the posterior stroma, with vacuoles and intra-cytoplasmic inclusions containing lipid-like material. On electron microscopy, there are membrane-bound intracellular vacuoles containing electron-dense material suggestive of secondary lysosomes and inclusions consistent with lipofuscin-like lipoprotein, suggesting a degenerative process.

CLINICAL FINDINGS   Focal, fine, gray opacities are seen in the deep stroma anterior to Descemet's membrane. Onset is usually after age 30, but it has been reported in children as young as 3 years. The rest of the cornea is normal. Vision is normal. Similar opacities have been described in pseudoxanthoma elasticum, X-linked and recessive ichthyosis, keratoconus, PPCD, EBMD, and CCDF (Fig 10-18).

MANAGEMENT   None indicated

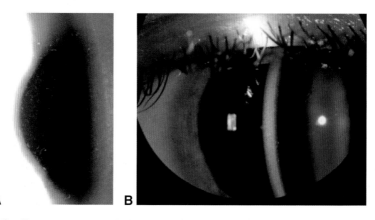

A   **B**

Figure 10-18   Pre-Descemet corneal dystrophy: punctate opacities anterior to Descemet's membrane demonstrated with **(A)** indirect illumination and **(B)** slit-lamp beam. *(Reproduced with permission from Weiss JS, Møller H, Lisch W, et al. The IC3D classification of the corneal dystrophies. Cornea. 2008;27(10:Suppl 2):S26.)*

Endothelial Dystrophies

Fuchs endothelial corneal dystrophy (FECD)

Alternative names   Endoepithelial corneal dystrophy, endothelial corneal dystrophy

Inheritance   Cases without known inheritance are most common; some cases with autosomal dominant inheritance have been reported

Genetics   Locus 13pTel-13q12.13, 15q, 18q21.2-q21.32; early-onset variant: 1p34.3-p32. Gene none (most commonly); early-onset variant: collagen type VIII alpha 2 *(COL8A2)*

Category   3 (FECD in patients with no known inheritance); 2 (FECD with known genetic loci but gene not yet localized); 1 (early-onset FECD)

PATHOLOGY   Microscopically, the endothelial cells are noted to be larger (polymegathism) and more polymorphic (pleiomorphism) than normal and are disrupted by excrescences of excess collagen, a product of the stressed endothelial cells. Primary dysfunction of the endothelial cells manifests as increased corneal swelling and deposition of collagen and extracellular matrix in Descemet's membrane, which is thickened. There is a reduction in the number of Na^+/K^+-ATPase pump sites or in pump function. It is not clear whether the reduction in the posterior nonbanded zone and the increase in thickness of the posterior banded zone (posterior collagenous layer) are primary effects of endothelial dysfunction or are secondary to chronic corneal edema.

CLINICAL FINDINGS   Findings vary with the severity of the disease. Cornea guttae are first evident centrally and spread toward the periphery (Fig 10-19). Descemet's membrane becomes thickened, and folds develop secondary to stromal edema (Fig 10-20). Increased endothelial pigmentation may also be seen. As the endothelium further decompensates, the central corneal thickness may approach 1 mm (0.52–0.56 mm is normal). Epithelial edema develops, leading to microcystic edema; this later progresses to epithelial bullae, which may rupture. Subepithelial fibrosis occurs in later stages.

Fuchs usually presents in the fifth or sixth decade (except for the early-onset variant, which may present in the third decade or earlier). Symptoms are rare before age 50 and are related to the edema, which causes a decrease in vision, as well as pain secondary to ruptured bullae. Symptoms are often worse upon awakening because of decreased surface evaporation during sleep. Painful episodes may subside once subepithelial fibrosis occurs.

MANAGEMENT   Initial treatment is aimed at reducing corneal edema and relieving pain. Use of sodium chloride drops and ointment (5%) and measures to lower IOP may temporarily help the edema. A soft bandage lens may be useful in treating ruptured bullae. In advanced cases, anterior stromal puncture, amniotic membrane, or a conjunctival flap may be considered to relieve pain, but restoration of vision requires corneal transplantation. In the past, full-thickness (penetrating) keratoplasty was the standard procedure, but this has been replaced by endothelial keratoplasty, as the latter targets the pathologic endothelial cells. In advanced cases where there has been anterior corneal scarring, a full-thickness

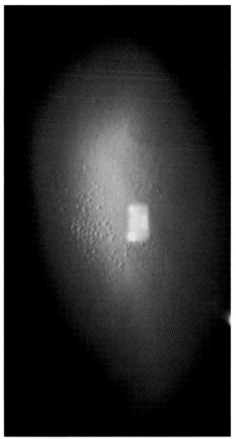

Figure 10-19 Fuchs endothelial dystrophy. Cornea guttae seen in retroillumination. *(Reproduced with permission from Krachmer JH, Mannis MJ, Holland EJ, eds. Cornea. 2nd ed. Vol 1. Philadelphia: Elsevier/Mosby; 2005:939.)*

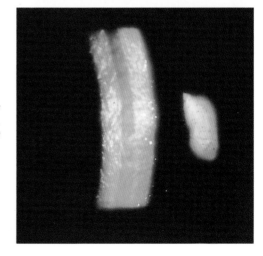

Figure 10-20 Fuchs endothelial dystrophy showing stromal edema, Descemet's folds, and endothelial guttae. *(Courtesy of Vincent P. deLuise, MD.)*

procedure may still be indicated. Prognosis for graft survival is good, especially if done before vascularization occurs. See Chapter 16 on corneal transplantation.

Gottsch JD, Sundin OH, Liu SH, et al. Inheritance of a novel COL8A2 mutation defines a distinct early-onset subtype of Fuchs corneal dystrophy. *Invest Ophthalmol Vis Sci.* 2005;46(6): 1934–1939.

Terry MA. Endothelial keratoplasty: history, current state, and future directions. *Cornea.* 2006; 25(8):873–878.

COMMENT Specular microscopy may be helpful in diagnosing Fuchs and following the clinical course for loss of endothelial cells. Corneal pachometry may indicate relative endothelial function and change with progression of the disease. Both procedures are useful in determining the relative safety of cataract or other intraocular surgery. Endothelial cell counts less than 1000/mm², corneal thickness greater than 640 μm, or the presence of epithelial edema suggests caution and the possibility that the cornea may decompensate with any intraocular surgery (see Chapter 2).

Seitzman GD, Gottsch JD, Stark WJ. Cataract surgery in patients with Fuchs' corneal dystrophy: expanding recommendations for cataract surgery without simultaneous keratoplasty. *Ophthalmology.* 2005;112(3):441–446.

Posterior polymorphous corneal dystrophy (PPCD)

Alternative names   Posterior polymorphous dystrophy (PPMD), Schlichting dystrophy

Inheritance   Autosomal dominant (Isolated unilateral cases with similar phenotype but no heredity have been reported.)

Genetics   Locus: PPCD1: 20p11.2-q11.2; PPCD2: 1p34.3-p32.3; PPCD3: 10p11.2. Gene: PPCD1: unknown; PPCD2: collagen type VIII alpha 2 *(COL8A2);* PPCD3: *ZEB1*

Category   PPCD1: 2; PPCD2: 1; PPCD3: 1

PATHOLOGY   The most distinctive microscopic finding is the appearance of abnormal, multilayered endothelial cells that look and behave like epithelial cells or fibroblasts. These cells

- show microvilli
- stain positive for keratin
- show rapid and easy growth in cell culture
- have intercellular desmosomes
- manifest proliferative tendencies

A diffuse abnormality of Descemet's membrane is common, including thickening, a multilaminated appearance, and polymorphous alterations. Similar changes that are not limited to the cornea are seen in iridocorneal endothelial (ICE) syndrome (see Chapter 12). ICE, however, is sporadic and unilateral. Specular microscopy may show typical vesicles and bands, in contrast to the involved cells in ICE syndrome, which appear as dark areas with central highlights and light peripheral borders. Opinion is divided on the value of relying on specular microscopy alone in making the diagnosis. Confocal microscopy reveals alterations in Descemet's membrane and polymegathism of the endothelial cells.

CLINICAL FINDINGS Careful examination of the posterior corneal surface will show any or all of the following:

- isolated grouped vesicles
- geographic-shaped, discrete, gray lesions
- broad bands with scalloped edges (Fig 10-21)

Variable amounts of stromal edema, corectopia, and broad iridocorneal adhesions may also be seen (Fig 10-22). Fine, glasslike iridocorneal adhesions may be seen goni-

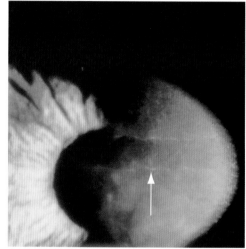

Figure 10-21 Posterior polymorphous dystrophy showing scallop-edged endothelial band *(arrow)*.

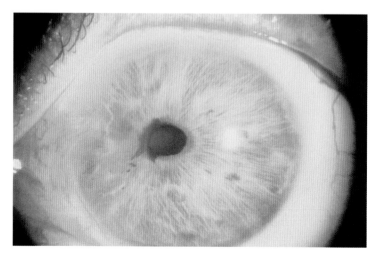

Figure 10-22 Posterior polymorphous dystrophy showing iridocorneal adhesion and corectopia.

oscopically. Both angle-closure and open-angle glaucoma can occur, and 14% of patients have elevated IOP.

MANAGEMENT Most patients are asymptomatic. Mild corneal edema may be managed as with early Fuchs dystrophy. To manage localized swelling, stromal micropuncture can be used to induce subepithelial pannus. With more severe disease, glaucoma must be managed, and corneal transplants may be required. Prognosis for PK is related to the presence of visible peripheral anterior synechiae and glaucoma. PPCD may recur in the graft. Endothelial keratoplasty is an alternative approach to targeting the abnormal endothelial cells in earlier cases without significant stromal opacification.

Weisenthal RW, Streeten BW. Posterior membrane dystrophies In: Krachmer JH, Mannis MJ, Holland EJ, eds. *Cornea*. 2nd ed. Vol 1. Philadelphia: Elsevier/Mosby; 2005:929–954.

Congenital hereditary endothelial dystrophy (CHED1)

Alternative names None

Inheritance Autosomal dominant

Genetics Locus 20p11.2-q11.2 (pericentromeric region); gene unknown

Category 2

PATHOLOGY There is diffuse thickening and lamination of Descemet's membrane with sparse, atrophic endothelial cells. Parts of the endothelium are replaced by keratin-containing stratified squamous epithelium. Multiple layers of basement membrane–like material are seen on the posterior part of Descemet's membrane along with degeneration of endothelial cells with many vacuoles. On electron microscopy, stromal thickening is seen, with severe disorganization and disruption of the lamellae.

CLINICAL FINDINGS CHED1 occurs congenitally or during the first or second year of life and shows diffuse corneal clouding and thickening. Symptoms include blurred vision, photophobia, and tearing that is worse in the morning. Some patients have only irregular peau d'orange–like endothelial changes. Clouding progresses over 1–10 years. Endothelial decompensation may occur over a prolonged period of time (Fig 10-23).

MANAGEMENT PK is used in advanced cases.

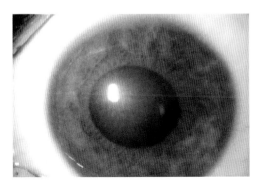

Figure 10-23 CHED1, showing milky appearance of the cornea with diffuse illumination. *(Reproduced with permission from Weiss JS, Møller H, Lisch W, et al. The IC3D classification of the corneal dystrophies. Cornea. 2008;27(10:Suppl 2):S29.)*

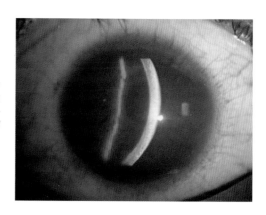

Figure 10-24 CHED2, showing diffuse stromal thickening. *(Reproduced with permission from Weiss JS, Møller H, Lisch W, et al. The IC3D classification of the corneal dystrophies. Cornea. 2008;27(10:Suppl 2):S29.)*

Congenital hereditary endothelial dystrophy (CHED2)

Alternative names   Maumenee corneal dystrophy

Inheritance   Autosomal recessive

Genetics   Locus 20p13 (telomeric portion); gene: solute carrier family 4, sodium borate transporter, member 11 *(SLC4A11)*

Category   1

PATHOLOGY   There is diffuse thickening and lamination of Descemet's membrane, with sparse atrophic endothelial cells. On electron microscopy, multiple layers of basement membrane–like material are seen on the posterior part of Descemet's membrane along with degeneration of the endothelial cells with many vacuoles. Stromal thickening with severe disorganization and disruption of the lamellar pattern is evident.

CLINICAL FINDINGS   CHED2 is congenital and stationary but more severe than CHED1. Corneal clouding ranges from a diffuse haze to ground glass, with occasional focal gray spots. Thickening of the cornea (2–3 times normal) occurs, with rare subepithelial band keratopathy and IOP elevation. Blurred vision and nystagmus occur with minimal to no tearing or photophobia (Fig 10-24).

MANAGEMENT   Because corneal clouding is more common and severe, PK is usually performed.

Ectatic Disorders

Keratoconus

Keratoconus is a common disorder (prevalence of about 50 per 100,000) in which the central or paracentral cornea undergoes progressive thinning and bulging, so the cornea takes on the shape of a cone (Fig 10-25). The hereditary pattern is not prominent or predictable,

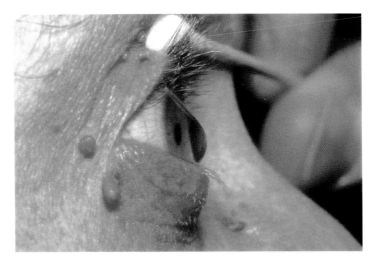

Figure 10-25 Keratoconus.

but positive family histories have been reported in 6%–8% of cases. Clinically unaffected first-degree relatives have a higher chance of showing subclinical topographic abnormalities associated with [ ] ple chromosomal loci have been repor elusive. The combination of genetic a flammation, and oxidative stress all p s.

> **Xalatan®**
> latanoprost ophthalmic solution

McMonnies CW. 007;33(6 Pt 1): 265–271.

Keratoconus

— *Scissoring of reflex on retinoscopy*

— *Rizzutti sign (conical reflection nasal on temporal light across cornea)*

PATHOLOGY Histop:

- fragmentatio
- thinning of th
- folds or break
- variable amo

— *Munson sign (protruding lower lid on downgaze)*

— *associated c Down's, atopy, Marfan, floppy eyelids, Leber's, MVP*

— *Vogt lines*

— *Fleischer ring*

CLINICAL FINDINGS more severely involved. Sometimes which may be considered the minima keratoscopy may show enantiomorpl ning in the other eye. The disease tends to progress during the adolescent years and into the mid-20s and 30s, although progression can occur at any time. Early biomicroscopic and histopathologic findings include fibrillation of Bowman layer, leading to breaks and followed by fibrous growth and dysplasia through the break. As progression occurs, the apical thinning of the central cornea worsens, and extreme degrees of irregular astigmatism can develop. No associated inflammation occurs.

Scissoring of the red reflex on ophthalmoscopy or retinoscopy is a very early sign of keratoconus. *Rizzutti sign,* a conical reflection on the nasal cornea when a penlight is shone from the temporal side, is another early finding (Fig 10-26). *Munson sign* is evident as a protrusion of the lower lid upon downgaze (Fig 10-27). Iron deposits are often present within the epithelium around the base of the cone and constitute a *Fleischer ring* (Fig 10-28). This ring is brown in color and best seen with the cobalt blue filter using a broad, oblique beam. Fine, relucent, and roughly parallel striations *(Vogt lines),* or stress lines, of the posterior stroma can be observed. Focal ruptures and flecklike scars occur in Bowman layer.

Spontaneous perforation in keratoconus is extremely rare. However, a tear can occur in Descemet's membrane at any time, resulting in the sudden development of corneal

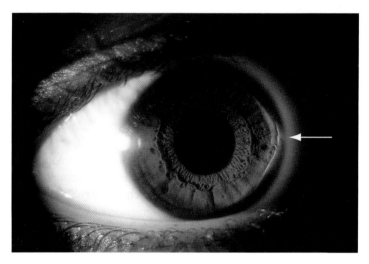

Figure 10-26 Rizzutti sign *(arrow).*

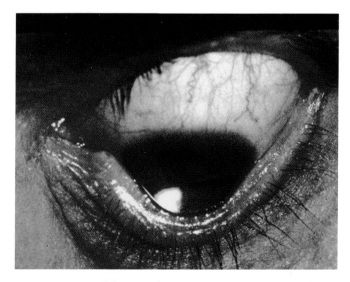

Figure 10-27 Munson sign. *(Courtesy of James R. Reidy, MD.)*

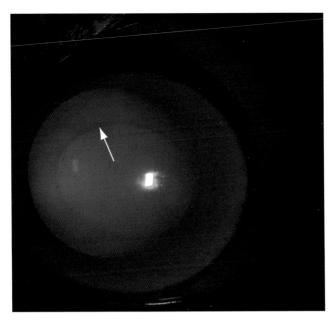

Figure 10-28 Keratoconus showing a Fleischer ring *(arrow)*. *(Courtesy of James J. Reidy, MD.)*

edema, or *acute hydrops*. Allergy and eye rubbing are risk factors for the development of hydrops. The break in the posterior cornea usually heals spontaneously in 6–12 weeks; the corneal edema then disappears, but stromal scarring may be left in its wake. Some patients regain good vision following the resolution of hydrops, depending largely on the extent and location of the scar.

An increased prevalence of keratoconus has been reported in Down syndrome, atopy, Marfan syndrome, floppy eyelid syndrome, Leber congenital hereditary optic neuropathy, and mitral valve prolapse. Keratoconus also occurs commonly in numerous congenital anomalies of the eye.

EVALUATION Computerized videokeratography is helpful in detecting early keratoconus, in following its progression, and in helping to fit contact lenses. Placido-based topography shows inferior steepening in the power map, but pachometry mapping shows the thin zone to be paracentral (Fig 10-29). Ultrasonic pachometry may be more accurate, however. Computerized videokeratography algorithms to diagnose forme fruste, or subclinical, keratoconus are continually being perfected to detect keratoconus suspects and screen them from prospective refractive surgery. Scanning slit and other elevation-based systems are being improved to measure deviation above a "best-fit sphere." (See Chapter 2 in this volume, as well as BCSC Section 3, *Clinical Optics,* and Section 13, *Refractive Surgery.*)

Belin MW, Rodila JF. Topographic analysis in keratorefractive surgery. In: Krachmer JH, Mannis MJ, Holland EJ, eds. *Cornea.* 2nd ed. Vol 2. Philadelphia: Elsevier/Mosby; 2005: 1909–1922.

Rao SN, Raviv T, Majmudar PA, Epstein RJ. Role of Orbscan II in screening keratoconus suspects before refractive corneal surgery. *Ophthalmology.* 2002;109(9):1642–1646.

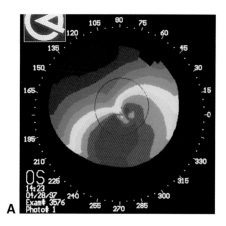
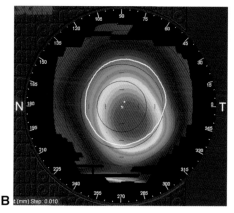

Figure 10-29 Keratoconus. **A,** Placido disk computerized videography showing inferior steepening. **B,** Orbscan computerized videography showing a pachometry map of the same eye as in **A.** Note that the thinnest zone is near the visual axis and not at the steepest point.

MANAGEMENT   Some cases of keratoconus are mild enough, at least for a time, that vision can be corrected adequately with glasses. However, rigid or gas-permeable contact lenses are far more helpful in all but the mildest cases. Their ability to neutralize the irregular corneal astigmatism often produces dramatic improvement in vision. The majority of patients with keratoconus without central corneal scarring can be fitted successfully with contact lenses using advanced techniques, and a central subepithelial scar can, on occasion, be removed (nodulectomy), allowing continued wear of contact lenses.

Indications for PK include the following:

- contact lens intolerance even with good vision
- poor vision even with a comfortable contact lens fit (usually due to scarring)
- unstable contact lens fit (even with good vision and tolerance)
- progressive thinning to the periphery approaching the limbus, requiring a very large graft (with increased risk)

The prognosis for keratoplasty in keratoconus is excellent. Deep anterior lamellar keratoplasty (DALK) has recently been reported as an alternate surgical modality. DALK leaves the host's endothelium untouched, thereby potentially decreasing rejection episodes. Intrastromal rings and collagen cross-linking (presently being investigated with riboflavin and UV light) are additional modalities to stabilize keratoconus. (See also Chapter 16.)

The disease is presently considered a contraindication for refractive procedures, except for intracorneal rings, because of unpredictability and the potential for poor results in either the short or long term in these patients. PK has been reported after LASIK in keratoconus patients because of long-term loss of best-corrected visual acuity.

Hydrops is treated conservatively with topical hypertonic agents and patching or a soft contact lens for several months. A cycloplegic agent may be needed for ciliary pain. Aqueous suppressants may decrease the flow of fluid into the cornea. Hydrops is not an indication for immediate surgery.

Pellucid Marginal Degeneration

Pellucid marginal degeneration is somewhat uncommon, nonhereditary, and bilateral. Pellucid (ie, transparent) inferior, peripheral corneal thinning takes place in the absence of inflammation. Etiology is unknown.

CLINICAL FINDINGS   Protrusion of the cornea occurs above the band of thinning. At times, a clear distinction between pellucid marginal degeneration and keratoconus is not possible. A cornea with keratoconus will show protrusion at the point of maximal thinning, but pellucid marginal degeneration can be superior or inferior and will show protrusion above the area of maximum thinning. No vascularization or lipid deposition occurs, but posterior stromal scarring has been noted within the thinned area. Most patients are diagnosed between 20 and 40 years of age, and men and women are affected equally. Decreased vision results from high irregular astigmatism (Figs 10-30, 10-31). Acute hydrops has been reported, and, although rare, spontaneous corneal perforation has also occurred.

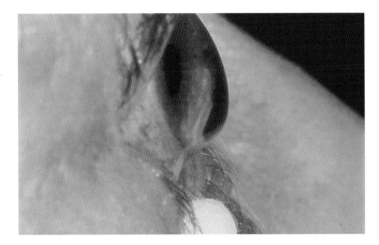

Figure 10-30   Pellucid marginal degeneration. *(Courtesy of Vincent P. deLuise, MD.)*

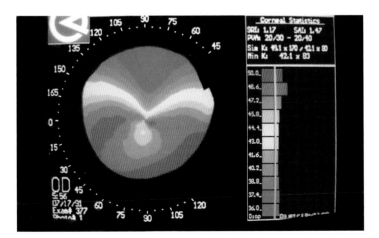

Figure 10-31   Topography of pellucid marginal degeneration. Note the inferior steepening and "lobster claw" pattern.

MANAGEMENT   Treatment consists of contact lenses early in the disease, although lens fitting is more difficult in pellucid marginal degeneration than in keratoconus. Hybrid (gas-permeable lenses with a soft lens "skirt") or scleral lenses may be options. Eventually, PK may be required to restore vision. Because of the location of the thinning, the grafts tend to be large and close to the limbus, making surgery technically more difficult and the graft more prone to rejection. Wedge resection and lamellar tectonic grafts have been advocated as alternative or adjunctive procedures.

> Rasheed K, Rabinowitz YS. Surgical treatment of advanced pellucid marginal degeneration. *Ophthalmology.* 2000;107(10):1836–1840.

Keratoglobus

Keratoglobus is a very rare, bilateral, noninflammatory condition that differs from keratoconus and pellucid marginal degeneration in typically being present at birth (Table 10-5). It is usually not hereditary. Keratoglobus is similar in appearance to keratoconus but manifests a globular rather than a conical deformation of the cornea (Fig 10-32).

PATHOLOGY   Keratoglobus is strongly associated with blue sclera and Ehlers-Danlos syndrome type VI (see Chapter 9), and it may represent a defect in collagen synthesis. Histopathologically, it is characterized by an absent or fragmented Bowman layer, thinned stroma with normal lamellar organization, and thin Descemet's membrane. Unlike keratoconus, keratoglobus is not associated with atopy, hard contact lens wear, or tapetoretinal degeneration.

CLINICAL FINDINGS   Both corneas have a globular shape with a very deep anterior chamber. The corneal curve may be as steep as 50–60 D, and generalized thinning appears, especially in the midperiphery; this is in contrast to keratoconus, which has maximal thinning at or near the apex of the protrusion. Spontaneous rupture of Descemet's membrane and corneal hydrops can occur, but iron lines, stress lines, and anterior scarring are not seen. The corneal diameter may be slightly increased. Fleischer rings are usually not present,

Table 10-5 Noninflammatory Ectatic Disorders Compared and Contrasted: Typical Clinical Presentation and Appearance

	Keratoconus	Pellucid Marginal Degeneration	Keratoglobus
Frequency	Most common	Less common	Rare
Laterality	Usually bilateral	Bilateral	Bilateral
Age at onset	Puberty	Age 20–40 years	Usually at birth
Thinning	Inferior paracentral	Inferior band 1–2 mm wide	Greatest in periphery
Protrusion	Thinning at apex	Superior to band of thinning	Generalized
Iron line	Fleischer ring	Sometimes	None
Scarring	Common	Only after hydrops	Mild
Striae	Common	Sometimes	Sometimes

Modified from Krachmer JH, Mannis MJ, Holland EJ, eds. *Cornea.* 2nd ed. Vol 1. Philadelphia: Elsevier/Mosby; 2005:955.

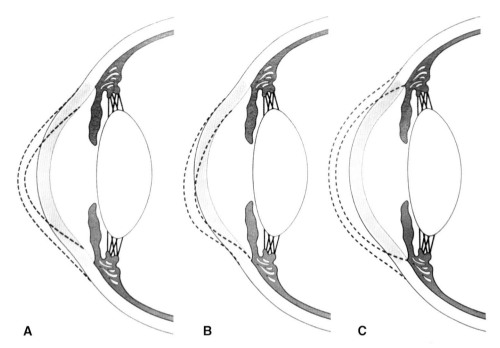

A **B** **C**

Figure 10-32 The presence of corneal thinning and the type of contour abnormality can be helpful in recognizing the type of ectatic disorder. **A,** Keratoconus. **B,** Pellucid marginal degeneration. **C,** Keratoglobus. *(Reproduced with permission from Krachmer JH, Mannis MJ, Holland EJ, eds. Cornea. 2nd ed. Vol 1. Philadelphia: Elsevier/Mosby; 2005:956.)*

but prominent folds and areas of thickening in Descemet's membrane are common. Keratoglobus may be associated with blue sclerae, hyperextensibility of the joints, sensorineural deafness, fractures, and corneal perforation with minimal trauma (fragile cornea).

MANAGEMENT   Contact lenses, especially scleral lenses, may be of benefit. Prognosis for successful PK is much poorer in keratoglobus than in the other ectasias. A lamellar tectonic graft followed by PK could be considered in cases requiring intervention to maintain functional vision. Spontaneous corneal rupture has been reported, so patients must be counseled regarding the importance of protective eyewear. High myopia is treated with spectacles to prevent amblyopia.

Feder RS, Kshettry P. Noninflammatory ectatic disorders. In: Krachmer JH, Mannis MJ, Holland EJ, eds. *Cornea.* 2nd ed. Vol 1. Philadelphia: Elsevier/Mosby; 2005:955–974.

CHAPTER 11

Metabolic Disorders With Corneal Changes

Many of the corneal manifestations of systemic disease are alterations in corneal clarity caused by abnormal storage of metabolic substances within the epithelium, stroma, or endothelium. Abnormal substances typically accumulate in lysosomes or lysosome-like intracytoplasmic structures as a result of a single enzyme defect. Most of these disorders are autosomal recessive, with the notable exceptions of Hunter syndrome (mucopolysaccharidosis type II) and Fabry disease, which are both X-linked recessive.

> Kenyon KR, Navon SE, Haritoglou C. Corneal manifestations of metabolic diseases. In: Krachmer JH, Mannis MJ, Holland EJ, eds. *Cornea.* 2nd ed. Vol 1. Philadelphia: Elsevier/Mosby; 2005:749–776.

Disorders of Carbohydrate Metabolism

Mucopolysaccharidoses

Systemic mucopolysaccharidoses (MPSs) are rare, inherited lysosomal storage diseases that result from the absence of lysosomal acid hydrolases, the enzymes that usually catabolize the glycosaminoglycans (GAGs) dermatan sulfate, heparan sulfate, and keratan sulfate.

PATHOGENESIS   Although there are at least 8 separate syndromes, several features are common to all. Heparan sulfate, dermatan sulfate, and keratan sulfate, the GAGs normally present in highest concentration, are the accumulated metabolites. All syndromes are autosomal recessive, with the exception of the X-linked recessive Hunter syndrome, which rarely involves the cornea until old age, if at all. Hurler (MPS I H), Scheie (MPS I S), and the intermediate (Hurler-Scheie, MPS I H/S) syndromes are all allelic for the enzyme α-L-iduronidase, with different nucleotide substitutions leading to different amino acid substitutions and markedly reduced enzyme activity (<0.1% of normal). Normally, GAGs constitute the ground substance of the cornea, but in these diseases, microscopic deposits of mucopolysaccharide are found in the keratocytes and stroma and, in some cases, in the corneal epithelium and endothelium.

CLINICAL FINDINGS   Differential findings are listed in Table 11-1. These various conditions are characterized by corneal clouding, retinopathy, and optic atrophy, although Sanfilippo

Table 11-1 Clinical Features of Mucopolysaccharidosis

I H: Hurler	VI: Maroteaux-Lamy	I S: Scheie	IV: Morquio	II: Hunter	III: Sanfilippo
Autosomal recessive	Autosomal recessive	Autosomal recessive	Autosomal recessive	X-linked recessive trait	Autosomal recessive
Severe corneal clouding within the first few years	Severe corneal clouding within the first few years	Corneal opacification from birth and slowly progresses to cause decreased vision by the second decade of life	Corneal opacities after 10 years old	Does not present as a congenital corneal opacity	Corneal opacity rarely develops
Diffuse punctate stromal opacities are present without involvement of the epithelium and endothelium	Narrow-angle glaucoma has been reported	Cornea appears thickened or edematous Corneal changes may be more prominent in the corneal periphery Glaucoma has also been reported		Corneal opacity may occur later in life in milder phenotypes	
Syndrome: mental retardation, dwarfism, large head with abnormal-appearing face, enlarged abdomen, and contractures of the joints Other abnormalities: hepatosplenomegaly; thickening of the skin, lips, and tongue; chest enlargement; hirsutism; deafness; neurologic defects; and cardiac defects Diagnosis confirmed by measuring the affected enzyme in peripheral leukocytes, cultured dermal fibroblasts, or amniotic cells	Mild facial abnormalities and multiple skeletal changes, dwarfism, kyphosis, protuberant sternum, and genu valgum Other abnormalities: optic neuropathy, hydrocephalus	Clawhand deformities, bony changes in the feet, and aortic valve abnormalities may be present	Dwarfism, aortic valvular disease, and laxity of the joints	Clinically it appears similar to Hurler syndrome Deafness and heart defects are common	

Reproduced with permission from Krachmer JH, Mannis MJ, Holland EJ, eds. *Cornea*. 2nd ed. Vol 1. Philadelphia: Elsevier/Mosby; 2005:320.

syndrome only occasionally has corneal opacities, and Hunter syndrome only rarely has corneal clouding. Clouding generally involves the entire cornea and may or may not be present at birth. It is often slowly progressive from the periphery toward the center and can cause serious reduction in visual acuity.

LABORATORY EVALUATION   Intracellular storage and extracellular accumulation of partially degraded GAGs are evident in tissues. The conjunctiva allows for a potential biopsy site. Numerous intracytoplasmic vacuoles in stromal fibroblasts and histiocytes contain fine fibrillogranular material. Vascular perithelial cells and lymphatic endothelial cells have similar inclusions. Schwann cells of conjunctival nerves have numerous membranous lamellar inclusions.

Although conjunctival biopsy can confirm classic histopathology, specific diagnosis requires biochemical assay for enzymes in tears, leukocytes, cultured fibroblasts, or amniotic cells and for elevated urinary GAG levels.

In the cornea, similar fibrillogranular accumulation is found in vacuoles of the basal epithelial cells, subepithelial histiocytes, and keratocytes. The degree of corneal clouding appears proportional to the amount of GAG accumulation.

Histiocytes laden with abnormally accumulated storage material (gargoyle cells) are found. Electron microscopic and x-ray diffraction studies show an abnormally large range of corneal stromal fibril size (2000–5200 angstroms [Å], in contrast to a normal 2600-Å size) with disruption of the extracellular matrix by sulfated GAG deposits. These factors cause significant light scattering and thus the clouding.

MANAGEMENT   These conditions, as well as those discussed in the following sections, are sometimes amenable to penetrating keratoplasty (PK), unless impairment of the patient's mental status or retinal or optic nerve abnormalities preclude visual improvement. The prognosis for successful keratoplasty is considered guarded, as the abnormal storage material may accumulate again in the graft. Some regression of corneal clouding following successful donor stem cell bone-marrow transplantation occurs in about one third of patients. Enzyme replacement therapy is being used for Scheie and Hurler syndromes, and gene transfer therapy is under investigation.

Diabetes Mellitus

The most common disorder of carbohydrate metabolism, diabetes mellitus (DM), has nonspecific corneal manifestations of punctate epithelial erosions, basement membrane changes resembling epithelial basement membrane dystrophy, Descemet's folds, and decreased corneal sensation. Diabetes is discussed at length in BCSC Section 12, *Retina and Vitreous,* although the emphasis is on retinal rather than corneal aspects of the disease.

PATHOGENESIS   Patients with DM have ultrastructural abnormalities of the basement membrane complex that contribute to problems of epithelial–stromal adhesion. These abnormalities include thickening of the multilaminar basement membrane, reduced hemidesmosome number, and decreased penetration of anchoring fibrils. Accumulation of polyols such as sorbitol by the action of aldose reductase on excess glucose may contribute to the alterations in the epithelium and endothelium and the corneal hypoesthesia seen in these patients.

CLINICAL FINDINGS   Corneal epithelial surface changes and hypoesthesia occur with increasing severity (eg, type 1 diabetes, or insulin-dependent diabetes mellitus, as opposed to type 2 diabetes, or non–insulin-dependent diabetes mellitus) and increasing duration of the disease. Removal of diabetic epithelium at surgery results in the loss of the basal cells and basement membrane, often leading to prolonged healing difficulties. Faint vertical folds in Descemet's membrane and deep stroma (Waite-Beetham lines) are not specific to DM but may represent early endothelial dysfunction and increased stromal hydration.

LABORATORY EVALUATION   Glycosolated hemoglobin is related to poor control of DM and may correlate with poor corneal healing in addition to progressive retinopathy.

MANAGEMENT   DM is not a contraindication to PK or other corneal surgery. Measures that can improve diabetic epitheliopathy include the following:

- perioperative management of meibomian gland dysfunction (increased comorbidity with DM)
- minimizing epithelial debridement at surgery
- increasing lubrication
- avoiding toxic medications
- using therapeutic contact lenses

Bartow, RM. Endocrine disease and the cornea. In: Krachmer JH, Mannis MJ, Holland EJ, eds. *Cornea*. 2nd ed. Vol 1. Philadelphia: Elsevier/Mosby; 2005:831–839.

Disorders of Lipid Metabolism and Storage

Hyperlipoproteinemias

Hyperlipoproteinemias are common conditions associated with premature coronary artery and peripheral vascular disease. Recognition of the ocular hallmarks of these diseases, such as xanthelasma and corneal arcus, can result in early intervention and reduced morbidity.

PATHOGENESIS   Extracellular deposits consist of cholesterol, cholesterol esters, phospholipids, and triglycerides.

CLINICAL FINDINGS   Corneal arcus is a very common degenerative change of older patients and does not require systemic evaluation. However, corneal arcus in individuals younger than 40 years of age or corneal arcus that is significantly asymmetric may suggest a lipid abnormality. These patients should have a systemic workup. Asymmetry may be secondary to carotid atherosclerotic disease on the less affected side.

Table 11-2 gives the Fredrickson classification of 5 types of hyperlipoproteinemia. Types II and III are associated with early-onset xanthelasma and corneal arcus, or arcus juvenilis. Type III has been linked to 19q13.2 (apolipoprotein E mutation).

Table 11-2 Genetically Determined Hyperlipoproteinemias (Frederickson Classification)

Type	Lipoprotein	Elevated Lipid	Clinical Findings	Ocular Findings	Inheritance
I	Chylomicrons	Triglycerides	Xanthoma/ pancreatitis	LR	AR
IIa	LDL	Cholesterol	Xanthoma/CAD	CA/XAN	AD
IIb	LDL and VLDL	Cholesterol	CAD	CA/XAN	AD
III	Chylomicron and VLDL remnants	Cholesterol and triglycerides	Xanthoma/CAD	LR/CA/XAN	AR
IV	VLDL	Triglycerides	Mild CAD/PAD	LR	AD
V	Chylomicrons and VLDL	Cholesterol and triglycerides	Xanthoma/ pancreatitis Mild CAD/PAD	LR	AD

AD = autosomal dominant, AR = autosomal recessive, CA = corneal arcus, CAD = coronary artery disease, LDL = low-density lipoprotein, LR = lipemia retinalis, PAD = pulmonary artery disease, VLDL = very low-density lipoprotein, XAN = xanthelasma.

Modified from Harrisons Online 2004–2005; and Bron AJ. Dyslipoproteinemias and their ocular manifestations. *Birth Defects Orig Artic Ser.* 1976;12:257–270.

Schnyder crystalline corneal dystrophy is thought to be a localized defect of lipid metabolism, but laboratory evaluation is needed to rule out concurrent systemic abnormality (see Chapter 10).

LABORATORY EVALUATION A fasting and alcohol-restricted lipid profile that includes cholesterol, triglycerides, and high- and low-density lipoproteins (HDL and LDL, respectively) is required. Patients can then be classified phenotypically to assess their risk for atherosclerotic disease.

MANAGEMENT Early detection gives the patient time to be referred for diet or drug treatment.

Hypolipoproteinemias

Abnormal reductions in serum lipoprotein levels occur in 5 disorders:

1. lecithin-cholesterol acyltransferase (LCAT) deficiency
2. Tangier disease
3. fish eye disease
4. familial hypobetalipoproteinemia
5. Bassen-Kornzweig syndrome

The last 2 disorders do not result in corneal disease; discussion here focuses on the other 3 disorders.

PATHOGENESIS LCAT facilitates the removal of excess cholesterol from peripheral tissues to the liver, and a deficiency leads to accumulation of unesterified cholesterol in the tissues. This, in turn, leads to atherosclerosis, renal insufficiency, early corneal arcus, and nebular corneal clouding composed of minute focal lipid deposits.

LCAT deficiency and fish eye disease are allelic variants of the same genetic locus on chromosome 16q22.1, but fish eye disease has normal levels of LCAT that do not function to help HDL in esterifying cholesterol. Tangier disease has a complete absence of serum high-density α-lipoproteins and maps to 9q22-q31.

CLINICAL FINDINGS   All 3 cornea-affecting hypolipoproteinemias are rare, autosomal recessive conditions. Familial LCAT deficiency is characterized by peripheral arcus and nebular stromal haze made up of myriad minute focal deposits of lipid that appear early in childhood but do not interfere with vision. Fish eye disease has obvious corneal clouding from minute gray-white-yellow dots that progress from the periphery to decrease vision. Tangier disease, named after the Chesapeake Bay island, features very large orange tonsils; enlarged liver, spleen, and lymph nodes; hypocholesterolemia; abnormal chylomicron remnants; and markedly reduced HDL in the plasma. Corneas show diffuse clouding and posterior focal stromal opacities but no arcus. Neuropathy leads to lagophthalmos and corneal sequelae.

LABORATORY EVALUATION AND MANAGEMENT   The serum lipid profile shows characteristic low levels of HDL. Recognition can allow the clinician to make appropriate referrals and encourage the patient to seek genetic counseling.

Sphingolipidoses

Sphingolipidoses are rare inherited disorders of complex lipids (gangliosides and sphingomyelin) that involve the cornea in 3 conditions:

1. Fabry disease (angiokeratoma corporis diffusum)
2. multiple sulfatase deficiency
3. generalized gangliosidosis (GM_1 gangliosidosis type I)

PATHOGENESIS   These disorders of lipid storage are autosomal recessive, with the exception of Fabry, which is X-linked recessive. They principally affect the retina or optic nerve and may lead to CNS dysfunction. Fabry disease is again an important exception. It is caused by a deficiency of α-galactosidase A, leading to the accumulation of ceramide trihexoside in the renal and cardiovascular systems. Multiple sulfatase deficiency combines features of metachromatic leukodystrophy and mucopolysaccharidosis. Affected children have subtle diffuse corneal opacities, macular changes, optic atrophy, and progressive psychomotor retardation. They die in the first decade. Generalized gangliosidosis is characterized by deficiencies of β-galactosidases and the accumulation of gangliosides in the CNS and keratan sulfate in somatic tissues. It has been linked to chromosome 3p12-3p13. Although Tay-Sachs disease (hexosaminidase A deficiency with accumulation of GM_2 ganglioside) primarily involves the retina, the corneal endothelial cells can appear distended and filled with single membrane–bound vacuoles.

CLINICAL FINDINGS   In these conditions, the cornea exhibits distinctive changes consisting of whorl-like lines (cornea verticillata) in the basal layers of the epithelium that appear to flow together to the inferior central corneal epithelium (Fig 11-1).

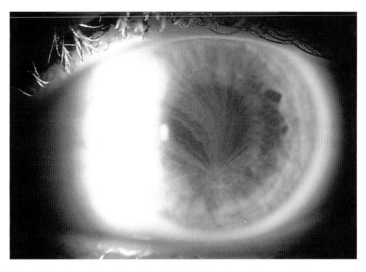

Figure 11-1 Whorl-like deposits of sphingolipid in the basal layer of the corneal epithelium in a patient with Fabry disease; identical deposits occur in otherwise asymptomatic female carriers of this disease.

Periorbital edema occurs in 25% of cases, posterior spokelike cataracts in 50%, and conjunctival aneurysms in 60%. Other ocular signs include papilledema, retinal or macular edema, optic atrophy, and retinal vascular dilation. The corneal changes resemble those seen in patients on long-standing oral chloroquine or amiodarone treatment. A careful drug history will help make this differentiation.

Hemizygous males with Fabry disease are more seriously affected and show the typical corneal changes. A heterozygous female is usually asymptomatic but still shows the same corneal changes. Fabry disease is also characterized by renal failure, peripheral neuropathy with painful dysesthesias in the lower extremities, and skin lesions. The skin lesions are small, round vascular eruptions that later become hyperkeratotic. They consist of an accumulation of sphingolipid within the vascular endothelium.

Corneal opacities have been reported in Gaucher disease, but this is a rare finding.

LABORATORY EVALUATION In Fabry disease, α-galactosidase A is markedly decreased in urine and plasma. Conjunctival biopsy may be positive before cornea verticillata are apparent. Prenatal diagnosis can be performed with chorionic villus sampling.

MANAGEMENT If a female patient is diagnosed as an asymptomatic heterozygous Fabry carrier, genetic counseling should be considered. The prognosis for successful PK in these conditions is generally poor. Enzyme replacement with infusion of α-galactosidase A is a therapeutic option.

Guemes A, Kosmorsky GS, Moodie DS, Clark B, Meisler D, Traboulsi EI. Corneal opacities in Gaucher disease. *Am J Ophthalmol.* 1998;126(6):833–835.

Masson C, Cissé I, Simon V, Insalaco P, Audran M. Fabry disease: a review. *Joint Bone Spine.* 2004;71(5):381–383.

Mucolipidoses

Mucolipidoses (MLs) are autosomal recessive conditions that have features common to both MPSs and lipidoses.

PATHOGENESIS   These diseases are inherited defects of carbohydrate and lipid metabolism combined. Consequently, they have something in common with the MPSs as well as the sphingolipidoses. Mucopolysaccharides accumulate in the cornea and viscera, and sphingolipids are deposited in the retina and CNS. Currently recognized diseases in this class are the following:

- ML I (dysmorphic sialidosis)
- ML II (inclusion-cell disease)
- ML III (pseudo-Hurler polydystrophy)
- ML IV
- Goldberg syndrome
- mannosidosis
- fucosidosis

These conditions are all autosomal recessive. ML IV has been mapped to chromosome 19p. Histopathologic examination of corneal scrapings has revealed the accumulation of intracytoplasmic storage material in the epithelium. In fucosidosis, histopathologic study has revealed that, in spite of clinically normal corneas, corneal endothelial cells show the presence of cytoplasmic, membrane-bound, confluent areas of fibrillar, granular, and multilaminated deposits. A retinal cherry-red spot and retinal degeneration are also associated with many of these disorders. All are caused by a defect in lysosomal acid hydrolase enzymes.

CLINICAL FINDINGS   With the exception of mannosidosis and fucosidosis, which are oligosaccharidoses, all of these conditions are characterized by varying degrees of corneal clouding, which can often be progressive.

LABORATORY EVALUATION   Plasma cells are vacuolated and plasma lysosomal hydrolases are elevated. In ML IV, with corneal clouding from birth, conjunctival biopsy shows fibroblast inclusion bodies that are

- single membrane–limited cytoplasmic vacuoles containing both fibrillogranular material and membranous lamellae
- lamellar and concentric bodies resembling those of Tay-Sachs disease

There is no evidence of mucopolysacchariduria or cellular metachromasia. Chorionic villus sampling has been reported in ML II for prenatal diagnosis.

MANAGEMENT   Both PK and lamellar keratoplasty (LK) have been associated with generally poor results, probably because resurfacing is impaired by the abnormal epithelial cells. Although donor limbal stem cell transplantation has been advocated, tissue matching may be required, as graft rejection in these vascularized recipient beds is possible. Bone-marrow transplantation has been reported.

Bietti Crystalline Corneoretinal Dystrophy

Bietti crystalline corneoretinal dystrophy is a very rare autosomal recessive condition that is characterized by peripheral corneal opacities and tapetoretinal dystrophy. It is presumed to be caused by a defect in lipid metabolism and has been mapped to chromosome 4q35-4qter.

PATHOGENESIS Lysosomes of fibroblasts in the choroid and skin and circulating lymphocytes contain crystalline deposits, but no abnormal accumulation of cholesterol or cholesterol esters has been documented.

CLINICAL FINDINGS Peripheral, sparkling, yellow-white spots are seen at the corneal limbus in the superficial stroma and subepithelial layers of the cornea in 75% of patients. These spots may fade with time. With progression, retinal crystals associated with retinal pigment epithelium atrophy and choroidal sclerosis result in nyctalopia, poor dark adaptation, peripheral visual field loss, or central visual acuity loss.

LABORATORY EVALUATION AND MANAGEMENT Visual fields, dark adaptation testing, and ERG may be normal in early cases, but advanced cases may have decreased ERG and retinal findings of atypical retinitis pigmentosa. No specific treatment is reported.

Palay DA. Corneal deposits. In: Krachmer JH, Mannis MJ, Holland EJ, eds. *Cornea.* 2nd ed. Vol 1. Philadelphia: Elsevier/Mosby; 2005:365–378.

Disorders of Amino Acid Metabolism

Table 11-3 summarizes the ocular and systemic findings in disorders of amino acid metabolism.

Cystinosis

Cystinosis is a rare autosomal recessive disorder characterized by the accumulation of the amino acid cystine within lysosomes. It affects 3.5 infants per 1 million births. Cystinosis has been mapped to chromosome 17p13; the defective gene is *CTNS*.

PATHOGENESIS A defect in transport across the lysosomal membrane leads to accumulation of cystine.

CLINICAL FINDINGS Cystinosis is a systemic metabolic defect that can present as an infantile, intermediate, or adult form. The age at diagnosis averages 1 year but can range into the teenage years. The *infantile,* or *nephropathic,* form features dwarfism and progressive renal dysfunction, with the deposition of fine polychromatic cystine crystals in the conjunctiva, corneal stroma, and other parts of the eye. The *intermediate,* or *adolescent,* form has less severe renal involvement. Systemic cysteamine treatment prevents or delays the negative consequences of the disease, which can include death. In the *adult* form, life expectancy is normal. Crystals can be seen in the corneal stroma on slit-lamp examination and in the trabecular meshwork on gonioscopy. These patients are often photophobic. The crystals, however, usually do not affect visual acuity.

Table 11-3 Disorders of Amino Acid Metabolism

Type	Heredity	Ocular Findings	Associated Conditions	Genetic Linkage
Cystinosis	Rare autosomal recessive	Polychromatic cystine crystals in conjunctiva, trabecular meshwork, and corneal stroma Photophobia	Dwarfism Renal dysfunction	Chromosome 17p13, gene *CTNS*
Tyrosinemia	Autosomal recessive	Photophobia; tearing; conjunctival injection; tarsal papillary hypertrophy; pseudodendrites Epithelial breakdown with secondary corneal neovascularization and scarring	Hyperkeratotic lesions of palms, soles, and elbows Mental retardation	Gene locus at 16q22.1-q22.3
Alkaptonuria	Rare autosomal recessive	Ochronosis (brownish) deposits of alkapton in corneal epithelium or in Bowman layer near limbus Rectus muscle tendons and adjacent sclera develop smudgelike pigmentation	Arthropathy, renal calculi, pigmentation of cartilaginous structures, including earlobes, trachea, nose, and tendons	Gene locus at 3q21-q23

LABORATORY EVALUATION   Cystine crystals may be seen in conjunctival biopsy, blood leukocytes, or bone marrow.

MANAGEMENT   Topical cysteamine drops reduce the density of the crystalline deposits and diminish corneal pain, possibly as a result of a decrease in the development of corneal erosions. Presumably, the topically administered cysteamine reacts with the intracellular cystine, forming a cysteine-cysteamine disulfide that resembles lysine and is transported through the lysosome by the normal lysine transport system. The crystals have been observed to recur in patients who have undergone PK for clouding associated with the corneal deposits. These refractile polychromatic crystals are densest in the peripheral cornea but are seen throughout the anterior stroma, even within the central cornea (Fig 11-2). Posterior manifestations such as pigmentary retinopathy and optic nerve elevation may be treated with oral cysteamine.

> Gahl WA, Kuehl EM, Iwata F, Lindblad A, Kaiser-Kupfer MI. Corneal crystals in nephropathic cystinosis: natural history and treatment with cysteamine eyedrops. *Mol Genet Metab.* 2000;71(1-2):100–120.

Tyrosinemia

Richner-Hanhart syndrome (tyrosinemia type II) is characterized by systemic findings, including hyperkeratotic lesions of palms, soles, and elbows, as well as eventual mental retardation.

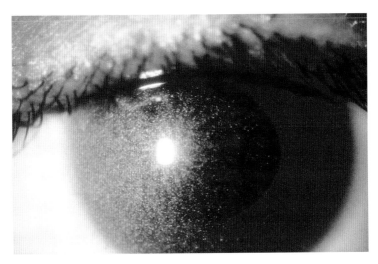

Figure 11-2 Cystinosis. Refractile polychromatic crystals are clustered in the peripheral cornea.

PATHOGENESIS This autosomal recessive disorder occurs secondary to an enzymatic defect of tyrosine aminotransferase that leads to excess tyrosine in the blood and urine. The elevated tyrosine probably has a direct action on lysosomal membranes, leading to release of their enzymes with characteristic changes. The gene locus is at 16q22.1-q22.3.

CLINICAL FINDINGS Ocular changes include marked photophobia, tearing, conjunctival injection, and tarsal papillary hypertrophy. Patients develop recurrent episodes of pseudo-dendrites, which usually do not stain well with fluorescein or rose bengal. Continued episodes of epithelial breakdown can result in corneal vascularization and scarring. It is important to consider this disorder in a young child who may carry a diagnosis of recurrent herpes simplex virus keratitis.

LABORATORY EVALUATION Hypertyrosinemia and tyrosinuria with normal phenylalanine level and biopsy showing soluble tyrosine aminotransferase (TAT) deficiency are diagnostic.

MANAGEMENT Restriction of dietary intake of tyrosine and phenylalanine can reduce both the corneal and systemic changes, including mental retardation. The institution of appropriate dietary restrictions even later in life can improve the mental status.

Alkaptonuria

Alkaptonuria is a rare autosomal recessive disorder with a defect of tyrosine metabolism that maps to gene locus 3q21-q23. An unusually high frequency occurs in the Dominican Republic and Slovakia.

PATHOGENESIS Homogentisate 1,2-dioxygenase, the enzyme necessary to degrade tyrosine and phenylalanine, is deficient. Phenylalanine and tyrosine cannot be metabolized beyond homogentisic acid, which is oxidized and polymerized into alkapton, a brown-black material similar to melanin. Alkapton then deposits in connective tissues as dark pigment known as *ochronosis.* Corneal lesions consisting of homogentisic acid are easily seen by light microscopy. Electron microscopic studies have shown extracellular deposits of finely granular ochronotic pigment in and around collagen fibrils. Intracellular membrane-bound ochronotic pigment granules were observed in macrophages in fibroblasts, along with 2 other forms of extracellular ochronotic pigment.

CLINICAL FINDINGS   Patients develop arthropathy, renal calculi, and pigmentation of cartilaginous structures, including earlobes, trachea, nose, tendons, dura mater, heart valves, and prostate. Eventually, medial and lateral rectus muscle tendons and the sclera adjacent to the tendon insertions develop smudgelike pigmentation. Darkly pigmented, dotlike opacities may appear in the corneal epithelium or in Bowman layer near the limbus.

LABORATORY EVALUATION   Urine turns dark on standing and alkalinization. Homogentisic acid oxidase deficiency can be shown.

MANAGEMENT   No specific therapy is available, although high-dose ascorbic acid is reported to reduce arthropathy in young patients. It is hoped that specific gene therapy will be available to treat this disorder in the future.

> Cheskes J, Buettner H. Ocular manifestations of alkaptonuric ochronosis. *Arch Ophthalmol.* 2000;118(5):724–725.

Disorders of Protein Metabolism

Amyloidosis

The amyloidoses are a heterogeneous group of diseases characterized by the accumulation of amyloid in various tissues and organs. Table 11-4 summarizes ocular findings in the amyloidoses.

PATHOGENESIS   Amyloid is an eosinophilic hyaline material with 5 basic staining characteristics:

1. positive staining with Congo red dye
2. dichroism and birefringence
3. metachromasia with crystal violet dye
4. fluorescence in ultraviolet light with thioflavine T stain
5. typical filamentous appearance by electron microscopy

Protein AP derives from α-globulin and is found in all amyloid fibrils. In addition, amyloid fibrils are composed of immunoglobulin light chains or fragments of light chains (especially of the variable region) and nonimmunoglobulin protein. Amyloid composed of immunoglobulin is designated *AL* for amyloid fibril protein and the L chain amyloid protein. Nonimmunoglobulin amyloid is designated *AA* for amyloid fibril protein and *SAA,* its serum-related protein. Protein AF has several subtypes found in the various dystrophies. These noncollagenous proteins can be deposited in the cornea and conjunctiva and in intraocular or adnexal structures.

Table 11-4 Amyloid in the Eye

Type	Heredity	Ocular Distribution	Associated Conditions	Genetic Linkage
Primary localized amyloidosis	Nonfamilial	Conjunctival plaque Polymorphic amyloid degeneration	None	
	Familial	Lattice corneal dystrophy types I and III Avellino and granular dystrophy Gelatinous droplike dystrophy		5q31 (keratoepithelin gene) 1p32-q12 (*M1S1* gene)
Primary systemic amyloidosis	Nonfamilial	Skin and conjunctiva (very rare)	Occult plasma cell dyscrasias	
	Familial	Ophthalmoplegia (orbital and muscle infiltrates), ptosis, vitreous veils, dry eye, pupil abnormalities	Cardiomyopathy Peripheral neuropathy Gastrointestinal disease Skin involvement	18q11.2-q12.1 (transthyretin gene)
		Lattice corneal dystrophy type II, cranial neuropathies	Meretoja syndrome (facial palsies, skin nodules, rarely renal involvement)	Many others 9q34 (gelsolin gene)
Secondary localized amyloidosis	Nonfamilial	Conjunctiva Skin Cornea	Trachoma, psoriasis, trauma, phlyctenulosis, retinopathy of prematurity, keratoconus, bullous keratopathy, interstitial keratitis, leprosy, contact lens wear, trichiasis, tertiary syphilis, uveitis, climatic droplet keratopathy	
Secondary systemic amyloidosis	Familial	None		
	Nonfamilial	Rarely vitreous body (corneal deposits are not amyloid)	Multiple myeloma	
		Conjunctiva, skin (rare)	Infectious diseases (tuberculosis, leprosy, syphilis) Inflammatory diseases (rheumatoid arthritis, other connective tissue disorders) Hodgkin disease	
	Familial	(Corneal nerve enlargement is not amyloid)	MEN type 2A	10q11.2 (*RET* oncogene)

CLINICAL FINDINGS Ocular amyloidosis is classified as either primary (idiopathic) or secondary (to some chronic disease) and either localized or systemic. A useful classification of amyloidosis considers these 4 types. Each type will be discussed separately:

1. primary localized amyloidosis
2. primary systemic amyloidosis
3. secondary localized amyloidosis
4. secondary systemic amyloidosis

Primary localized amyloidosis is the most common form of ocular amyloidosis. Conjunctival amyloid plaques occur in the absence of systemic involvement (Fig 11-3). Primary familial amyloidosis of the cornea (gelatinous droplike dystrophy), in which pudding-like translucent nodules occur as cobblestone masses on the central corneal surface (Fig 11-4), and lattice corneal dystrophy, a special form of primary localized

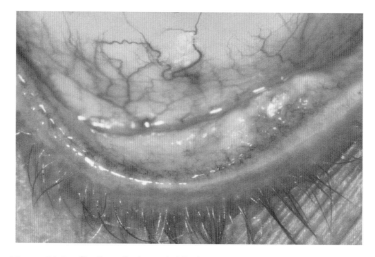

Figure 11-3 Conjunctival amyloidosis. *(Courtesy of Vincent P. deLuise, MD.)*

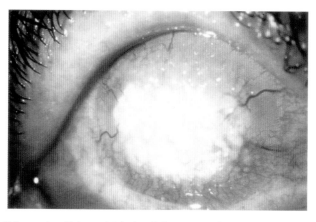

Figure 11-4 Primary familial amyloidosis of the cornea (*gelatinous droplike dystrophy*).

amyloidosis, are discussed in Chapter 10. Polymorphic amyloid degeneration is discussed in Chapter 12.

Primary systemic amyloidosis is a heterogeneous group of diseases in which waxy ecchymotic eyelid papules occur in association with vitreous veils and opacities as well as pupillary anomalies such as light–near dissociation. Orbital involvement, extraocular muscle involvement with ophthalmoplegia, and scleral infiltration with uveal effusion have been reported. The most common form of primary systemic amyloidosis is an auto-somal dominant group of diseases linked to 18q11.2-q12.1, with more than 40 different mutations of the transthyretin (TTR, prealbumin) gene described. Corneal involvement occurs in lattice dystrophy type II (Meretoja syndrome), as discussed in Chapter 10.

Secondary localized amyloidosis is the most common form of amyloidosis of the cornea. It develops in eyes with long-standing chronic inflammatory disease such as trachoma; interstitial keratitis; tumors; or connective tissue disorders, usually rheumatoid arthritis. Corneal involvement may be seen in keratoconus, trachoma, phlyctenulosis, bullous keratopathy, interstitial keratitis, leprosy, contact lens wear, trichiasis, tertiary syphilis, uveitis, and climatic droplet keratopathy. Secondary deposition takes the form of a degenerative pannus, lamellar deposits in the deep stroma, or perivascular deposits. Deposits are typically yellowish pink or yellow-gray, depending on the associated disease.

Secondary systemic amyloidosis features amyloid AA and is seen in association with rheumatoid arthritis, Mediterranean fever, bronchiectasis, and Hansen disease (leprosy). The eyelids can be affected but less commonly than with primary systemic amyloidosis. Amyloid does not deposit in the cornea in secondary systemic amyloidosis.

Chang RI, Ching SST. Corneal and conjunctival degenerations. In: Krachmer JH, Mannis MJ, Holland EJ, eds. *Cornea.* 2nd ed. Vol 1. Philadelphia: Elsevier/Mosby; 2005:987–1004.

Disorders of Immunoglobulin Synthesis

The excess synthesis of immunoglobulins by plasma cells in multiple myeloma, Waldenström macroglobulinemia, and benign monoclonal gammopathy may be associated with crystalline corneal deposits.

PATHOGENESIS Monoclonal proliferation of plasma cells (B lymphocytes) leads to over-production of both light (K or λ) chains and heavy (α, γ, ε, δ, or μ) chains (together, M proteins), overproduction of light chains with or without production of heavy chains (Bence Jones protein), or overproduction of heavy chains without light chains (heavy chain disease). Pathogenesis is related either to direct tissue invasion, particularly of the bone marrow, or to hyperviscosity syndrome. Secondary hypercalcemia may occur. Deposition of paraproteins in the cornea is very rare and is related to diffusion of the proteins, probably from the limbal vessels or, alternatively, from the tears or aqueous humor, followed by precipitation perhaps related to corneal temperature or local tissue factors.

CLINICAL FINDINGS Ophthalmic findings include the following:

- crystalline deposition in all layers of the cornea or in the conjunctiva
- copper deposition in the cornea

- sludging of blood flow in the conjunctiva and retina
- pars plana proteinaceous cysts
- infiltration of the sclera
- orbital bony invasion with proptosis

Corneal deposits are numerous, scintillating, and polychromatic. They are typical of IgG K chain deposition and possibly related to the size of the paraprotein and the chronicity of the disease.

Waldenström macroglobulinemia is characterized by malignant proliferation of plasma cells generating IgM, causing hyperviscosity syndrome, principally in older men. It has been associated with needlelike crystals and amorphous deposits subepithelially and in deep stroma.

Benign monoclonal gammopathy is a frequent finding in people over age 60 (up to 6%). The systemic evaluation in these cases is negative, but a mild increase in paraprotein is detected (<3 g/dL). Slit-lamp findings of iridescent crystals resemble myeloma and are also very infrequent (about 1%–2% of affected patients).

Cryoglobulins are proteins that precipitate on exposure to cold. They occur nonspecifically in autoimmune disorders, immunoproliferative disorders, or hepatitis B infection. Ophthalmic findings include retinal hyperviscosity signs, occasional crystalline corneal deposits, amorphous limbal masses, and signs of autoimmune disease.

LABORATORY EVALUATION   Corneal crystalline deposits have many causes, and evaluation depends on appearance and location in the cornea. Table 11-5 summarizes the differential diagnosis of corneal deposits based on the depth of corneal involvement, color and refractile character, and conjunctival involvement.

Serum protein electrophoresis, complete blood count (CBC), and general screening for albumin/globulin and calcium levels are performed when clinical suspicion of immunoglobulin excess arises. Further testing for systemic evaluation depends on clinical suspicion and the initial findings.

MANAGEMENT   No ophthalmic treatment is needed unless the amorphous depositions interfere with vision and need to be removed with LK. Crystals will resolve slowly after successful treatment of an underlying malignancy.

Noninflammatory Disorders of Connective Tissue

Table 11-6 summarizes the connective tissue disorders associated with corneal changes.

Ehlers-Danlos Syndrome

Ehlers-Danlos syndrome (EDS), a heterogeneous group of diseases, is characterized by hyperextensibility of joints and skin, easy bruisability, and formation of "cigarette paper" scars. It was discussed briefly in Chapter 9 in connection with blue sclera.

PATHOGENESIS   The many (more than 20) known types of Ehlers-Danlos syndrome are classified as autosomal dominant and recessive and X-linked recessive. Eight genetic loci

Table 11-5 Corneal Deposits in Differential Diagnosis

Type	Superficial	Stromal	Deep Stromal/Endothelial	Conjunctiva
Pigmented	Cornea verticillata (Fabry disease, amiodarone)	Phenothiazines	Mercury	Tetracycline
	Striate melanokeratosis	Blood staining	Wilson disease (copper)	Adrenochrome
	Iron lines	Bilirubin	Chalcosis (copper)	
	Pigmented (noncalcific) band keratopathy	Siderosis (iron)	Chrysiasis (systemic gold)	Argyriasis
	Spheroidal degeneration	Corneal tattoo	Argyriasis (topical silver)	
	Adrenochrome		Krukenberg spindle	
	Alkaptonuria			
Nonpigmented	Subepithelial mucinous dystrophy	Granular dystrophy	Cornea farinata	Gout (urate)
	Coats white ring	Macular dystrophy	Pre-Descemet's dystrophy	
	Calcific band keratopathy	Fleck dystrophy	X-linked ichthyosis	
	Ciprofloxacin	Lipid deposition	Argyriasis (silver)	
		Mucopolysaccharidoses		
Refractile/ crystalline	Meesmann dystrophy	Lattice dystrophy	Polymorphic amyloid degeneration	Cystinosis
	Superficial amyloid	Schnyder dystrophy		
	Tyrosinemia type II	Bietti crystalline corneoretinal dystrophy		
	Intraepithelial ointment	Immunoglobulin deposition		
	Gout (urate)	Cystinosis		
		Infectious crystalline keratopathy		

From Palay DA. Corneal deposits. In: Krachmer JH, Mannis MJ, Holland EJ, eds. *Cornea.* 2nd ed. Vol 1. Philadelphia: Elsevier/Mosby; 2005:365–378.

Table 11-6 Skeletal/Connective Tissue Disorders of Interest to the Ophthalmologist

Name (OMIM #)	Corneal Findings	Other Ocular Findings	Genetics/Map/Other Information
Albright hereditary osteodystrophy (300800)	None	Zonular cataracts with multicolored flecks in 25% of patients	AD; sex-influenced 1 male:2 female
Apert syndrome (101200)	Exposure keratitis with severe proptosis Keratoconus (very rare) Megalocornea (very rare)	Strabismus (exotropia with V pattern) Absence of extraocular muscles, proptosis, ocular hypopigmentation, optic atrophy Rare: nystagmus, ptosis, cataract, ectopia lentis, coloboma of iris	AD Gene maps to 10q26 Mutations in *FGFR2*
Carpenter syndrome; acrocephalopolysyndactyly type II (201000)	Exposure keratitis secondary to severe proptosis Microcornea (rare) Corneal leukoma (rare)	Epicanthal folds, antimongoloid slant, hyper- or hypotelorism, optic atrophy, strabismus Rare: coloboma of the iris and choroid, congenital cataract, lens subluxation, nystagmus, retinal detachment	AR
Cockayne syndrome (Type I: 216400 Type B: 133540 Type III: 216411)	Raised inferior corneal lesion, band keratopathy, recurrent erosions	Cataracts, retinal dystrophy, nystagmus, iris atrophy, hyperopia, enophthalmos, strabismus	AR Type I: Chromosome 5 Type II: 10q11
Crouzon syndrome (123500)	Exposure keratitis with severe proptosis Keratoconus (very rare) Microcornea (very rare)	Strabismus (exotropia with V pattern) Exophthalmos, hypertelorism, optic atrophy in 30% Rare: nystagmus, glaucoma, cataract, ectopia lentis, aniridia, anisocoria, myelinated nerve fibers	AD Gene maps to 10q26 Mutations in *FGFR2*
Ehlers-Danlos syndrome (EDS I: 130000 EDS II: 130010 EDS III: 130020 EDS IV: 130050 EDS V: 305200 EDS VI: 225400 EDS VII: AD–130060 EDS VII: AR–225410 EDS VIII: 130080)	Brittle cornea in type VI Keratoconus in types I and VI Keratoglobus in type VI	Epicanthal folds, blue sclerae, retinal detachment, glaucoma, ectopia lentis, angioid streaks (rare)	See text

Syndrome	Ocular Features	Inheritance/Genetics
Goldenhar-Gorlin syndrome; oculoauriculovertebral sequence; hemifacial microsomia (164210)	Limbal dermoid	Upper > lower lid coloboma, strabismus (25%), Duane retraction syndrome, microphthalmia, anophthalmia, lacrimal system dysfunction, optic nerve hypoplasia, tortuous retinal vessels, macular hypoplasia and heterotropia, choroidal hyperpigmentation, iris and retinal colobomas	Sporadic Rarely AD and AR
Hallermann-Streiff-François syndrome; oculomandibulo-dyscephaly (234100)	One case of sclerocornea	Congenital cataracts, spontaneous resorption of lens cortex with secondary membranous cataract formation, glaucoma, uveitis, retinal folds, optic nerve dysplasia, microphthalmia	Sporadic Rarely AD Increases anesthetic risk secondary to tracheomalacia
Hypophosphatasia (Infantile: 241500 Childhood: 241510 Adult: 146300)	Band keratopathy with conjunctival calcifications in infantile form	Blue sclerae, cataracts, optic atrophy secondary to craniostenosis, atypical retinitis pigmentosa; ocular complications present only in infantile and childhood forms, not in adult form	Infantile: AR Childhood: AR, AD Adult: AD *ALPL* gene maps to 1p36-p34
Marfan syndrome (154700)	Megalocornea Flat cornea Keratoconus (uncommon)	Ectopia lentis, strabismus, cataracts, myopia, retinal detachment, glaucoma	AD Gene maps to 15q21.1 Mutations in *FBN-1*
Nail-patella syndrome; onychoosteodysplasia (161200)	Microcornea	Cataracts, microphthalmia	AD Gene maps to 9q34.1
Oculodentoosseous dysplasia (AD: 164200 AR: 257850)	Microcornea	Hypotelorism, convergent strabismus, anterior segment dysgenesis, glaucoma, cataracts, remnants of the hyaloid system	AD; mutations in connexin-43 (*GJA1*) gene on 6q21-23.2
Osteogenesis imperfecta (Type I: 259400 Type II: 166200 Type III: 259420 Type IV: 166220)	Decreased central corneal thickness Keratoconus Megalocornea (rare) Posterior embryotoxon (rare)	Blue sclerae Rare: congenital glaucoma, cataract, choroidal sclerosis, subhyaloid hemorrhage, hyperopia, ectopia lentis	See text

(Continued)

Table 11-6 *(continued)*

Name (OMIM #)	Corneal Findings	Other Ocular Findings	Genetics/Map/Other Information
Parry-Romberg syndrome; progressive facial hemiatrophy (141300)	Neuroparalytic keratitis	Enophthalmos, oculomotor palsies, pupillary abnormalities, Horner syndrome, heterochromia, intraocular inflammation, optic nerve hypoplasia, choroidal atrophy	Sporadic 5% bilateral, left > right
Pierre Robin malformation (261800)	Megalocornea (rare)	Congenital glaucoma, high myopia, vitreoretinal degeneration, retinal detachment, esotropia, congenital cataracts, microphthalmia	Sporadic Stickler syndrome in 1/3 of cases Other syndromes *NB*: increased anesthetic risk secondary to glossoptosis
Rothmund-Thomson syndrome (268400)	Degenerative lesions of cornea	Cataracts	AR 70% female Mutations in DNA helicase (*RECQL4*) on 8q24.3
Treacher Collins syndrome; mandibulofacial dysostosis (154500)	Microcornea	Coloboma of lower lids, dysplasia of bony orbit, absent lower lid cilia, absent lower lid lacrimal punctae, iris coloboma, microphthalmia, strabismus, antimongoloid slant	AD Mutations in treacle (*TCOF1*) gene on 5q32-q33.1
Werner syndrome (277700)	Corneal edema secondary to endothelial decompensation following cataract surgery Poor wound healing	Presenile posterior subcapsular cataracts (20s–30s), proptosis, blue sclerae Rare: nystagmus, astigmatism, telangiectasia of iris, macular degeneration, pigmentary retinopathy	AR Mutations in DNA helicase (*RECQL2*) gene on 8p12-p11

For more information and bibliography on disorders listed in this table, consult Online Mendelian Inheritance in Man (OMIM) at http://www.ncbi.nlm.nih.gov/omim/. The numbers given in column 1 after the disease name(s) are the OMIM entry numbers.

AD = autosomal dominant, AR = autosomal recessive.

Reproduced with permission from Krachmer JH, Mannis MJ, Holland EJ, eds. *Cornea*. 2nd ed. Vol 1. Philadelphia: Elsevier/Mosby; 2005:779–780.

have been identified. Specific defects occur in collagen type I and III synthesis, and there can be lysyl hydroxylase deficiency.

CLINICAL FINDINGS Ehlers-Danlos syndrome VI (EDS VI), or the ocular-scoliotic type, is autosomal recessive and associated with only moderate joint and skin extensibility, brittle cornea easily ruptured on minor trauma, blue sclera, keratoconus and keratoglobus, and severe scoliosis. Type VIA shows lysyl hydroxylase deficiency, but type VIB shows normal production of lysyl hydroxylase.

LABORATORY EVALUATION Traditionally, the clinical diagnosis is confirmed by an insufficiency of hydroxylysine on analysis of hydrolyzed dermis and/or reduced enzyme activity in cultured skin fibroblasts. However, it can also be confirmed by the altered urinary ratio of lysyl pyridinoline to hydroxylysyl pyridinoline that is characteristic for EDS VI.

MANAGEMENT Recognition of the syndrome and awareness of its association with mitral valve prolapse, spontaneous bowel rupture, and complications of strabismus surgery, and of potential confusion of the brittle cornea with child abuse, are essential. Scleral patch grafts for ruptures have been successful. Genetic counseling should be considered.

Marfan Syndrome

Marfan syndrome is a common autosomal dominant disorder associated with disorders of the eye (ectopia lentis), heart (dilation of the aortic root and aneurysms of the aorta), and skeletal system (arachnodactyly, pectus excavatum, and kyphoscoliosis). It maps to chromosome 15q21.1 (fibrillin gene).

PATHOGENESIS Fibrillin and glycoprotein make up the microfibrillar system of the extracellular matrix. Fibrillin is found in corneal basement membrane, zonular fibers of the lens and capsule, and sclera. Defects in fibrillin synthesis lead to thinning of the sclera (blue sclera), lens subluxation, and flattening of the cornea. BCSC Section 11, *Lens and Cataract,* discusses and illustrates the lens subluxation caused by Marfan syndrome.

CLINICAL FINDINGS Megalocornea and keratoconus are uncommon, but excessive flattening (35 D range) occurs in up to 20% of patients.

MANAGEMENT Cardiac evaluation should be completed, as premature mortality is associated with aortic complications. Open-angle glaucoma and cataract occur at a higher rate and earlier age than in the normal population. Lens subluxation may require advanced cataract techniques such as corneal tension rings or scleral fixation.

Disorders of Nucleotide Metabolism

Gout

Hyperuricemia is a heterogeneous group of disorders of purine metabolism that result in increased uric acid. Discrete deposits of urate crystals into the joints or kidney is called *gout.*

PATHOGENESIS Hyperuricemia may be familial, as a result of an enzyme deficiency (eg, hypoxanthine phosphoribosyltransferase in Lesch-Nyhan syndrome). More commonly, it is polygenic or secondary to obesity, cytotoxic chemotherapy, myeloproliferative disease, diuretic therapy, or excessive alcohol consumption.

CLINICAL FINDINGS Acute inflammation of the sclera, episclera, or conjunctiva can occur. Fine corneal epithelial and stromal deposits may appear in the absence of inflammation. See Table 11-5 for differential diagnosis of corneal deposits. An orange-brown band keratopathy or a typical whitish band keratopathy is seen in rare cases.

LABORATORY EVALUATION Serum uric acid level is typically elevated. However, in urate keratopathy, uric acid level may be normal in the presence of keratopathy if there is no concurrent inflammation.

MANAGEMENT Acute treatment is with indomethacin, colchicine, or phenylbutazone; long-term reduction in uric acid levels should be pursued with drugs such as allopurinol. Superficial deposits can be removed mechanically with scraping or keratectomy.

Porphyria

The porphyrias are a group of disorders characterized by excess production and excretion of porphyrins, pigments involved in the synthesis of heme.

PATHOGENESIS *Porphyria cutanea tarda,* the form most commonly associated with ocular surface problems, is either sporadically or autosomal dominantly inherited (chromosome 1p34). The enzyme uroporphyrinogen decarboxylase is deficient, resulting in an accumulation of porphyrins in the liver and in the circulation. Typically, a second insult to the liver such as alcoholism or drug metabolism brings on the condition in late middle age.

The pathogenesis is related to porphyrin accumulation in the skin and mucous membranes and to significant iron overload. A severe form of porphyria, called *hepatoerythropoietic porphyria (HEP),* is a homozygous presentation of the same enzymatic defect, but the onset of the disease occurs in infancy.

CLINICAL FINDINGS Sun-exposed surfaces develop hyperpigmentation, erythema, scleroderma-like changes, increased fragility, and vesicular and ulcerative lesions. Interpalpebral injection occurs, and the conjunctiva may develop vesicles, necrosis, scarring, and symblepharon mimicking bullous pemphigoid. Necrotizing scleritis has been reported. The cornea may be affected by exposure or by thinning and perforation at the limbus. Skin and ocular lesions may fluoresce.

LABORATORY EVALUATION Urine turns dark on standing. Reduced liver and red cell uroporphyrinogen decarboxylase is confirmatory, and hepatic biopsy shows liver parenchyma cells filled with porphyrins that fluoresce bright red in ultraviolet light.

MANAGEMENT Protection from ultraviolet light and reduction of iron by phlebotomy are the principal treatments. No specific ocular treatment is available, and corneal thinning and perforation are treated in standard ways.

Disorders of Mineral Metabolism

Wilson Disease

Inherited as an autosomal recessive metabolic defect linked to chromosome 13q14.3-q21.1, Wilson disease, or *hepatolenticular degeneration,* is caused by multiple allelic substitutions or deletions in DNA coding for an ATPase, Cu^{2+}-transporting, β-polypeptide.

PATHOGENESIS   Copper is deposited in the liver, then in the kidneys, and eventually in the brain and the cornea at Descemet's membrane.

CLINICAL FINDINGS   Muscular rigidity increases, and tremor and involuntary movement gradually occur in a fluctuating course resembling parkinsonism. Unintelligible speech and mild dementia usually occur concomitantly. Equal numbers of patients (40%) present with hepatic or nervous system symptoms. In the cornea, a golden brown, ruby red, or green pigment ring (Kayser-Fleischer ring) appears in peripheral Descemet's membrane (Fig 11-5). Not all patients with bona fide Wilson disease will manifest a Kayser-Fleischer ring, which appears first superiorly, gradually spreading and widening to meet deposits inferiorly. It consists of deposits of copper in the posterior lamella of Descemet's membrane. Gonioscopy may assist in visualizing the ring. A "sunflower" cataract may be present.

The differential diagnosis includes primary biliary cirrhosis, chronic active hepatitis, exogenous chalcosis, and progressive intrahepatic cholestasis of childhood. These and other non-Wilsonian hepatic disorders can also be associated with Kayser-Fleischer rings, but only Wilson disease has decreased serum ceruloplasmin and neurologic symptoms.

LABORATORY EVALUATION   Patients with Wilson disease can be differentiated from patients with other diseases that show Kayser-Fleischer rings by their inability to incorporate radioactive copper into ceruloplasmin. Low serum ceruloplasmin, high nonceruloplasmin-bound serum copper, and high urinary copper suggest the diagnosis, which can be established with liver biopsy. Nonspecific findings of proteinuria, aminoaciduria, glycosuria, uricaciduria, hyperphosphaturia, and hypercalciuria are seen.

MANAGEMENT   Wilson disease can be treated with penicillamine. The Kayser-Fleischer ring disappears gradually with therapy, including liver transplantation, and the disappearance

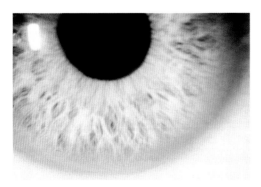

Figure 11-5 Deposits of copper in Descemet's membrane in Kayser-Fleischer ring of Wilson hepatolenticular degeneration. *(Reproduced with permission from Krachmer JH, Mannis MJ, Holland EJ, eds.* Cornea. *2nd ed. Vol 1. Philadelphia: Elsevier/Mosby; 2005:375.)*

of the rings can be used to help monitor therapy. Recently, electrophysiologic abnormalities from retinal dysfunction have been shown to reverse after disease treatment.

Hypercalcemia

Disorders of calcium and phosphate metabolism are associated with formation of *band keratopathy*. See Chapter 12.

Hemochromatosis

Systemic iron overload is not associated with corneal deposits or changes. In rare cases, congenital spherocytosis has been associated with deep intraepithelial reddish brown deposits in an oval shape of unknown pathogenesis. Iron depositions are discussed further in Chapter 12.

Corneal and External Disease Signs of Systemic Neoplasia

Chapter 8 discusses neoplastic disorders in greater depth. See also BCSC Section 7, *Orbit, Eyelids, and Lacrimal System*.

Enlarged Corneal Nerves

Several conditions feature enlarged corneal nerves (Fig 11-6). The most important is multiple endocrine neoplasia (MEN) type 2B. This autosomal dominant (chromosome 10q11.2) disease is characterized by medullary carcinoma of the thyroid gland,

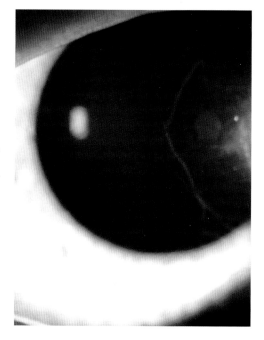

Figure 11-6 Prominent corneal nerve. *(Reproduced with permission from Krachmer JH, Mannis MJ, Holland EJ, eds. Cornea. 2nd ed. Vol 1. Philadelphia: Elsevier/Mosby; 2005:836.)*

Table 11-7 Prominent Corneal Nerves

Enlarged Corneal Nerves	More Visible Corneal Nerves
Multiple endocrine neoplasia type IIB (Sipple-Gorlin syndrome)	Keratoconus
Phytanic acid storage disease (Refsum syndrome)	Ichthyosis
Hansen disease (leprosy, beading of nerves)	Fuchs corneal dystrophy
Familial dysautonomia (Riley-Day syndrome)	Corneal edema
Neurofibromatosis	Congenital glaucoma
Acanthamoeba perineuritis	

pheochromocytoma, and mucosal neuromas in patients who frequently have a marfanoid habitus. Besides the thickened corneal nerves, conjunctival and eyelid neuromas and keratoconjunctivitis sicca may occur. Patients with MEN type 2A also have been noted to have enlarged corneal nerves. Other causes of prominent corneal nerves from either true enlargement or increased visibility are listed in Table 11-7.

CHAPTER 12

Clinical Approach to Depositions and Degenerations of the Conjunctiva, Cornea, and Sclera

Degeneration of a tissue refers to decomposition of tissue elements and deterioration of tissue functions. Degenerations of the ocular surface may occur from physiologic changes associated with aging, or they may follow chronic environmental insults to the eye, such as exposure to ultraviolet light.

Degenerative Changes of the Conjunctiva

Age-related (Involutional) Changes

As a result of aging, the conjunctiva loses transparency. The epithelium thickens and may become keratinized in exposed zones. The substantia propria (stroma) becomes thinner and less elastic. In older persons, the conjunctival vessels can become more prominent. Saccular telangiectasias, fusiform dilatory changes, or tortuosities may appear in the vessels. These changes are not necessarily uniform and tend to be more pronounced in the area of the interpalpebral fissure, corresponding to the area most commonly exposed to the environmental elements.

Pinguecula

A *pinguecula* is a common conjunctival condition that occurs typically at the nasal and temporal anterior bulbar conjunctiva as a result of the effects of ultraviolet (UV) light (actinic exposure), although it may also be related to other insults, such as welding. The epithelium overlying a pinguecula may be normal, thick, or thin. Calcification occurs occasionally.

Pingueculae appear adjacent to the limbus in the interpalpebral zone, more often nasally, and have the appearance of yellow-white, amorphous subepithelial deposits. They may enlarge gradually over long periods of time. Recurrent inflammation and ocular irritation may be encountered.

Lubricant therapy to alleviate ocular irritation is the mainstay of treatment. Excision is indicated only when pingueculae cause cosmetic problems or in the rare instances in which they become chronically inflamed or interfere with successful contact lens wear. Judicious use of topical corticosteroids can be considered in patients with chronic inflammation, but they are strongly discouraged as a chronic therapy for pingueculae due to their side effects.

Pterygium

A *pterygium* is a wing-shaped fold of conjunctiva and fibrovascular tissue that has invaded the superficial cornea (Fig 12-1). As with a pinguecula, the pathogenesis of a pterygium is strongly correlated with UV exposure, although dryness, inflammation, and exposure to wind and dust or other irritants may also be factors. The histopathology of pterygium shows elastotic degeneration of the stromal collagen with subepithelial fibrovascular tissue. Further discussion of the histopathology of both pinguecula and pterygium can be found in BCSC Section 4, *Ophthalmic Pathology and Intraocular Tumors.*

Pterygia are nearly always preceded and accompanied by pingueculae, although why some patients develop pterygia whereas others have only pingueculae is not known. The prevalence of pterygia increases steadily with proximity to the equator. Regular and irregular astigmatism occurs in proportion to pterygium size. A pigmented iron line *(Stocker line)* may be seen at the central anterior edge of the pterygium on the cornea when long-standing and stable. Excision is indicated if the pterygium approaches the visual axis, causing loss of vision from irregular astigmatism or in cases of considerable irritation. See Chapter 15.

Conjunctival Concretions

Concretions appear histopathologically to be epithelial inclusion cysts filled with epithelial and keratin debris. Yellow-white deposits are sometimes found in the palpebral conjunctiva of older patients or patients who have had chronic conjunctivitis. Secondary calcification occurs occasionally, in which case the lesions are sometimes referred to as

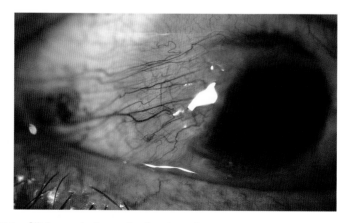

Figure 12-1   Slit-lamp photograph of a pterygium. *(Courtesy of Robert W. Weisenthal, MD.)*

conjunctival lithiasis. The subconjunctival deposition of oral tetracyclines mimics concretions. Concretions are almost always asymptomatic but may erode the overlying epithelium to cause foreign-body sensation. If symptomatic, concretions can be easily removed under topical anesthesia.

Conjunctivochalasis

Conjunctivochalasis is a loose adherence of the lower conjunctiva; it occurs commonly with chronic inflammation or aging and is often overlooked and asymptomatic. Occasionally, the redundant conjunctiva overlies the lower eyelid margin to such an extent that various clinical problems appear (Fig 12-2A, B). These range from the aggravation of dry eye in the mild stages (from exposure of the redundant conjunctiva due to uneven wetting), to secondary tearing due to occlusion of the lower punctum when the chalasis is prominent medially, to exposure-related pain and irritation in its severe stages.

Lubricants, anti-inflammatory agents, antihistamines, and nocturnal patching have been offered as treatments, although none besides lubrication is offered as a long-term potential solution. If these modalities fail, then cautious surgical excision, conjunctival fixation to the sclera, amniotic membrane grafts, or cauterization of the redundant folds may be required.

Di Pascuale MA, Espana EM, Kawakita T, Tseng SC. Clinical characteristics of conjunctivochalasis with or without aqueous tear deficiency. *Br J Ophthalmol.* 2004;88(3):388–392.

Haefliger IO, Vysniauskiene I, Figueiriedo AR, Piffaretti JM. Superficial conjunctiva cauterization to reduce moderate conjunctivochalasis. *Klin Monatsbl Augenheilkd.* 2007;224(4): 237–239.

Maskin SL. Effect of ocular surface deconstruction by using amniotic membrane transplant for symptomatic conjunctivochalasis on fluorescein clearance test results. *Cornea.* 2008;27(6):644–649.

Meller D, Tseng SC. Conjunctivochalasis: literature review and possible pathophysiology. *Surv Ophthalmol.* 1998;43(3):225–232.

Otaka I, Kyu N. A new surgical technique for management of conjunctivochalasis. *Am J Ophthalmol.* 2000;129(3):385–387.

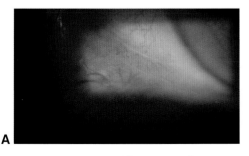
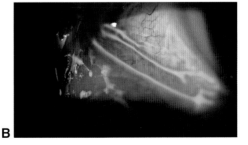

A
B

Figure 12-2 **A** and **B,** "Redundant," or extra, conjunctival tissue inferotemporally overlying the lid, causing foreign-body sensation due to interruption of the tear film, highlighted with fluorescein. *(Courtesy of Robert W. Weisenthal, MD.)*

Degenerative Changes in the Cornea

Age-related (Involutional) Changes

As a result of aging, the cornea gradually becomes flatter, thinner, and slightly less transparent. Its refractive index increases, and Descemet's membrane becomes thicker, increasing from 3 µm at birth to 10 µm in adults as a result of the increased thickness of its posterior nonbanded zone. Occasional peripheral endothelial guttae, sometimes known as *Hassall-Henle bodies,* can form with age (see the discussion later in the chapter). Age-related attrition of corneal endothelial cells results in a loss of about 100,000 cells during the first 50 years of life, from a cell density of about 4000 cells/mm^2 at birth to a density of 2500–3000 cells/mm^2 in older adults. The average rate of endothelial cell density decrease throughout adult life is approximately 0.6% per year. It is important to differentiate corneal degenerations from corneal dystrophies (Table 12-1).

> Bourne WM, Nelson LR, Hodge DO. Central corneal endothelial cell changes over a ten-year period. *Invest Ophthalmol Vis Sci.* 1997;38(3):779–782.

Epithelial and Subepithelial Degenerations

Coats white ring

A small (1 mm or less in diameter) circle or oval-shaped area of discrete gray-white dots is sometimes seen in the superficial stroma. Referred to as *Coats white ring,* it represents iron-containing fibrotic remnants of a metallic foreign body; once these lesions mature and are free of any associated inflammation, they do not change; hence, therapy with corticosteroids or other anti-inflammatories is not indicated (Fig 12-3).

Spheroidal degeneration

Spheroidal degeneration is a common degeneration; it is often bilateral and interpalpebral and is more common in males. It is characterized by the appearance in the cornea, and sometimes in the conjunctiva, of translucent, golden brown, spheroidlike deposits in the superficial stroma (Fig 12-4). The condition has been reported under different names, including *corneal elastosis, keratinoid degeneration, climatic droplet keratopathy, Bietti nodular dystrophy, proteinaceous degeneration,* and *Labrador keratopathy.*

In *primary spheroidal degeneration,* the deposits are bilateral and initially located in the nasal and temporal cornea. With advancing age, they can extend onto the conjunctiva. The degeneration is unrelated to the coexistence of other ocular disease. In rare cases,

---

Table 12-1 Differences Between Corneal Degenerations and Corneal Dystrophies

Degeneration	Dystrophy
Opacity often peripherally located	Often centrally located
May be asymmetric	Bilateral and symmetric
Presents later in life, associated with aging	Presents early in life, hereditary
Progression can be very slow or rapid	Progression usually slow

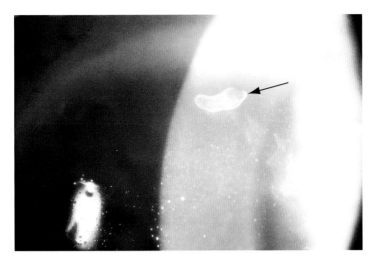

Figure 12-3 Coats white ring *(arrow)* (not to be confused with map-dot-fingerprint dystrophy). *(Courtesy of W. Craig Fowler, MD.)*

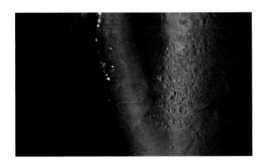

Figure 12-4 Spheroidal degeneration at the corneal limbus *(Courtesy of Robert W. Weisenthal MD.)*

generally in childhood, the spheroidal deposits extend across the interpalpebral zone of the cornea, producing a noncalcific band-shaped keratopathy. *Secondary spheroidal degeneration* is associated with ocular injury or inflammation. The deposits aggregate near the area of corneal scarring or vascularization. All cases show extracellular proteinaceous deposits with characteristics of elastotic degeneration, which are thought to be secondary to the combined effects of genetic predisposition, actinic exposure, age, and perhaps various kinds of environmental trauma other than sunlight, such as wind. The pattern is similar to that of other UV light-associated degenerations, such as pingueculae. The composition is not lipid despite its "oil droplet" appearance. No medical therapy is of much value, although lubrication is recommended to address uneven layering of the tear film over affected areas. In cases of central involvement, superficial keratectomy or excimer excision may be indicated. Recurrence after conjunctival resection is common.

Iron deposition

A *Fleischer ring,* representing iron deposition in keratoconus, is one of many corneal iron lines associated with epithelial irregularities (see Fig 10-28). This sign is extremely useful in the diagnosis of mild or early cases of keratoconus. Often it can be seen only by using red-free or cobalt blue illumination prior to instilling fluorescein. The Hudson-Stähli line, generally located at the junction of the upper two thirds and lower third of the cornea, is ubiquitous. Most iron lines are related to abnormalities of tear pooling related to surface irregularities (Fig 12-5). Iron lines are also associated with keratorefractive procedures. Following radial keratotomy, visually insignificant iron lines are noted centrally in approximately 80% of patients and are commonly characterized as a "tear star." Common conditions associated with corneal iron lines are listed in Table 12-2.

> Palay DA. Corneal deposits. In: Krachmer JH, Mannis MJ, Holland EJ. *Cornea*. 2nd ed. Vol 1. Philadelphia: Elsevier/Mosby; 2005:chap 26, pp 365–378.

Stromal Degenerations

Age-related (involutional) changes

White limbal girdle Two forms of the white limbal girdle of Vogt have been described. Type I is a narrow, concentric, whitish superficial band running along the limbus in the palpebral fissure. A lucid interval appears between the limbus and the girdle. This girdle is a degenerative change of the anterior limiting membrane, with chalklike opacities and small clear areas like the holes in Swiss cheese. Type II consists of small white, flecklike, and needlelike deposits that are often seen at the nasal and temporal limbus in older patients. No clear interval separates this girdle from the limbus. The histopathologic picture represents epithelial elastotic degeneration of collagen, sometimes with particles of calcium.

Corneal arcus Corneal arcus, or arcus senilis, is most often an involutional change modified by genetic factors. However, arcus is sometimes indicative of a hyperlipoproteinemia (involving low-density lipoproteins) with elevated serum cholesterol, especially in patients under 40 years of age (see Chapter 11). It can be a prognostic factor for coronary artery disease in this age group. Arcus occurs occasionally as a congenital anomaly (arcus juvenilis), usually involving only a sector of the peripheral cornea and not associated with abnormalities of serum lipid.

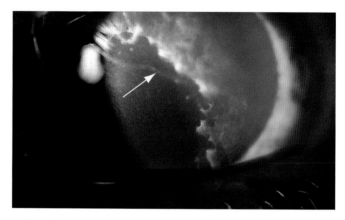

Figure 12-5 Iron deposition (iron line) *(arrow)* due to irregularity of the tear film from subepithelial fibrosis. *(Courtesy of Robert W. Weisenthal, MD.)*

Table 12-2 Corneal Pigmentations

Pigment	Clinical Condition	Location in Cornea
Melanin	Krukenberg spindle	Endothelium, in a vertically oriented ellipse; sometimes associated with pigmentary glaucoma
Melanin-like pigment (oxidized epinephrine)	Adrenochrome deposition	Between basement membrane and Bowman layer or in conjunctival cysts; occurs in patients using topical epinephrine compounds for glaucoma
Melanin-like pigment (alkapton)	Ochronosis	Epithelium and superficial stroma, peripherally; occurs in the metabolic disease alkaptonuria
Iron	Blood staining	Chiefly stroma; epithelium in some cases; occurs in some cases of hyphema
Iron (foreign body)	Siderosis	Chiefly stroma; epithelium in some cases
Iron	Ferry line	Corneal epithelium anterior to filtering bleb
Iron	Fleischer ring (or line)	Corneal epithelium surrounding base of cone in keratoconus
Iron	Hudson-Stähli line	Corneal epithelium at junction of upper two thirds with lower one third of the aging cornea
Iron	Stocker line	Corneal epithelium anterior to head of pterygium
Copper	Kayser-Fleischer ring	Descemet's membrane peripherally, in patients with Wilson hepatolenticular degeneration
Copper	Chalcosis	Descemet's membrane
Silver	Argyriasis	Deep stroma and Descemet's membrane
Gold	Chrysiasis	Deep stroma (more in periphery)
Carbon	Corneal tattoo	Stroma

Arcus is a deposition of lipid in the peripheral corneal stroma. It starts at the inferior and superior poles of the cornea and in the late stages encircles the entire circumference. The incidence is 60% in individuals between the ages of 50 and 60; it approaches 100% in individuals over 80. The frequency is higher in the black population. The arcus has a hazy white appearance, a sharp outer border, and an indistinct central border; it is denser superiorly and inferiorly (Fig 12-6). A lucid interval is usually present between the peripheral edge of the arcus and the limbus. The lipid is found to be concentrated mainly in 2 areas of the peripheral corneal stroma: one adjacent to Bowman layer and another near Descemet's membrane. Unilateral arcus is a rare condition associated with contralateral carotid artery disease or ocular hypotony. Arcus is also seen in Schnyder central crystalline dystrophy.

Crocodile shagreen   Anterior crocodile shagreen, or mosaic degeneration, is a central corneal opacity at the level of Bowman layer characterized by mosaic, polygonal, gray opacities separated by clear zones. Histologically, the Bowman layer is thrown into ridges and may be calcified. Posterior crocodile shagreen shows similar changes in the deep stroma near Descemet's membrane. The posterior variety of crocodile shagreen resembles central cloudy dystrophy of François (see Fig 10-17).

Cornea farinata   Cornea farinata, an involutional change, probably depends on a dominantly transmitted genetic predisposition. The deep corneal stroma shows many dot- and comma-shaped opacities (Fig 12-7). They are very nebulous and subtle and often are best

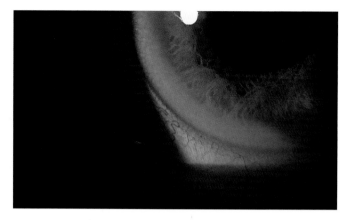

Figure 12-6 Corneal arcus. *(Courtesy of Robert W. Weisenthal, MD.)*

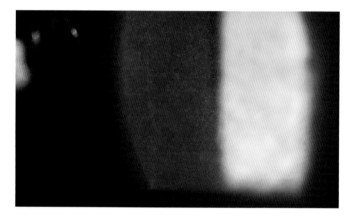

Figure 12-7 Corneal farinata. *(Courtesy of Robert W. Weisenthal, MD.)*

seen with retroillumination. The condition does not affect vision and has no clinical significance, except that it is sometimes mistaken for a progressive dystrophy. The deposits may consist of lipofuscin, a degenerative pigment that appears in some aged cells. Pre-Descemet's dystrophy is probably a morphologic variant of cornea farinata. Although these conditions are most likely related, it is unclear whether they are degenerations or dystrophies.

Polymorphic amyloid degeneration Polymorphic amyloid degeneration is a bilaterally symmetric, slowly progressive corneal degeneration that appears late in life. The corneal opacities emerge as either stellate flecks in mid- to deep stroma or irregular filaments. Both forms may occur together, but usually 1 predominates. These deposits are usually axial, polymorphic, and filamentous. The opacities are gray to white and somewhat refractile but appear translucent in retroillumination (Fig 12-8). The intervening stroma appears clear, and visual acuity is usually normal. The corneal deposits consist of amyloid and can resemble some of the deposits seen in early lattice corneal dystrophy type III.

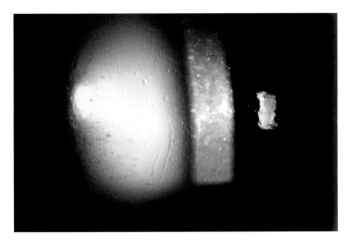

Figure 12-8 Polymorphic amyloid degeneration. *(Courtesy of Robert W. Weisenthal, MD.)*

Peripheral cornea

The peripheral cornea differs from the central cornea in several unique anatomical and physiologic features. Contiguity with the limbal vasculature is the most important difference. Thus, compared to the central cornea, the peripheral cornea is much more susceptible to the adverse effects of pathologies associated with blood vessels, such as inflammatory infiltrations and depositions of serum proteins or other substances. Because of this proximity to limbal vessels, the peripheral cornea is also inevitably involved in the early stage of any condition causing corneal vascularization.

The peripheral cornea is also close to the surrounding conjunctiva, episclera, and sclera and is thus secondarily affected by primary diseases of these adjacent tissues. For example, conjunctival inflammatory conditions such as pterygium and trachoma often involve the peripheral cornea. Mechanical disruption of normal corneal wetting by the adjacent swollen conjunctiva can lead to drying of the peripheral cornea and dellen formation. Autoimmune scleral inflammation (eg, scleritis) may be seen contiguous with peripheral corneal ulceration, in a process called *peripheral ulcerative keratitis (PUK)*.

Senile furrow degeneration Senile furrow degeneration is an appearance of thinning that is seen in older people in the lucid interval of a corneal arcus. There is no inflammation, vascularization, or tendency to perforate. Vision is rarely affected unless astigmatism occurs because of the thinning. Although slight thinning is occasionally present, it is usually more apparent than real. The epithelium is intact. No treatment is required.

Terrien marginal degeneration The cause of Terrien marginal degeneration is unknown. This condition is a quiet, essentially noninflammatory, unilateral or asymmetrically bilateral, slowly progressive thinning of the peripheral cornea. Sex prevalence is roughly equal, and cases usually occur in the second or third decade of life. The corneal thinning can be localized or involve extensive portions of the peripheral cornea.

Terrien marginal degeneration begins superiorly, spreads circumferentially, and rarely involves the inferior limbus. The central wall is steep, and the peripheral wall slopes

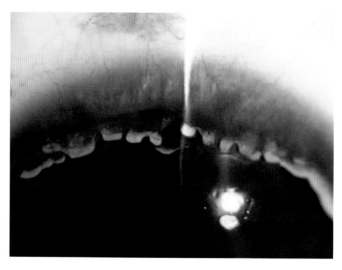

Figure 12-9 Terrien marginal degeneration with superior thinning. *(Courtesy of J. Judelson, MD.)*

gradually. The epithelium remains intact, and a fine vascular pannus traverses the area of stromal thinning. A line of lipid deposits appears at the leading edge of the pannus (central edge of the furrow) (Fig 12-9). Spontaneous perforation is rare, although perforation can easily occur with minor trauma. Corneal topography reveals flattening of the peripheral thinned cornea, with steepening of the corneal surface approximately 90° away from the midpoint of the thinned area. This pattern usually results in high against-the-rule or oblique astigmatism. Spontaneous ruptures in Descemet's membrane can result in interlamellar fluid or even a corneal cyst.

An inflammatory condition of the peripheral cornea that may resemble Terrien marginal degeneration occurs, in rare instances, in children and young adults. Also known as *Fuchs superficial marginal keratitis,* it features progressive thinning without epithelial ulceration and can lead to perforation.

Surgical correction is indicated when perforation is imminent due to progressive thinning or when marked astigmatism significantly limits visual acuity. Crescent-shaped lamellar or full-thickness corneoscleral patch grafts may be used and have been reported to arrest the progression of severe against-the-rule astigmatism for up to 20 years. Annular lamellar keratoplasty grafts may be required in severe cases of 360° marginal degeneration.

Postinflammatory changes

Salzmann nodular degeneration   Salzmann nodular degeneration is a noninflammatory corneal degeneration that sometimes occurs as a late sequela to old, long-standing keratitis, or it may often be idiopathic. Causes include phlyctenulosis, trachoma, and interstitial keratitis. The degeneration may not appear until years after the active keratitis has subsided. It can be bilateral and is more common in middle-aged and older women. The nodules are gray-white or blue-white and elevated (Fig 12-10), and they may be associated with recurrent erosion. They often develop in a roughly circular configuration in the central or paracentral cornea and at the ends of vessels of a pannus. Histopathologic examination

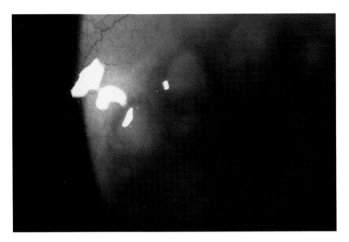

Figure 12-10 Salzmann corneal nodules in the superonasal periphery of the cornea. *(Courtesy of Robert W. Weisenthal, MD.)*

reveals localized replacement of Bowman layer by hyaline and fibrillar material, probably representing basement membrane and material similar to that found in spheroidal degeneration. Treatment for mild cases is lubrication, although superficial keratectomy may be indicated in more severe cases causing decreased vision secondary to irregular astigmatism. This degeneration may recur after removal; however, treatment with mitomycin C at the time of surgery has been shown to reduce the incidence of recurrence.

> Bowers PJ Jr, Price MO, Zeldes SS, Price FW Jr. Superficial keratectomy with mitomycin C for the treatment of Salzmann's nodules. *J Cataract Refract Surg.* 2003;29(7):1302–1306.

Amyloid degeneration   Acquired (secondary localized) corneal amyloidosis may be associated with corneal inflammation (such as trachoma, keratoconus, Hansen disease [leprosy], or phlyctenulosis) or intraocular disease (such as uveitis, retinopathy of prematurity, or glaucoma) or may be secondary to trauma. Clinically, amyloid deposits usually occur as raised, yellow-pink nodular masses in the cornea. Less commonly, they may appear as perivascular deposits. In most cases, corneal vascularization is associated with the amyloid. The deposits may be refractile with retroillumination. See the discussion on amyloidosis in Chapter 11. Amyloid deposits of the conjunctiva are described in BCSC Section 4, *Ophthalmic Pathology and Intraocular Tumors.*

Corneal keloid   Corneal keloids are white, sometimes protuberant, glistening corneal masses that often resemble dermoids and can involve the entire corneal surface. They are thought to be secondary to a vigorous fibrotic response to corneal perforation or injury. The resemblance to corneal dermoids can make diagnosis difficult. Subtle differences between corneal keloids and dermoids include the glistening and jellylike quality of the keloids. Definitive diagnosis can be made by corneal biopsy. Study of enucleation specimens has revealed associated findings, including cataract, anterior staphyloma, ruptured lens capsule with lens fragments in the wound, buphthalmos, chronic glaucoma, and angle-closure glaucoma.

Lipid keratopathy   In lipid keratopathy, yellow or cream-colored lipids containing cholesterol, neutral fats, and glycoproteins are deposited in the superficial or deeper cornea, usually in areas of vascularized corneal scars. The epithelium is involved secondarily, after prolonged corneal inflammation with corneal vascularization (eg, herpes simplex or herpes zoster keratitis or trachoma). This form is best described as secondary lipid keratopathy (Fig 12-11). Argon laser treatment with and without fluorescein and subconjunctival and topical bevacizumab have been reported to reduce corneal neovascularization and lipid deposition. Lipid keratopathy has been reported, in rare instances, with no evidence of an antecedent infection, inflammatory process, or corneal damage. These cases are best described as primary lipid keratopathy.

Doctor PP, Bhat PV, Foster CS. Subconjunctival bevacizumab for corneal neovascularization. *Cornea.* 2008;27(9):992–995.

Gordon YJ, Mann RK, Mah TS, Gorin MB. Fluorescein-potentiated argon laser therapy improves symptoms and appearance of corneal neovascularization. *Cornea.* 2002;21(8): 770–773.

You IC, Kang IS, Lee SH, Yoon KC. Therapeutic effect of subconjunctival injection of bevacizumab in the treatment of corneal neovascularization. *Acta Ophthalmol.* 2009;87(6): 653–658.

Calcific band keratopathy   Calcific band keratopathy (calcium hydroxyapatite deposition) is a calcific degeneration of the superficial cornea that involves mainly Bowman layer. It is often idiopathic. There are 6 main known causes:

1. chronic ocular disease (usually inflammatory) such as uveitis in children, interstitial keratitis, severe superficial keratitis, and phthisis bulbi
2. hypercalcemia caused by hyperparathyroidism, vitamin D toxicity, milk–alkali syndrome, sarcoidosis, and other systemic disorders
3. hereditary transmission (primary hereditary band keratopathy, with or without other anomalies)
4. elevated serum phosphorus with normal serum calcium, which sometimes occurs in patients with renal failure
5. chronic exposure to mercurial vapors or to mercurial preservatives (phenylmercuric nitrate or acetate) in ophthalmic medications (the mercury causes changes in corneal collagen that result in the deposition of calcium)
6. silicone oil instillation in an aphakic eye

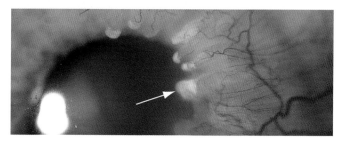

Figure 12-11   Lipid keratopathy secondary to corneal vascularization *(arrow points to lipid).* *(Courtesy of Robert W. Weisenthal, MD.)*

Other rare associated disorders have been reported, including iris melanoma. Band keratopathy may also result from the deposition in the cornea of urates, which appear brown, unlike the gray-white calcific deposits, and may be associated with gout or hyperuricemia.

Calcific band keratopathy begins as fine, dustlike, basophilic deposits in Bowman layer. These changes are usually first seen peripherally. A peripheral clear zone representing a lucid interval is seen between the limbus and the peripheral edge of the keratopathy. Eventually, the deposits may coalesce to form a horizontal band of dense calcific plaques across the interpalpebral zone of the cornea (Fig 12-12).

A reasonable first step in managing this condition would be a workup (eg, serum electrolytes and urinalysis) to rule out associated metabolic/renal disease. Underlying conditions, such as keratoconjunctivitis sicca or renal failure, should be treated or controlled as much as possible, which may reduce or control the deposition of calcium or at least help reduce the recurrence of band keratopathy. The calcium can usually be removed from Bowman layer by chelation with a neutral solution of disodium ethylenediaminetetraacetic acid (EDTA; usual concentration 0.5%–1.5%), which can be warmed to speed up the chemical chelation of calcium. (Disodium EDTA is no longer commercially available but can be obtained through a compounding pharmacy.) The epithelium overlying the calcium needs to be removed prior to applying the chelating solution. Any cylindrical tube that approximates the corneal diameter can facilitate the process by acting as a reservoir to confine the chelating solution to the desired treatment area, although this is not always necessary. With the reservoir in place, very gentle surface agitation with truncated Weck-Cel sponges may further enhance the release of the impregnated calcium. If used at all, scraping should be gentle so as to prevent damage to Bowman layer. A fibrous pannus may be present along with extensive calcific band keratopathy, especially if silicone oil is responsible, and neither EDTA nor scraping will remove such fibrous tissue. A soft contact lens can be helpful postoperatively until the epithelium has healed. The problem can recur but may not do so for years, at which time the treatment may be repeated.

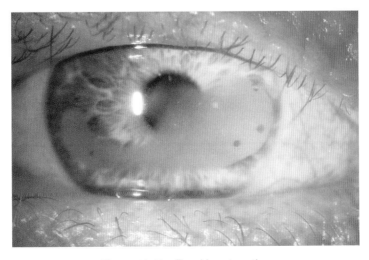

Figure 12-12 Band keratopathy.

Phototherapeutic keratectomy (PTK) using excimer laser is not advised as a primary treatment because calcium ablates at a different rate from stroma, which could produce a severely irregular surface. If residual opacification remains after the initial EDTA chelation, then PTK may be employed.

Roy FH. Corneal and conjunctival calcification. In: Roy FH, Fraunfelder FW, Fraunfelder FT. *Roy and Fraunfelder's Current Ocular Therapy*. 6th ed. Current Therapy series. Philadelphia: Elsevier/Saunders; 2008:337–338.

Endothelial Degenerations

Iridocorneal endothelial syndrome

Iridocorneal endothelial (ICE) syndrome is a spectrum of disorders characterized by varying degrees of corneal edema, glaucoma, and iris abnormalities (Fig 12-13).

The pathogenesis of ICE syndrome is unknown but appears to involve an abnormal clone of endothelial cells that takes on the ultrastructural characteristics of epithelial cells. The condition appears to represent an acquired maldifferentiation of a group of endothelial cells, although the abnormal clone could originate at birth or before. Varying degrees of endothelialization take place in the anterior chamber angle and on the iris surface. Herpesvirus DNA has been identified in some corneal specimens following keratoplasty and in the aqueous humor of some patients. This raises the intriguing possibility that a herpes simplex virus infection may induce these changes.

When the pathology is confined to the inner corneal surface, corneal edema may result from subnormal endothelial pump function, producing the Chandler variant of ICE syndrome. Frequently, the border between the abnormal and normal endothelium can be seen at the slit lamp using specular reflection. When the abnormal endothelium migrates over the anterior chamber angle, the resultant peripheral anterior synechiae and outflow obstruction produce glaucoma. When the abnormal endothelium spreads onto the surface of the iris, the resulting contractile membrane may produce iris atrophy, corectopia, and polycoria, hallmarks of the essential iris atrophy variant of ICE syndrome (see Fig 12-13).

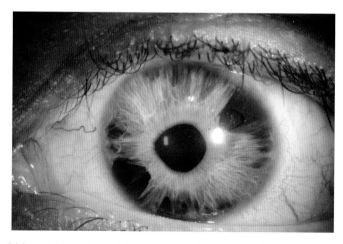

Figure 12-13 Iridocorneal endothelial syndrome with corectopia. *(Courtesy of Stephen Orlin, MD.)*

The Cogan-Reese (or iris nevus) variant shows multiple pigmented iris nodules, also produced by the contracting endothelial membrane.

This syndrome becomes apparent most commonly in middle-aged females and is almost always unilateral. Asymmetric posterior polymorphous dystrophy, as well as other causes of unilateral corneal edema, must be included in the differential diagnosis of ICE syndrome.

Penetrating keratoplasty and endothelial keratoplasty are effective treatments for the corneal component of this syndrome. Glaucoma is an important feature of the ICE syndrome. Long-term graft clarity depends on the successful control of IOP, which can be difficult (see BCSC Section 10, *Glaucoma*).

Alvarado JA, Underwood JL, Green WR, et al. Detection of herpes simplex viral DNA in the iridocorneal endothelial syndrome. *Arch Ophthalmol.* 1994;112(12):1601–1609.

Carpel EF. Iridocorneal endothelial syndrome. In: Krachmer JH, Mannis MJ, Holland EJ. *Cornea.* 2nd ed. Vol 1. Philadelphia: Elsevier/Mosby; 2005:chap 79, pp 975–985.

Groh MJ, Seitz B, Schumacher S, Naumann GO. Detection of herpes simplex virus in aqueous humor in iridocorneal endothelial (ICE) syndrome. *Cornea.* 1999;18(3):359–360.

Herde J. Iridocorneal endothelial syndrome (ICE-S): classification, clinical picture, diagnosis. *Klin Monatsbl Augenheilkd.* 2005;222(10):797–801.

Price MO, Price FW Jr. Descemet stripping with endothelial keratoplasty for treatment of iridocorneal endothelial syndrome. *Cornea.* 2007;26(4):493–497.

Peripheral cornea guttae

Peripheral cornea guttae (Hassall-Henle bodies) are small, wartlike excrescences that appear in the peripheral portion of Descemet's membrane as a normal aging change. They occur on the posterior aspect of the membrane and protrude toward the anterior chamber. With the slit lamp, Hassall-Henle bodies have the appearance of small, dark dimples within the endothelial mosaic; these are best seen by specular reflection. Rarely seen before age 20, they then increase steadily in number with age. They are pathologic when they appear in the central cornea and are then referred to as *cornea guttae*. Central cornea guttae associated with progressive stromal and eventually epithelial edema represent Fuchs endothelial dystrophy (see Chapter 10). They are the result of localized overproduction of basement membrane by endothelial cells and so have the same collagenous structure as does normal Descemet's membrane.

Melanin pigmentation

Deposits of melanin on the corneal endothelium can be observed in patients with glaucoma associated with pigment dispersion syndrome. Typically, the cluster of vertically oriented pigments is known as *Krukenberg spindle* (see Table 12-2).

Scleral Degenerations

Scleral rigidity increases in older people, and there is a relative decrease in scleral hydration and the amount of mucopolysaccharide. These changes are accompanied by subconjunctival deposition of fat, which gives the sclera a yellowish appearance. Calcium may also be deposited either diffusely among the scleral collagen fibers in granular or crystalline form or focally in a plaque anterior to the horizontal rectus muscle insertions. These senile

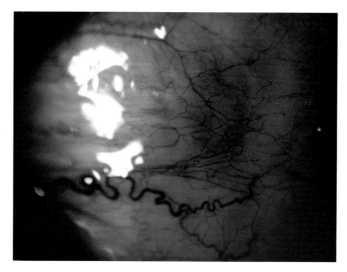

Figure 12-14 Senile scleral plaque anterior to horizontal rectus muscle insertions. *(Courtesy of Robert W. Weisenthal, MD.)*

plaques are visible as ovoid or rectangular zones of grayish translucency (Fig 12-14). Histologically, the midportion of the involved sclera contains a focal calcified plaque surrounded by relatively acellular collagen. The plaques do not elicit inflammation and rarely extrude. If sufficiently dense, they may be visualized on CT scan.

Drug-Induced Deposition and Pigmentation

Ocular medications deposit within the cornea as a result of their concentration within the tear film, limbal vasculature, or aqueous humor; or due to a specific affinity of the chemical properties of the medication to corneal tissue. Specific drugs deposit in characteristic fashion and corneal layer. The deposition of the drug may reduce visual acuity, produce photosensitivity, or cause ocular irritation. Its cessation often eliminates the symptoms and resolves the drug deposits. Most drug-induced deposition is not symptomatic, however, and does not require cessation of the medication (Table 12-3).

Corneal Epithelial Deposits

Corneal verticillata

Corneal verticillata, or *vortex keratopathy,* manifests as a whorl-like pattern of golden brown or gray deposits in the inferior interpalpebal portion of the cornea in a clockwise fashion (Fig 12-15). A variety of medications bind with the cellular lipids of the basal epithelial layer of the cornea due to their cationic, amphiphilic properties. Amiodarone, an antiarrhythmic, is the most common cause of corneal verticillata, followed by chloroquine, hydroxychloroquine, indomethacin, and phenothiazines. A comprehensive list of systemic drugs associated with corneal verticillata is given in Table 12-3.

Table 12-3 Systemic Drugs Associated With Corneal Deposits

Corneal Verticillata	Stromal Deposits
Aminoquinolones (chloroquine, hydroxychloroquine, amodiaquine)	Antacids
Amiodarone	Clofazimine
Atovaquone	Gold
Biaxin (clarithromycin)	
Clofazimine	Immunoglobulins
Phenothiazine (chlorpromazine)	Indomethacin
Gentamicin (subconjunctival)	Phenothiazines
Gold	Phenylbutazone
Ibuprofen	Practolol
Indomethacin	Retinoids (isotretinoin)
Mepacrine	Silver
Monobenzone (topical skin ointment)	
Naproxen	
Perhexiline maleate	
Suramin	
Tamoxifen	
Thioxanthines (chlorprothixine, thiothixine)	
Tilorone hydrochloride	

Adapted from Hollander DA, Aldave AJ. Drug-induced corneal complications. *Curr Opin Ophthalmol.* 2004;15:541-548; and Tyagi AK, Kayarkar VV, McDonnell PJ. An unreported side effect of topical clarithromycin when used successfully to treat Mycobacterium avium-intracellulare keratitis. *Cornea.* 1999;18(5):606–607.

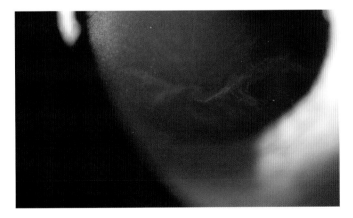

Figure 12-15 Corneal verticillata. *(Courtesy of Robert W. Weisenthal, MD.)*

It is unusual for these deposits to result in reduction of visual acuity or ocular symptoms, although this has occurred in some patients. The deposits typically resolve with discontinuation of the responsible agents. If there is reduced vision with the use of amiodarone and tamoxifen, the possibility of optic neuropathy should be considered. Retinal toxicity associated with the chloroquine family and tilorone hydrochloride can also reduce vision. The differential diagnosis of corneal verticillata should also include Fabry disease, a disorder of sphingolipid metabolism.

Epithelial cysts

Due to the rapid turnover of epithelial cells, drugs that inhibit DNA synthesis may be toxic to the epithelium when used in high doses systemically. Cytarabine (Ara-C), for example, may cause punctate keratopathy and refractile epithelial microcysts that are associated with pain, photophobia, foreign-body sensation, and reduced vision.

Ciprofloxacin deposits

Topical ciprofloxacin therapy can result in the deposition within an epithelial defect of a chalky white precipitate composed of ciprofloxacin crystals. Although white plaques predominate, a crystalline pattern may also be observed. The deposits resolve after discontinuation of the medication.

Adrenochrome

Long-standing administration of epinephrine compounds may lead to black or very dark brown deposits in the conjunctiva and cornea. Composed of adrenochrome, an oxidation product of the basic epinephrine compound, these melanin-like deposits can accumulate in conjunctival cysts and concretions in the conjunctiva (Fig 12-16). They may discolor the cornea or contact lenses as well. The deposits are harmless, although they are occasionally misdiagnosed as conjunctival melanoma or other conditions.

Arffa RC. *Grayson's Diseases of the Cornea.* 4th ed. St Louis: Mosby; 1997.

Kaiser PK, Pineda R, Albert DM, Shore JW. "Black cornea" after long-term epinephrine use. *Arch Ophthalmol.* 1992;110(9):1273–1275.

Stromal and Descemet's Membrane Pigmentation

Chlorpromazine, a member of the phenothiazine family, may cause corneal pigmentation in 18%–33% of patients on chronic therapy. It probably enters the cornea through the aqueous, and, therefore, the brown opacities are first found in the posterior stroma,

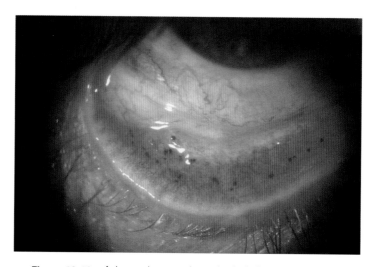

Figure 12-16 Adrenochrome deposits in inferior cul-de-sac.

Descemet's membrane, and endothelium; it later spreads to the anterior stroma and epithelium. Chlorpromazine can also deposit on the anterior lens capsule. Clofazimine may produce anterior stromal opacities or crystalline deposition. Isotretinoin is typically associated with fine, diffuse gray deposits in the central and peripheral cornea.

Certain classes of metallic compounds can produce characteristic deep stromal or Descemet opacities. Silver compounds were commonly used in the preantibiotic era to treat external infections. Their chronic use can result in a condition known as *argyriasis,* which consists of a slate-gray or silver discoloration involving the bulbar and palpebral conjunctiva. Argyriasis can also occur after inadvertent excessive application of silver nitrate to the bulbar conjunctiva for the treatment of superior limbic keratoconjunctivitis. This condition can be permanent. Gold salts are used for the treatment of rheumatoid arthritis. With chronic usage and cumulative dosages exceeding 1 g, a high percentage of patients develop posterior stromal deposits that spare Descemet's membrane and endothelium.

Table 12-2 lists pigments that may be of diagnostic importance, with their locations and associated conditions. See also Chapter 11, Table 11-5.

Endothelial Manifestations

Although rare, rifabutin has been described as causing stellate, refractile endothelial deposits initially in the periphery that may extend to the central cornea.

Frauenfelder FT, Frauenfelder FW. *Drug-induced Ocular Side-Effects.* 5th ed. Boston: Butterworth-Heinemann; 2001:647–648.

Hollander DA, Aldave AJ. Drug-induced corneal complications. *Curr Opin Ophthalmol.* 2004; 15(6):541–548.

Clinical Aspects of Toxic and Traumatic Injuries of the Anterior Segment

Injuries Caused by Temperature and Radiation

Thermal Burns

Heat

Rapid-reflex eyelid closure, Bell phenomenon, and reflex movement away from the source of intense heat usually limit damage to the globe from flames. Burns from molten metal that stays in contact with the eye are more likely to cause corneal injuries that result in permanent scarring. Heat is a major inducer of inflammation and stromal protease expression and can lead to collagen melt if severe. The major objectives of therapy for burns caused by heat are the following:

- Relieve discomfort.
- Prevent secondary corneal inflammation, ulceration, and perforation from infection or from exposure caused by eyelid damage.
- Minimize eyelid scarring and resultant malfunction.

A cycloplegic agent can help relieve discomfort from secondary ciliary spasm or iridocyclitis. Prophylactic antibiotics (topical and/or systemic) can help prevent infection of burned eyelids and/or reduce the chances of infectious corneal ulceration. Limited debridement of devitalized tissues and granulation tissue, used with full-thickness skin grafts and tarsorrhaphy, helps minimize eyelid scarring and ectropion. Burned ocular tissue can be protected temporarily by covering the eye with a lubricant and a piece of sterile plastic wrap. Topical corticosteroids help suppress any associated iridocyclitis, but they can also inhibit corneal wound healing and must be used with caution and, in general, for short periods of time.

Hair-curling irons are a common household cause of corneal burns. Fortunately, burns caused by curling irons are usually limited to the epithelium and generally require only a brief period of antibiotic and cycloplegic therapy.

Freezing

Transient corneal stromal edema induced by cold has been reported in a variety of settings, including individuals with Raynaud disease. Associated conjunctival vascular changes consistent with the Raynaud phenomenon have been documented under cold stress. Transient cold-induced corneal edema has also been reported in several patients with corneal nerve V (trigeminal) dysfunction. Research suggests that sensory denervation of the eye influences ocular temperature regulation, as well as altering the morphologic characteristics—and likely the function—of corneal cells, including the endothelium.

Ultraviolet Radiation

The corneal epithelium is highly susceptible to injury from ultraviolet (UV) radiation. Initially, there may be no symptoms; symptoms usually occur a few hours after exposure, when the injured epithelial cells are shed. The condition, although painful, is generally self-limited, and the epithelium heals within 24 hours.

The most common causes of ocular UV injuries are unprotected exposure to sunlamps, arc welding, and prolonged outdoor exposure to reflected sunlight. *Snow blindness,* which occurs in skiers and mountain climbers, is caused by UV light reflected from snow. Appropriate protection with UV-filtering eyewear can prevent such injuries. Treatment consists of patching to minimize discomfort from eyelid movement, topical antibiotic ointment, and cycloplegia. If discomfort is severe, patients may require systemic analgesics.

Ionizing Radiation

Exposure to ionizing radiation may be associated with nuclear explosions, x-rays, and radioisotopes. The amount of exposure is related to the amount of energy, the type of rays emitted, and proximity to the ionizing source. Tissue destruction may be the result of direct killing of cells; cellular DNA changes that produce lethal or other mutations; or radiation damage to blood vessels, with secondary ischemic necrosis. Longer wavelengths penetrate less deeply, causing a more intense reaction in superficial layers. Shorter wavelengths penetrate to deeper tissues and may not cause extensive damage to superficial tissues.

Most cases of ocular exposure to ionizing radiation involve both the conjunctiva and cornea and possibly the lacrimal glands. Conjunctival edema and chemosis occur acutely, often followed by scarring, shrinkage, loss of tear production, and alterations in conjunctival blood vessels with telangiectasia. Necrosis of the conjunctiva and underlying sclera can occur if radioactive material (or radiomimetic chemicals such as mitomycin C) is embedded in the conjunctiva. Punctate epithelial erosions typify acute corneal changes. Explosions involving ionizing radiation may lead to perforation of ocular tissues with immediate radiation necrosis.

Management of acute problems includes removal of all foreign bodies. Depending on the severity of the injury, a bandage soft contact lens, tissue adhesive, or tectonic graft may be necessary. Poor wound healing is a hallmark of ionizing radiation injuries. Late complications are related to lack of tears, loss of corneal sensation, loss of corneal epithelium and its failure to heal, secondary microbial keratitis, vascularization, and keratitis. Management of these sequelae includes the use of artificial tears and tarsorrhaphy. Late changes in the conjunctiva preclude its use for a conjunctival flap. If the fellow eye has not been injured, a contralateral autologous conjunctival flap may be helpful. The prognosis for penetrating keratoplasty in these situations is poor due to chronic ocular surface disease.

Miller D, ed. *Clinical Light Damage to the Eye*. New York: Springer-Verlag; 1987.

Chemical Injuries

Chemical trauma to the external eye is a common problem that can range in severity from mild irritation to complete destruction of the ocular surface epithelium, corneal opacification, loss of vision, and even loss of the eye. The offending chemical may be in the form of a solid, liquid, powder, mist, or vapor. Chemical injuries can occur in the home, most commonly from detergents, disinfectants, solvents, cosmetics, drain cleaners, oven cleaners, ammonia, bleach, and other common household alkaline agents. Fertilizers and pesticides are common offending agents in agricultural chemical injuries. In the workplace, plaster and cement products are frequent causes of alkali burns due to calcium hydroxide. Chemical injuries occurring in industry are usually caused by caustic chemicals and solvents. Some of the worst ocular chemical injuries result when strong alkalis (eg, lye) or acids are used for assault.

Whenever possible, the offending chemical agent should be identified, because the severity of a chemical injury depends on the pH, the volume and duration of contact, and the inherent toxicity of the chemical. The most severe chemical injuries are caused by strong alkalis and, to a lesser extent, acids. These solutions cause damage by drastically altering the concentration of highly reactive hydrogen and hydroxyl ions in affected tissues.

Alkali Burns

Strong alkalis raise the pH of tissues and cause saponification of fatty acids in cell membranes and ultimately cellular disruption. Once the surface epithelium is damaged, alkaline solutions readily penetrate the corneal stroma, where they rapidly destroy the proteoglycan ground substance and collagen fibers of the stromal matrix. Strong alkaline substances may also penetrate into the anterior chamber, producing severe tissue damage and intense inflammation.

The visual prognosis is often determined by the extent of ocular surface injury (Table 13-1) and the presence and degree of skin burns and their effect on eyelid function.

Table 13-1 The Hughes Classification of Ocular Alkali Burns

Grade I	Grade II	Grade III	Grade IV
Corneal epithelial defect without limbal ischemia.	Corneal epithelial defect with stromal haze and ischemia affecting less than one third of the limbus	Total corneal epithelial defect, with stromal haze obscuring iris details and ischemia affecting one third to one half of the limbus	Opaque cornea obscuring view of iris or pupil; ischemia of greater than one half of the limbus

The most unfavorable visual prognosis is associated with extensive limbal epithelial damage and intraocular chemical penetration. The limbus contains corneal epithelial stem cells; hence, damage to this area can lead to a disruption in the normal repopulation of the corneal epithelium. Severe damage to the limbal area can be appreciated as limbal "blanching"—as the vascular supply to this critical area is disrupted via death of vascular endothelial cells. Resultant ischemia to the limbus and anterior segment can have dire consequences for eyes thus affected (Figs 13-1, 13-2, 13-3). Repopulation of the corneal

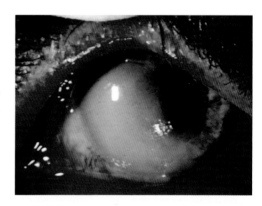

Figure 13-1 Mild, grade II alkali burn. Note inferior scleral ischemia. *(Courtesy of James J. Reidy, MD.)*

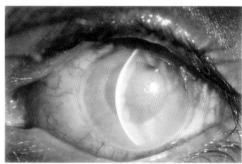

Figure 13-2 Moderate, grade III alkali burn with corneal edema and haze.

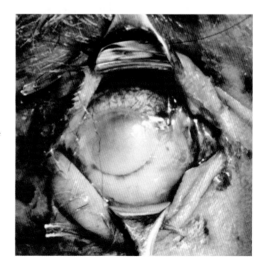

Figure 13-3 Severe, grade IV alkali burn with epithelial loss and stromal necrosis. *(Courtesy of James J. Reidy, MD.)*

surface epithelium with cells that do not have the proper degree of differentiation leads to "conjunctivalization" of the cornea, which is associated with vascularization, persistence of goblet cells in the cornea (easily discernible with PAS staining), poor epithelial adhesion and recurrent breakdown, and possibly chronic inflammation if the original trauma is severe. Intraocular chemical penetration is often accompanied by cataract formation and secondary glaucoma; the latter is thought to result from damage to the outflow tract and conjunctival cicatrization, which can affect outflow facility. In the most severe cases, phthisis of the globe may occur.

Colby KA. Chemical injuries of the eye. *Focal Points: Clinical Modules for Ophthalmologists.* San Francisco: American Academy of Ophthalmology; 2010, module 1.

Wagoner MD, Kenyon KR. Chemical injuries of the eye. In: Albert DM, Jakobiec FA, eds. *Principles and Practice of Ophthalmology.* 2nd ed. Vol 2. Philadelphia: Saunders; 2000:943–959.

Acid Burns

Acids denature and precipitate proteins in the tissues they contact. Acidic solutions tend to cause less severe tissue damage than alkaline solutions because of the buffering capacity of tissues as well as the barrier to penetration formed by precipitated protein. Acids do not directly cause loss of the proteoglycan ground substance in the cornea, although they too can incite severe inflammation with secondary up-regulation in protease expression that can damage the corneal matrix.

Management of Chemical Injuries

Beyond the immediate steps that need to be taken to minimize ongoing exposure to the offending agent (see the following discussion), there is no general consensus regarding the optimal management of chemical injuries. Few clinical trials have been performed in humans, and many of the current recommendations for management are based on animal models of acute alkaline injury (Table 13-2).

The most important step in the management of chemical injuries is *immediate and copious irrigation* of the ocular surface with water or balanced saline solution. If these liquids are not available, any other generally nontoxic and unpolluted solutions (eg, carbonated beverages) can also be used to avoid delaying treatment. If possible, irrigation should be initiated at the site of the chemical injury and continued until an ophthalmologist evaluates the patient. The eyelid should be immobilized with a retractor or eyelid speculum, and topical anesthetic should be instilled. Irrigation may be accomplished using handheld intravenous tubing, an irrigating eyelid speculum, or a Morgan medi-FLOW Lens (Mor-Tan, Missoula, MT), a special scleral contact lens that connects to IV tubing. Irrigation should continue until the pH of the conjunctival sac normalizes. The conjunctival pH can be checked easily with a urinary pH strip. If this is not available, it is better to "overtreat" for prolonged periods of irrigation than to "guess" that the pH has normalized.

Because they can continue to release the toxic chemical, particulate chemicals should be removed from the ocular surface with cotton-tipped applicators and forceps. Eversion of the upper eyelid should be performed to search for material in the upper fornix (Fig 13-4).

Table 13-2 Management of Ocular Chemical Injuries

Emergent management
Pain management
  Topical tetracaine
  Topical 2% lidocaine jelly
  Systemic analgesics
Copious irrigation with 2–3 liters of normal saline
  Morgan lens or by hand
Removal of all particulate matter on the ocular surface
  Saline flush of fornices
  Gentle sweep of fornices with sterile Dacron swab
  Removal of adherent particles with jeweler's forceps
Debridement of devitalized corneal epithelium
  Surgical sponge or Dacron swab
Cycloplegia
  Atropine 1%/scopolamine 0.25% bid or homatropine 5% tid
Control of IOP
  Mannitol 20% 1–2 g/kg ideal body weight IV over 1–2 h
  Acetazolamide 5–10 mg/kg IV q 6–8 h
  Anterior chamber paracentesis
Acute management (first 1–2 weeks)
Antimicrobial therapy
  Polymyxin/bacitracin ointment qid or fourth-generation fluoroquinolone qid
Topical lubrication
  Preservative-free tears q 2 h
  Preservative-free ointment
Anti-inflammatory therapy
  Prednisolone acetate 1% qid to q 1 h for 7–10 days with rapid taper thereafter
Inhibitors of matrix metalloprotease (MMP)
  Doxycycline 50–100 mg PO bid
  Ascorbate 500–1000 mg q 12 h
  10% sodium citrate qid (compounded)
Cycloplegia
  Atropine 1%/scopolamine 0.25% bid or homatropine 5% tid
Control of IOP
  Timolol 0.5% q 12 h
  Brimonidine 0.1%–0.2% tid
  Dorzolamide/brinzolamide bid
  Diamox 250 mg PO q 12 h–q 6 h
  Methazolamide 25–50 mg PO q 12 h
Management of persistent epithelial defect
  Therapeutic bandage contact lens
  Temporary lateral tarsorrhaphy
  Punctal occlusion
  Amniotic membrane grafting for large, persistent epithelial defects
Chronic management (week 3 and beyond)
Topical lubrication
  Preservative-free tears and ointment
Anti-inflammatory therapy
  Ideally, corticosteroid use should be stopped or minimized
Antimicrobial therapy
  Continue qid and discontinue when surface epithelium is intact
Control intraocular pressure
Inhibitors of matrix metalloprotease (MMP)
  Continue until surface epithelium is intact
Surgical therapy
  Advancement of Tenon fascia
  Limbal stem cell transplantation when inflammation is controlled
  Rotational tarsoconjunctival graft for scleral necrosis

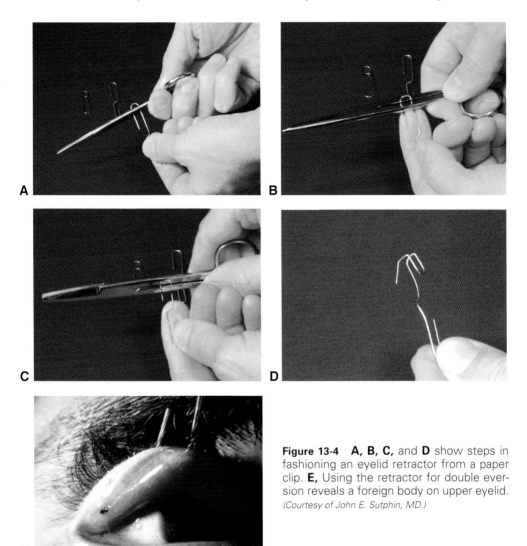

Figure 13-4 **A, B, C,** and **D** show steps in fashioning an eyelid retractor from a paper clip. **E,** Using the retractor for double eversion reveals a foreign body on upper eyelid. *(Courtesy of John E. Sutphin, MD.)*

The next phase of management should be directed at *decreasing inflammation, monitoring IOP, limiting matrix degradation,* and *promoting reepithelialization of the cornea.* An intense polymorphonuclear (PMN) leukocyte infiltration of the corneal stroma has been noted in histologic sections of corneas subjected to acute alkali burns. PMNs may be a major source of proteolytic enzymes capable of dissolving corneal stromal collagen and ground substance. Corticosteroids are excellent inhibitors of PMN function, and intensive topical corticosteroid administration is recommended for the acute phase (first 10–14 days) following chemical injuries. The dosage should be markedly reduced after 10–14 days, because corticosteroids can inhibit wound healing and possibly exacerbate sterile stromal melting. Corticosteroids also increase the risk of secondary infection by means of inhibition of normal ocular surface immune mechanisms; thus, their untoward side effects in the chronic phase may exceed the beneficial effects.

A deficiency of calcium in the plasma membrane of PMNs inhibits their ability to degranulate, and both tetracycline and citric acid are potent chelators of extracellular calcium. Therefore, oral tetracyclines and topical 10% sodium citrate have theoretical benefits for inhibiting PMN-induced collagenolysis. In addition, topical 1% medroxyprogesterone is effective in suppressing collagen breakdown.

Topical cycloplegics are recommended for patients with significant anterior chamber reaction. IOP is best controlled by use of oral carbonic anhydrase inhibitors in order to avoid toxicity from topical glaucoma medications. However, if the corneal epithelium is healing normally, topical therapies may be used as well. BCSC Section 10, *Glaucoma*, discusses medications for IOP control in depth.

Measures to promote wound healing and inhibit collagenolytic activity may help prevent stromal ulceration. Severe alkali burns in rabbit eyes have been found to reduce aqueous humor ascorbate levels to one third of normal levels. Reduced aqueous humor ascorbate has been correlated with corneal stromal ulceration and perforation. Systemic administration of ascorbic acid to rabbits with acute corneal alkaline injuries has restored the aqueous humor ascorbate level to normal and significantly reduced the incidence of ulceration. High-dose ascorbic acid is believed to promote collagen synthesis in the alkali-burned eye because ascorbic acid is required as a cofactor for this synthesis. There is currently no widely accepted standard for administration of ascorbate to corneas after chemical injury, but one recommendation is for patients to receive 1–2 g of oral ascorbic acid (vitamin C) per day. However, because this therapy is potentially toxic to the kidneys, patients with compromised renal function are not good candidates for this approach.

There are several strategies for promoting epithelial healing in acute and chronic chemical injury. Patients should be treated initially with intensive nonpreserved lubricants. Necrotic corneal epithelium should be debrided to minimize the release of inflammatory mediators produced by damaged epithelial cells and to promote reepithelialization. A bandage contact lens or temporary tarsorrhaphy may be beneficial for protecting ocular surface epithelium once it has begun to move onto the peripheral cornea. A tarsorrhaphy has the advantage of not increasing the risk of corneal infection, which is a concern with contact lens use in eyes with poor epithelium. Avascular sclera will usually not epithelialize until revascularization occurs. If scleral melting occurs, then a rotational tarsoconjunctival graft from the adjacent eyelid can be performed to promote revascularization.

Autologous conjunctival or limbal transplants from a patient's uninvolved fellow eye may restore the integrity of the damaged corneal epithelium. Amniotic membrane transplantation may be helpful in suppressing inflammation and thereby promoting reepithelialization and prevention of symblepharon formation. Limbal stem cell transplantation may be performed as soon as 2 weeks after chemical injury if no signs of corneal epithelialization have appeared. However, in general, the prognosis of limbal grafts is better when the eye is not very inflamed. Corneal transplantation is often delayed for years after a severe alkali injury to allow the surface inflammation to quiet down or until after the surface inflammation has quieted as a result of limbal stem cell grafting (ocular surface reconstruction). Even when there is no active inflammation in the ocular surface, stromal vascularization in the host bed is associated with a much higher risk of rejection in these keratoplasty cases. Keratoprosthesis surgery has also been used in eyes with a history of chemical injury; as with other types of surgery in these eyes, the prognosis is best when the inflammation has been brought under control.

Colby K. Chemical injuries of the cornea. *Focal Points: Clinical Modules for Ophthalmologists.* San Francisco: American Academy of Ophthalmology; 2010, module 1.

Rao SK, Rajagopal R, Sitalakshmi G, Padmanabhan P. Limbal autografting: comparison of results in acute and chronic phases of ocular surface burns. *Cornea.* 1999;18(2):164–171.

Tejwani S, Kolari RS, Sangwan VS, Rao GN. Role of amniotic membrane graft for ocular chemical and thermal injuries. *Cornea.* 2007;26(1):21–26.

Toxic Keratoconjunctivitis From Medications

A commonly encountered and frequently unrecognized clinical problem is that of epithelial keratopathy secondary to topically applied ocular medications. One of the most toxic ingredients in these preparations is the preservative, usually benzalkonium chloride. The corneal and conjunctival epithelium absorbs and retains preservatives. Residual amounts of preservatives are detectable in the epithelium days after a single topical application. Toxic effects on the epithelium include loss of microvillae, plasma membrane disruption, and subsequent cell death.

Topical anesthetics have repeatedly been shown to be toxic if used for prolonged periods. Prolonged use can lead to frank epithelial loss, stromal edema, infiltration, and corneal opacities. However, sometimes even a single application of a topical anesthetic may cause transient epithelial irregularity. Medical personnel with easy access to anesthetics are especially susceptible to this factitious disorder.

PATHOGENESIS Toxic conjunctivitis or keratoconjunctivitis may occur as a complication of exposure to various substances (Table 13-3). Topically applied ophthalmic medications can result in a dose-dependent cytotoxic effect on the ocular surface. The epithelium of the conjunctiva and cornea may show punctate staining or erosive changes indicative of

Table 13-3 Toxic Reactions Associated With Topical Ophthalmic Medications

Toxic Keratoconjunctivitis	Toxic Follicular Conjunctivitis
Aminoglycosides	Antiglaucoma agents
Neomycin	*Miotics*
Gentamycin	Pilocarpine
Tobramycin	Carbachol
Antiviral agents	Echothiophate iodide
Trifluorothymidine	*α-Agonists*
Antineoplastic agents	Brimonidine
Mitomycin C	Apraclonidine
Topical Anesthetics	Dipivefrin
Proparacaine	Epinephrine
Tetracaine	Cycloplegics
Preservatives	Atropine
Benzalkonium chloride	Homatropine

direct toxicity. A conjunctival reaction may be observed in the form of either a papillary reaction (vascular dilation) or a follicular response. An immune response can also produce subepithelial corneal infiltrates.

CLINICAL PRESENTATION   Although these reactions generally occur after long-term use (weeks to months) of a drug, they may take place sooner in individuals with delayed tear clearance from aqueous tear deficiency or tear drainage obstruction. Toxic reactions of the ocular surface can take different forms. A generalized injection of the tarsal and bulbar conjunctiva may be associated with a mild to severe papillary reaction of the tarsal conjunctiva, mucopurulent discharge, and punctate keratopathy. Occasionally, the discharge may be severe and mimic bacterial conjunctivitis. Infrequently, the reaction occurs in only 1 eye even though the medication has been applied to both.

In its mildest form, *toxic keratitis* consists of punctate epithelial erosions of the inferior cornea. A diffuse punctate epitheliopathy, occasionally in a whorl pattern, may be observed in more severe cases. This pattern is sometimes called *vortex* or *hurricane* keratopathy. The most severe cases may involve a corneal epithelial defect of the inferior or central cornea, stromal opacification, and neovascularization. This severe type of corneal disease is seen with extensive damage to the limbal stem cells. A sign of limbal stem cell deficiency is effacement of the palisades of Vogt. Prolonged use of preservative-containing medications or administration of antifibrotic agents (eg, topical mitomycin C drops, which have a radiomimetic effect on surrounding cells) may be the cause. Even when used in correct dosages for brief periods, mitomycin has been associated with prolonged, irreversible stem cell damage with resultant chronic keratopathy. Localized application of mitomycin using a cellulose surgical sponge to the surgical field (as in trabeculectomy or pterygium excision) is believed to incur a lower risk than more widespread topical administration and is the preferred method of antifibrotic therapy.

A different type of toxic keratitis manifests as peripheral corneal infiltrates located in the epithelium and anterior stroma, leaving a clear zone between them and the limbus. Conjunctival and/or corneal toxic reactions are typically seen following use of aminoglycoside antibiotics, antiviral agents, or medications preserved with benzalkonium chloride or thimerosal.

Chronic follicular conjunctivitis is another manifestation of external ocular toxicity. Generally, the follicular reaction involves both the upper and lower palpebral conjunctivae, but the follicles are usually most prominent on the inferior tarsus and fornix. Bulbar follicles are uncommon but highly suggestive of a toxic etiology when present (Fig 13-5). The medications most commonly associated with toxic follicular conjunctivitis include atropine, antiviral agents, miotics (particularly phospholine iodide), sulfonamides, epinephrine (including dipivefrin), apraclonidine (Iopidine), α_2-adrenergic agonists (eg, brimonidine), and vasoconstrictors. Inferior punctate epithelial erosions may occasionally accompany toxic follicular conjunctivitis.

With ongoing use of topical medications, the conjunctiva shows an increased number of chronic inflammatory cells and fibroblasts. Although any medication may potentially cause this low-grade inflammatory response, it is most common with the chronic use of miotics for treatment of glaucoma. Asymptomatic subconjunctival fibrosis is not

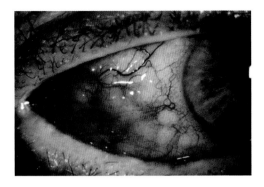

Figure 13-5 Drug-induced chronic follicular conjunctivitis induced by topical dipivefrin. *(Courtesy of James J. Reidy, MD.)*

uncommon with chronic topical drug use, but a small minority of affected patients will develop an insidiously progressive and more severe type of subconjunctival scarring that can lead to contraction of the conjunctival fornix, symblepharon formation, and corneal pannus formation. This entity is called *pseudopemphigoid,* or *drug-induced cicatricial pemphigoid.*

MANAGEMENT   Treatment of toxicity requires discontinuation of the offending topical medications. Severe cases may take months to resolve completely; thus, the failure of symptoms and signs to resolve within a period of days to a few weeks is not inconsistent with a toxic etiology. Patients who are experiencing significant ocular irritation may find relief with nonpreserved topical lubricant drops or ointment. It is important to stress that toxic reactions to ocular medications can lead to irreversible changes, as may occur rarely with use of cholinergic (pilocarpine-like) and other medications.

Pseudopemphigoid should be confirmed with a conjunctival biopsy, which often (but not always) demonstrates the characteristic diffuse, nonlinear immunofluorescent staining indicative of antibody deposition. Withdrawal of the medication is generally followed by a lag of weeks to months before progressive scarring can be stabilized. If clinical observation and photographic documentation demonstrate clinical progression despite discontinuation of the medication, chemotherapy may be necessary (see Chapter 7).

Grant WM, Schuman JS. *Toxicology of the Eye: Effects on the Eyes and Visual System from Chemicals, Drugs, Metals and Minerals, Plants, Toxins, and Venoms; Also, Systemic Side Effects from Eye Medications.* 4th ed. Springfield, IL: Thomas; 1993.

Liesegang TJ. Conjunctival changes associated with glaucoma therapy: implications for the external disease consultant and the treatment of glaucoma. *Cornea.* 1998;17(6):574–583.

Animal and Plant Substances

Insect Injuries

Bee and wasp stings to the cornea and/or conjunctiva are rare. Conjunctival hyperemia and chemosis usually occur acutely, sometimes associated with severe pain, corneal edema, and infiltration with subsequent decreased vision. The variability of the acute response is thought to reflect differences in the quantity of the venom injected and whether the reaction to the venom is primarily toxic or immunologic. In rare instances, other sequelae have been documented, including hyphema, lenticular opacities, iritis, secondary glaucoma, and heterochromia. Initial therapy with cycloplegics and topical, and occasionally systemic, corticosteroids has been beneficial. Removal of externalized stingers may be attempted. After the acute episode, retained stingers may remain inert in the cornea for years. Caterpillar and tarantula hairs (urticating hairs) may also become embedded in the cornea and conjunctiva. These hairs are very fine and usually cannot be removed manually. Because of their structure, these urticating hairs tend to migrate more deeply into ocular tissues and elicit a localized granulomatous inflammatory response (ophthalmia nodosum). Inflammatory sequelae usually respond to topical corticosteroids.

Spraul CW, Wagner P, Lang GE, Lang GK. Ophthalmia nodosa caused by the hairs of the bird spider (family Theraphosidae) or hairy megalomorph (known in the US as tarantula): case report and review of the literature. *Klin Monatsbl Augenheilkd.* 2003;220(1-2):20–23.

Vegetation Injuries

Ocular contact with the sap (latex) from a variety of trees can cause toxic reactions manifested by acute keratoconjunctivitis, epithelial defects, and stromal infiltration. The pencil tree and the manchineel tree, widely distributed in tropical regions, are known offenders. The dieffenbachia, which is a common houseplant, is known to cause keratoconjunctivitis and deposition of calcium oxalate crystals in the cornea. Corneal foreign bodies from coconut shell, sunflower stalk, and ornamental cactus have all been documented.

Initial management for all such plant materials should include irrigation removal of foreign bodies when possible and administration of topical cycloplegics with prophylactic antibiotic coverage, as indicated by the clinical situation. Corticosteroids are best avoided, as they suppress immunity to microbes in general and may promote fungal infection specifically, which is of concern in all cases involving vegetation matter. Surgical removal of foreign bodies may be required in the setting of uncontrolled inflammatory response or associated secondary microbial infections. Clinicians should be aware that plant sources are common causes of fungal keratitis. Hence, in a patient with a severe injury from plant sources or in cases that fail to improve after supportive therapy, the possibility of infection should be entertained and appropriate workup (including culturing and/or biopsy) is indicated. For additional discussion of microbial keratitis, see Chapters 4, 5, and 16.

Concussive Trauma

Conjunctival Hemorrhage

Blood under the conjunctiva creates a dramatic appearance that can alarm the patient. Most frequently, patients present with subconjunctival hemorrhage without a history of antecedent trauma. When trauma has occurred, damage to deeper structures of the eye must be ruled out. Subconjunctival hemorrhage is usually not associated with an underlying systemic disease and rarely has an identifiable cause. Occasionally, a history of vomiting, coughing, or other forms of the Valsalva maneuver can be elicited.

Most patients simply require reassurance that things are not as bad as they appear to be. However, if a patient suffers from repeated episodes of spontaneous subconjunctival hemorrhage or indicates the presence of a possible bleeding diathesis (easy bruising, frequent bloody noses), a careful medical evaluation may be warranted. Recurrent subconjunctival hemorrhages can be seen in association with systemic illness such as uncontrolled hypertension, diabetes mellitus, or a bleeding diathesis. No therapy is necessary for the hemorrhage, as it usually resolves in 7–12 days. Patients should be warned that the hemorrhage might spread around the circumference of the globe before it resolves and that it may change in color from red to yellow during its dissolution.

Corneal Changes

Blunt trauma to the cornea can result in abrasions, edema, tears in Descemet's membrane, and corneoscleral lacerations, usually located at the limbus. Traumatic posterior annular keratopathy or traumatic corneal endothelial rings have also been described. The rings, composed of disrupted and swollen endothelial cells, are whitish gray in appearance and occur directly posterior to the traumatic impact. The endothelial rings appear within several hours of a contusive injury and usually disappear within a few days.

Traumatic Mydriasis and Miosis

Blunt injury to the globe may result in traumatic mydriasis or, less commonly, miosis. Traumatic mydriasis is often associated with iris sphincter tears that can permanently alter the shape of the pupil. Miosis tends to be associated with anterior chamber inflammation (traumatic iritis; see the following section). Pupillary reactivity may be sluggish in both situations. Cycloplegia is essential to prevent formation of posterior synechiae.

Traumatic Iritis

Photophobia, tearing, and ocular pain may occur within the first 24 hours after injury. The inflammation of traumatic iritis is often associated with diminished vision and perilimbal conjunctival injection. The anterior chamber reaction can be surprisingly minimal but is usually present if carefully sought.

Treatment should consist of, at the very least, a topical cycloplegic agent to relieve patient discomfort. Topical corticosteroids may be used if significant inflammation is present and if compliance can be expected. Once the iritis has diminished, cycloplegia may be discontinued, and topical corticosteroids should be tapered off to prevent rebound iritis. See BCSC Section 9, *Intraocular Inflammation and Uveitis,* for a more detailed discussion of uveitis.

Rosenbaum JT, Tammaro J, Robertson JE Jr. Uveitis precipitated by nonpenetrating ocular trauma. *Am J Ophthalmol.* 1991;112(4):392–395.

Iridodialysis and Cyclodialysis

Iridodialysis

Blunt trauma may cause traumatic separation of the iris root from the ciliary body (Fig 13-6). Frequently, anterior segment hemorrhage ensues, and the iridodialysis may not be recognized until the hyphema has cleared. A small iridodialysis requires no treatment. A large dialysis may cause polycoria and monocular diplopia, necessitating surgical repair.

Cyclodialysis

Traumatic cyclodialysis is characterized by a separation of the ciliary body from its attachment to the scleral spur, resulting in a cleft. Gonioscopically, this cleft appears at the junction of the scleral spur and the ciliary body band. Sclera may be visible through the disrupted tissue. Ultrasound biomicroscopy is useful in identifying the location and extent of the cyclodialysis (Fig 13-7). A cyclodialysis cleft can cause increased uveoscleral outflow and aqueous hyposecretion, leading to chronic hypotony and macular edema. If treatment with topical cycloplegics does not suffice, closure may be attempted by using argon laser, diathermy, cryotherapy, or direct suturing. If repair is necessary, it should be done after the resolution of the hyphema.

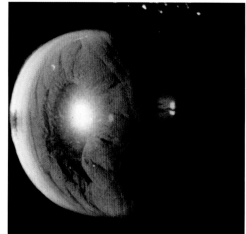

Figure 13-6 Severe iridodialysis resulting from blunt trauma. *(Courtesy of James J. Reidy, MD.)*

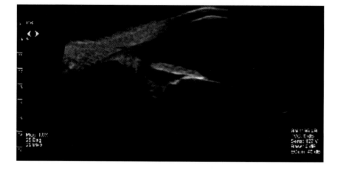

Figure 13-7 Ultrasound biomicroscopy of cyclodialysis. *(Courtesy of James J. Reidy, MD.)*

Traumatic Hyphema

Traumatic hyphema occurs most commonly in young males. It results from injury to the vessels of the peripheral iris or anterior ciliary body. Trauma causes posterior displacement of the lens–iris diaphragm and scleral expansion in the equatorial zone, which leads to disruption of the major iris arterial circle, arterial branches of the ciliary body, and/or recurrent choroidal arteries and veins (Fig 13-8). Anterior segment bleeding can often be seen on penlight examination as a layering of blood inferiorly in the anterior chamber (Fig 13-9). At other times, the bleeding is so subtle that it can be detected only as a few circulating red blood cells on slit-lamp examination (microscopic hyphema). At presentation, more than 50% of hyphemas occupy less than one third of the height of the anterior chamber; fewer than 10% fill the whole chamber. The prognosis is good in patients who do not develop complications, but it is not dependent on the size of the hyphema itself. Even total, or "eight-ball," hyphemas can resolve without sequelae, unless secondary complications result (Fig 13-10). Hyphema is frequently associated with corneal abrasion, iritis, and mydriasis, as well as with significant injuries to the angle structures, lens, posterior segment, and orbit.

Spontaneous hyphema is much less common and should alert the examiner to the possibility of rubeosis iridis, clotting abnormalities, herpetic disease, or intraocular lens (IOL) problems. Juvenile xanthogranuloma, retinoblastoma, and leukemia are associated with spontaneous hyphema in children.

Rebleeding

The major concern after a traumatic hyphema is rebleeding. Complications associated with secondary hemorrhage include glaucoma, optic atrophy, and corneal blood staining

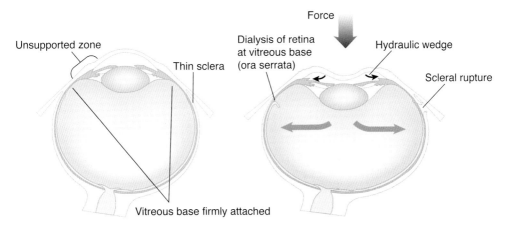

Figure 13-8 Mechanism of hyphema and blunt force injury to the eye. Blunt force applied to the eye displaces the aqueous volume peripherally, causing an increase in hydraulic pressure at the lens, iris root, and trabecular meshwork. If this "wedge of pressure" exceeds the tensile strength of ocular structures, the vessels in the peripheral iris and face of the ciliary body may rupture, leading to hyphema. The force may cause scleral ruptures, typically at the limbus and posterior to the muscle insertions, where the sclera is thinner and unsupported by the orbital bones. Severe trauma leads to subluxation of the lens, retinal dialysis, optic nerve avulsion, and/or vitreous hemorrhage. *(Illustration by C.H. Wooley.)*

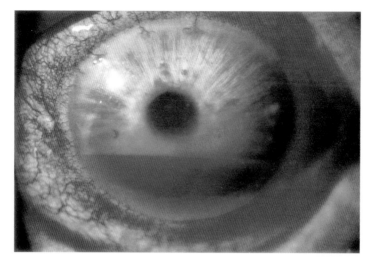

Figure 13-9   Layered hyphema from blunt trauma.

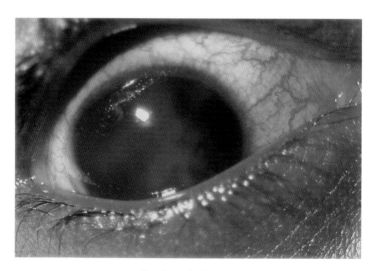

Figure 13-10   Total, or "eight-ball," hyphema.

(Fig 13-11). The rate of rebleeding reported in different studies varies; however, most studies report an incidence of less than 5%.

Rebleeding may complicate any hyphema, regardless of size, and occurs most frequently between 2 and 5 days after injury. The timing of the rebleeding may be related to the lysis and clot retraction that occur during this period. Numerous studies have documented the importance of rebleeding as a prognostic factor for poor visual outcome.

Approximately 50% of patients with rebleeding develop elevated IOP. The combination of elevated IOP, endothelial dysfunction, and anterior chamber blood predisposes the eye to corneal blood staining, which is difficult to detect when blood is in apposition to the endothelium. Red blood cells within the anterior chamber release hemoglobin

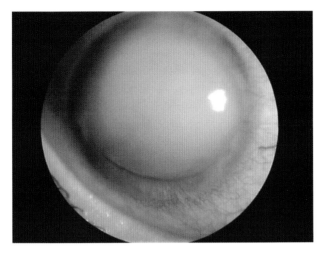

Figure 13-11 Dense corneal blood staining after a traumatic hyphema. *(Courtesy of Vincent P. deLuise, MD.)*

that penetrates into the posterior corneal stroma, where it is absorbed by keratocytes. Hemoglobin is converted to hemosiderin within the keratocytes, which in turn causes keratocyte death. On slit-lamp examination, early blood staining is detected by yellow granular changes and reduced fibrillar definition in the posterior corneal stroma. Blood staining leads to a reduction in corneal transparency that may persist for years and can lead to the development of amblyopia in children. Histologically, red blood cells and their breakdown products can be seen within the corneal stroma. Corneal blood staining often slowly clears in a centripetal pattern starting in the periphery.

Medical management
The overall treatment plan for traumatic hyphema should be directed at minimizing the possibility of secondary hemorrhage. Elevated IOP may require treatment in order to reduce the chances of corneal blood staining and optic atrophy. Specifics of medical management remain controversial; however, most patients are treated with the following:

- protective shield over the injured eye
- restriction of physical activity
- elevation of the head of the bed
- frequent observation

Analgesics that do not contain aspirin should be used for pain relief, because aspirin has been demonstrated to increase the risk of rebleeding due to its antiplatelet effects. Nonsteroidal anti-inflammatory medications can also increase the risk of rebleeding. Hospitalization often facilitates daily examination and is necessary if satisfactory home care and outpatient observation cannot be ensured.

Most ophthalmologists administer long-acting topical cycloplegic agents initially for comfort, to facilitate posterior segment evaluation, and to eliminate iris movement. Topical corticosteroids are beneficial in controlling anterior chamber inflammation and preventing synechiae formation, and they may play a role in preventing rebleeding. Oral corticosteroids may be used to facilitate the resolution of severe inflammation and/or to prevent rebleeding. Topical antihypertensives (β-blockers and α-agonists) are the mainstay of therapy, although occasionally intravenous or oral hyperosmotic agents may be required.

Prospective studies have supported the efficacy of antifibrinolytic agents (aminocaproic acid [Amicar]; tranexamic acid; prednisone) in reducing the incidence of rebleeding; however, these studies have failed to show any statistical improvement in visual outcome. It is postulated that these agents inhibit fibrinolysis at the site of the injured blood vessel. Significant side effects are associated with some of these agents, including nausea, vomiting, postural hypotension, muscle cramps, conjunctival suffusion, nasal stuffiness, headache, rash, pruritus, dyspnea, toxic confusional states, and arrhythmias, as well as the risk of increased IOP on discontinuation. Patients on aminocaproic acid should be hospitalized; but patients using oral corticosteroids, which may also reduce the rate of rebleeding, may be treated as outpatients. Aminocaproic acid is used in an oral dosage of 50 mg/kg every 4 hours for 5 days (up to 30 g/day). Studies have suggested that a topical preparation containing 30% aminocaproic acid is equally effective as systemic Amicar, with a much better side-effect profile. Unfortunately, a commercial preparation is not currently available. Evidence-based medical analysis would argue against the routine use of these agents due to potential adverse side effects, medical risks, cost, and lack of evidence for improved visual outcomes.

Surgery

Surgery (to evacuate blood) may be required to prevent irreversible corneal blood staining and optic atrophy from persistently elevated IOP. The timing of surgery is controversial, but surgery is generally recommended at the earliest definitive detection of blood staining. Some authors suggest that surgery may be indicated if the IOP averages greater than 25 mm Hg for 5 days with a total hyphema. Surgical intervention should be considered when the IOP is greater than 60 mm Hg despite maximal medical management for 2 days to prevent optic atrophy. Patients with preexisting optic nerve damage or hemoglobinopathies may require earlier intervention. Table 13-4 has guidelines on surgical intervention.

Surgical techniques are multiple and varied. The simplest technique is paracentesis and anterior chamber irrigation with balanced salt solution. The goal is to remove circulating red blood cells that may obstruct the trabecular meshwork; removal of the entire clot is neither necessary nor wise. This procedure can be repeated. If the patient is being treated with aminocaproic acid, then clot dissolution will not occur until the medication is discontinued. Large limbal incision techniques with clot expression, if necessary, are best performed 4–7 days after the initial injury, when clot consolidation is at its peak. Automated cutting/aspiration instruments can be used to remove blood and debulk clots through small incisions. Care must be taken to avoid damage to the iris and lens, as well as the corneal endothelium, when using automated cutting devices. Intraocular diathermy may also be used to control active intraoperative bleeding. Iris damage, lens injury, and additional bleeding are the major complications of surgical intervention.

Table 13-4 Guidelines for Surgical Intervention in Traumatic Hyphema

To prevent optic atrophy
  IOP averages >60 mm Hg for 2 days
  IOP averages >35 mm Hg for 7 days
To prevent corneal blood staining
  IOP averages >25 mm Hg for 5 days
  Evidence of early corneal blood staining
To prevent peripheral anterior synechiae
  Total hyphema that persists for 5 days
  Any hyphema failing to resolve to a volume of less than 50% by 8 days
In hyphema patients with sickle hemoglobinopathies
  IOP averages ≥25 mm Hg for 24 hours
  IOP has repeated transient elevations >30 mm Hg for 2–4 days

Adapted with permission from Deutsch TA, Goldberg MF. Traumatic hyphema: medical and surgical management. *Focal Points: Clinical Modules for Ophthalmologists*. San Francisco: American Academy of Ophthalmology; 1984, module 5.

Sickle cell complications

When an African-American patient develops a traumatic hyphema, a sickle cell workup should be performed to evaluate the patient for the possibility of sickle cell hemoglobinopathy. Sickle cell patients and carriers of the sickle cell trait are predisposed to sickling of red blood cells in the anterior chamber. Sickle cells are restricted in their outflow through the trabecular meshwork and may raise the IOP dramatically. In addition, the optic nerve appears to be at greater risk for damage in sickle cell patients, even with modest IOP elevations (presumably due to decreases in blood flow to the optic nerve).

All efforts must be made to normalize IOP in these patients. Carbonic anhydrase inhibitors and osmotic agents must be used with caution because of their tendency to reduce pH and lead to hemoconcentration, both of which may exacerbate sickling of red blood cells. Surgical intervention has been recommended if the average IOP remains 25 mm Hg or higher after the first 24 hours or after repeated, transient elevations greater than 30 mm Hg for 2–4 days, despite medical intervention.

Campagna JA. Traumatic hyphema: current strategies. *Focal Points: Clinical Modules for Ophthalmologists*. San Francisco: American Academy of Ophthalmology; 2007, module 10.

Walton W, Von Hagen S, Grigorian R, Zarbin M. Management of traumatic hyphema. *Surv Ophthalmol*. 2002;47(4):297–334.

Nonperforating Mechanical Trauma

Conjunctival Laceration

In managing conjunctival lacerations associated with trauma, the physician must be certain that the deeper structures of the eye have not been damaged and that no foreign body is present. It is often useful to explore the limits of a conjunctival laceration using sterile forceps or cotton-tipped applicators. The slit lamp is used following the instillation of a topical anesthetic. If any question remains as to whether the globe has been penetrated, consideration must be given to performing a peritomy in the operating room to better explore and examine the injured area. In general, conjunctival lacerations do not need to be sutured.

Conjunctival Foreign Body

Foreign bodies on the conjunctival surface are best recognized with slit-lamp examination. Foreign bodies can lodge in the inferior cul-de-sac or can be located on the conjunctival surface under the upper eyelid (Fig 13-12). It is imperative to evert the upper eyelid to examine the superior tarsal plate and eyelid margin in all patients with a history that suggests a foreign body. If several foreign bodies are suspected or particulate matter is present, double eversion of the eyelid with a Desmarres retractor or a bent paperclip is advised to allow the examiner to effectively search the entire arc of the superior cul-de-sac (see Fig 13-4).

Following eversion of the upper eyelid, copious irrigation should be used to cleanse the fornix. This procedure should then be repeated using a Desmarres retractor for the upper and lower eyelids. Glass particles, cactus spines, and insect hairs are often difficult to see, but a careful search of the cul-de-sac with high magnification aids in identification and removal. With slit-lamp magnification, the clinician can gently use a moistened cotton-tipped applicator to remove superficial foreign material. Occasionally, saline lavage of the cornea or cul-de-sac washes out debris that is not embedded in tissue.

When a patient complains of foreign-body sensation, topical fluorescein should be instilled to check for the fine, linear, vertical corneal abrasions that are characteristic of retained foreign bodies on the eyelid margin or superior tarsal plate. Foreign matter embedded in tissue is removed with a sterile, disposable hypodermic needle. Glass or particulate matter may be removed with a fine-tipped jeweler's forceps or blunt spatula. If a foreign body is suspected but not seen, the cul-de-sac should be irrigated and wiped with a moistened cotton-tipped applicator.

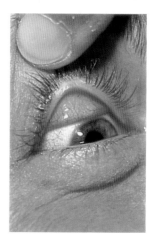

Figure 13-12 Foreign bodies seen on the everted surface of the upper eyelid.

Corneal Foreign Body

Identifying the probable composition of a foreign body based on a detailed history is important due to the increased risk of infection associated with vegetable matter. Occult intraocular foreign bodies must be identified when there is a history of exposure to high-speed metallic foreign bodies, most commonly produced by high-speed grinding tools and metal-on-metal hammering.

Corneal foreign bodies are identified most effectively during slit-lamp examination. Before removing the corneal foreign body, the clinician should assess the depth of corneal penetration. If anterior chamber extension is present or suspected, the foreign body should be removed in a sterile operating-room environment with sufficient microscopic magnification and coaxial illumination, adequate anesthesia, and appropriate instruments. Overly aggressive attempts to remove deeply embedded foreign bodies at the slit lamp may result in leakage of aqueous humor and collapse of the anterior chamber. If such a leak occurs and cannot be adequately tamponaded with a therapeutic bandage contact lens, tissue adhesive and/or urgent surgical repair is required.

If several glass foreign bodies are present, all of the exposed fragments should be removed. Fragments that are deeply embedded in the cornea are often inert and can be left in place. Careful gonioscopic evaluation of the anterior chamber is essential to ensure that the iris and the angle are free of any retained glass particles.

When an iron foreign body has been embedded in the cornea for more than a few hours, an orange-brown "rust ring" results (Fig 13-13). Corneal iron foreign bodies and rust rings can usually be removed at the slit lamp under topical anesthesia with a disposable (25- or 26-gauge) hypodermic needle, resulting in minimal tissue disruption. A battery-powered dental burr with a sterile tip may also be used; however, caution must be taken to cause minimal tissue disruption and thus minimize scar formation. A metallic foreign body that enters the corneal stroma beyond the Bowman layer always results in

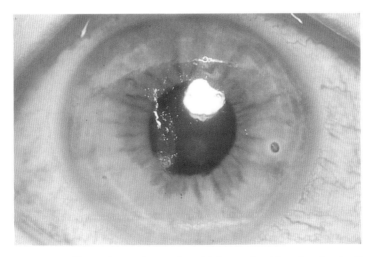

Figure 13-13   Corneal rust ring and multiple retained iron foreign bodies.

some degree of scar formation. When they occur in the visual axis, these scars may result in glare and decreased visual acuity from irregular astigmatism. Corneal perforation is a rare complication of foreign-body removal. Judicious decision making is mandatory; if multiple, very small foreign bodies are seen in the deep stroma (as may occur after an explosion) with no resultant inflammation or sign of infection, the patient may be monitored closely, because aggressive surgical manipulation of the cornea in search of the very last particle may be unnecessary.

Therapy following the removal of a corneal foreign body includes topical antibiotics, cycloplegia, and occasionally the application of a firm pressure patch or bandage contact lens to help the healing process. Close observation is usually indicated. If the residual corneal abrasion does not heal or if additional curettage is needed to remove a rust ring, cycloplegic and antibiotic drops are instilled before a new pressure patch is applied.

Corneal Abrasion

Corneal abrasions are usually associated with immediate pain, foreign-body sensation, tearing, and discomfort with blinking. Abrasions may be caused by contact with a finger, fingernail, fist, or even the edge of a piece of paper. The abrasion can also be caused by a propelled foreign body or by contact lens wear, because of either improper fit or excessive wear. Occasionally, a patient may not recall a definite history of trauma but still present with signs and symptoms suggestive of a corneal abrasion. Herpes simplex virus keratitis must be excluded as a possible diagnosis in such cases.

A slit-lamp examination is essential in determining the presence, extent, and depth of the corneal defect. It is very important to make a distinction between a "clean" corneal abrasion, which generally has sharply defined edges and little to no associated inflammation (when seen acutely), and a true corneal ulcer, which is characterized by an inflammation-mediated breakdown of the stromal matrix and possible thinning. Foreign-body sensation is an exceedingly specific localizing symptom for a corneal epithelial defect. It is important to evert the upper eyelid and examine the superior cul-de-sac to rule out a retained foreign body.

Patching is not necessary for most abrasions; many patients find patches uncomfortable. Abrasions may be managed with antibiotic ointment in combination with topical cycloplegia alone. Topical nonsteroidal anti-inflammatory agents have anesthetic properties and may be used for the first 24–48 hours for pain relief in selected patients. In addition, oral pain management for the first 24–48 hours can be helpful for many patients. Alternatively, a therapeutic contact lens in conjunction with antibiotic prophylaxis is also very effective, but this should be reserved for eye care professionals and patients being closely followed. Abrasions caused by organic material require closer follow-up to monitor for infection.

Patients with contact lens–associated epithelial defects should never be patched because of the possibility of promoting a secondary infection. These patients should be treated with topical antibiotic drops or ointment.

Posttraumatic Recurrent Corneal Erosion

A corneal abrasion can precipitate future recurrent corneal erosions. See Chapter 3 for a discussion of the pathogenesis, diagnosis, and treatment of recurrent corneal erosions.

Perforating Trauma

It is important to differentiate a *penetrating* wound from a *perforating* wound. A penetrating wound passes *into* a structure; a perforating wound passes *through* a structure. For example, an object that passes through the cornea and lodges in the anterior chamber perforates the cornea but penetrates the eye.

Evaluation

History

If a patient presents with both eye and systemic trauma, diagnosis and treatment of any life-threatening injury take precedence over evaluation and management of the ophthalmic injury. Once the patient is medically stable, the ophthalmologist should elicit a complete presurgical history (Table 13-5). Even though the diagnosis of perforating injury in many cases may be obvious from casual eye examination, a detailed history of the nature of the injury should include questions about factors known to predispose to ocular penetration so that this diagnosis will not be overlooked in more subtle cases. Such factors include

- metal-on-metal strike
- high-velocity projectile
- high-energy impact on globe
- sharp injuring object
- lack of eye protection

Examination

Evaluation of a patient with suspected perforating injury to the eye should include a complete general and ophthalmic examination. As soon as possible, the examiner should

---

Table 13-5 Penetrating/Perforating Ocular Injury History

Nature of injury
  Concomitant life-threatening injury
  Time and circumstances of injury
  Suspected composition of intraocular foreign body (brass, copper, iron, vegetable, soil
    contamination)
  Use of eye protection
  Prior treatment of injury
Past ocular history
  Refractive history
  Eye diseases
  Current eye medications
  Previous surgery
Medical history
  Diagnoses
  Current medications
  Drug allergies
  Risk factors for HIV/hepatitis
  Currency of tetanus prophylaxis
  Previous surgery
  Recent food ingestion

determine visual acuity, which is the most reliable predictor of final visual outcome in traumatized eyes, and perform a pupillary examination to detect the presence of an afferent pupillary defect (including a reverse Marcus Gunn response). Busy emergency room staff may omit these "ocular vital signs"; therefore, it is incumbent on the ophthalmologist to check both visual acuity and pupils, as well as educate nonophthalmologic practitioners about the importance of these assessments. The ophthalmologist should then look for key signs that are suggestive or diagnostic of perforating ocular injury (Table 13-6).

If a significant perforating injury is suspected, forced duction testing, gonioscopy, tonometry, and scleral depression should be avoided. Ancillary tests that may be useful in this setting are summarized in Table 13-7. Regardless of the results of laboratory tests, all cases should be managed with safeguards appropriate for patients known to have blood-borne infections (see universal precautions, Chapter 2).

Management

Preoperative management

If surgical repair is required, the timing of the operation is crucial. Although studies have not documented any disadvantage in delaying the repair of an open globe for up to

Table 13-6 Signs of Perforating Ocular Trauma

Suggestive	Diagnostic
Deep eyelid laceration	Exposed uvea, vitreous, retina
Orbital chemosis	Positive Seidel test
Conjunctival laceration/hemorrhage	Visualization of intraocular foreign body
Focal iris–corneal adhesion	Intraocular foreign body seen on x-ray or
Shallow anterior chamber	ultrasonography
Iris defect	
Hypotony	
Lens capsule defect	
Acute lens opacity	
Retinal tear/hemorrhage	

Table 13-7 Ancillary Tests in Perforating Eye Trauma

Useful in many cases (to assess extent of injury and provide needed information for preoperative assessment of patient)
    CT scan
    Plain-film x-rays (generally not as useful as CT scans)
    CBC, differential, platelets
    Electrolytes, blood urea nitrogen, creatinine
    Test for HIV status, hepatitis

Useful in selected cases
    MRI (especially in cases of suspected organic foreign objects in the eye or orbit; this should
      never be used if a metallic foreign object is suspected)
    Prothrombin time, partial thromboplastin time, bleeding time
    Sickle cell
    Drug and/or ethanol levels

36 hours, intervention ideally should occur as soon as possible. Prompt repair can help minimize numerous complications, including

- pain
- prolapse of intraocular structures
- suprachoroidal hemorrhage
- microbial contamination of the wound
- proliferation of the microbes projected into the eye
- migration of epithelium into the wound
- intraocular inflammation
- lens opacity

The following temporizing measures can be taken during the preoperative period:

- Apply a protective shield.
- Avoid administering topical medications or other interventions that require prying open the eyelids.
- Keep the patient on NPO status.
- Provide appropriate medications for sedation and pain control, as well as antiemetics.
- Initiate intravenous antibiotics.
- Provide tetanus prophylaxis.
- Seek anesthesia consultation.

Injuries associated with soil contamination and/or retained intraocular foreign bodies require attention to the risk of *Bacillus* endophthalmitis. Because this organism can destroy the eye within 24 hours, intravenous and/or intravitreal therapy with an antibiotic effective against *Bacillus* species, usually fluoroquinolones (such as levofloxacin, moxifloxacin, gatifloxacin), clindamycin, or vancomycin, should be considered. Surgical repair should be undertaken with minimal delay in cases at risk for contamination with this organism.

Nonsurgical options

Some penetrating injuries are so minimal that they spontaneously seal prior to ophthalmic examination, with no intraocular damage, prolapse, or adherence. These cases may require only systemic and/or topical antibiotic therapy along with close observation. If a corneal wound is leaking (see Chapter 2, Fig 2-6), but the chamber remains formed, the clinician can attempt to stop the leak with pharmacologic suppression of aqueous production (topical [eg, β-blocker] or systemic), patching, and/or a therapeutic contact lens. Generally, if these measures fail to seal the wound in 2–3 days, surgical closure with sutures is recommended.

Surgical repair

The eye can sustain severe internal damage with even a small, seemingly insignificant wound. The management of a typical corneoscleral laceration with uveal prolapse generally requires surgery (Fig 13-14). The primary goal of initial surgical repair of a corneoscleral laceration is to restore the integrity of the globe. The secondary goal, which may be accomplished at the time of the primary repair or during subsequent procedures, is to restore vision through repair of both external and internal damage to the eye.

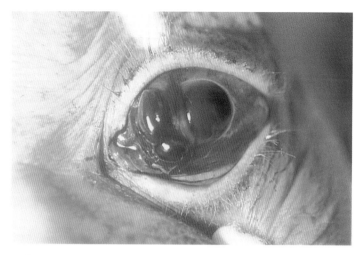

Figure 13-14 Scleral laceration with prolapse of uveal tissue secondary to blunt trauma.

If the prognosis for vision in the injured eye is hopeless and the patient is at risk for sympathetic ophthalmia, enucleation must be considered. Primary enucleation should be performed only for an injury so devastating that restoration of the anatomy is impossible, when it may spare the patient another procedure. In the overwhelming majority of cases, however, the advantages of delaying enucleation for a few days far outweigh any advantage of primary enucleation. This delay (which should not exceed the 12–14 days thought necessary for an injured eye to incite sympathetic ophthalmia) allows for assessment of postoperative visual function, vitreoretinal or ophthalmic plastic consultation, and stabilization of the patient's medical condition. Most important, delay in enucleation following unsuccessful repair and loss of light perception allows the patient time to acknowledge that loss and accompanying disfigurement and to consider enucleation in a nonemergency setting.

Castiblanco CP, Adelman RA. Sympathetic ophthalmia. *Graefes Arch Clin Exp Ophthalmol.* 2009;247(3):289–302.

Anesthesia General anesthesia is almost always required for repair of an open globe because retrobulbar or peribulbar anesthetic injection increases orbital pressure, which may cause or exacerbate the extrusion of intraocular contents. After the surgical repair is complete, a periocular anesthetic injection may be used to control postoperative pain.

Steps in the repair of a corneoscleral laceration All attempts at repairing a corneoscleral laceration should be performed in the operating room with use of the operating microscope and trained ophthalmic personnel. Table 13-8 summarizes the basic steps in restoring the integrity of the globe with a corneoscleral laceration. No attempt should be made to fixate an open globe with rectus muscle sutures. Repair of adnexal injury should follow repair of the globe itself because eyelid surgery can put pressure on an open globe and certain eyelid lacerations may actually improve globe exposure.

Table 13-8 Essential Steps in Surgical Repair of a Corneoscleral Laceration

1. General anesthesia
2. Excision of anteriorly prolapsed vitreous, lens fragments, corneal foreign bodies
3. Repositioning of anteriorly prolapsed uvea, retina
4. Closure of corneal component of laceration at limbus, landmarks
5. Completion of watertight corneal closure (10-0 nylon)
6. Peritomy as necessary for exposure of scleral component
7. Stepwise excision of posteriorly prolapsed vitreous
8. Stepwise repositioning of posteriorly prolapsed uvea, retina
9. Stepwise closure of scleral component (9-0 nylon or 8-0 silk)
10. Conjunctival closure
11. Subconjunctival antibiotics, corticosteroids

The corneal component of the injury is approached first. If vitreous or lens fragments have prolapsed through the wound, these should be cut flush with the cornea, taking care not to exert traction on the vitreous or zonular fibers. If uvea or retina (seen as translucent, tan tissue with extremely fine vessels) protrudes, it should be reposited using a gentle sweeping technique through a separate limbal incision, with the assistance of viscoelastic injection to temporarily re-form the anterior chamber (Fig 13-15). If epithelium has obviously migrated onto a uveal surface or into the wound, an effort should be made to peel this tissue off. Only in cases of frankly necrotic uveal prolapse should uveal tissue be excised.

Points at which the laceration crosses landmarks such as the limbus are then closed with 9-0 or 10-0 nylon suture, followed by closure of the remaining corneal components of the laceration. It may be necessary to reposit iris tissue repeatedly after each suture is placed to avoid entrapment of iris in the wound. Despite these efforts, uvea may still remain apposed to the posterior corneal surface. Many surgeons place very shallow sutures at this stage of the closure to avoid impaling uvea with the suture needle. Then, after the closure is watertight, the uvea can be definitively separated from the cornea with viscoelastic injection, followed by replacement of shallow sutures with new ones of ideal, near-full-thickness depth. Suture knots should be buried in the corneal stroma, not in the wound.

If watertight closure of the wound proves difficult to achieve because of unusual laceration configuration or loss of tissue, X-shaped or "purse-string" sutures or other customized techniques may suffice. Cyanoacrylate glue or even primary lamellar keratoplasty may be required in extremely difficult cases. A conjunctival flap should not be used to treat a wound leak.

When the anatomy of the wound allows, a topographic closure is best for reducing long-term complications. Wider-spaced, longer sutures are used in the peripheral cornea to flatten locally and steepen centrally. Closer, shorter sutures are used centrally, avoiding the visual axis, to close the wound without excessive flattening (Fig 13-16); however, care should be taken that sutures are long enough to minimize their "cheese wiring" through the inflamed stroma.

The scleral component of the laceration is then approached with gentle peritomy and conjunctival separation only as necessary to expose the wound. Prolapsed vitreous is

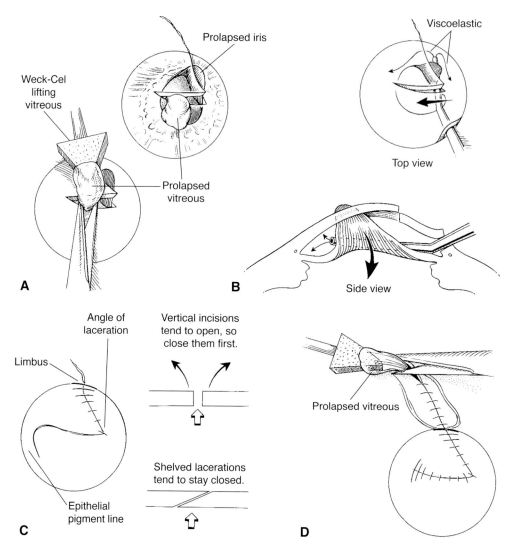

Figure 13-15 Restoring anatomical relationships in corneoscleral laceration repair. **A,** Prolapsed vitreous or lens fragments are excised. **B,** Iris is reposited by means of viscoelastic and a cannula inserted through a separate paracentesis. **C,** Landmarks such as limbus, laceration angles, or epithelial pigment lines are closed. Vertical lacerations are closed first to create a watertight globe more quickly, followed by shelved lacerations. **D,** The scleral part of the wound is exposed, prolapsed vitreous is severed, and the wound is closed from the limbus, working posteriorly. *(Reproduced with permission from Hamill MB. Repair of the traumatized anterior segment. Focal Points: Clinical Modules for Ophthalmologists. San Francisco: American Academy of Ophthalmology; 1992, module 1. Illustrations by Christine Gralapp.)*

excised, and prolapsed nonnecrotic uvea and retina are reposited with a spatula or similar instrument (Fig 13-17). The scleral wound is closed with 9-0 nylon or 8-0 silk sutures. Often, dissection of Tenon capsule and management of prolapsed tissue must be repeated incrementally after each suture is placed.

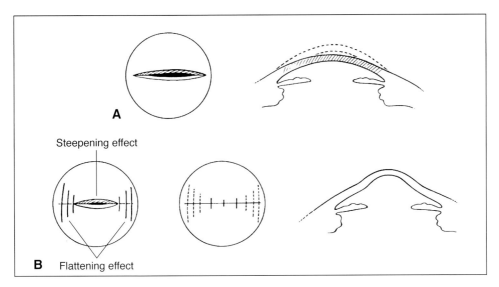

A

Steepening effect

B Flattening effect

Figure 13-16 Restoring functional architecture in corneal wound closure. **A,** Laceration has a flattening effect on the cornea. **B,** Long, compressive sutures are taken in the periphery to flatten the peripheral cornea and steepen the central cornea. Subsequently, short, minimally compressive sutures are taken in the steepened central cornea to preserve sphericity despite the flattening effect of the sutures. *(Reproduced with permission from Hamill MB. Repair of the traumatized anterior segment. Focal Points: Clinical Modules for Ophthalmologists. San Francisco: American Academy of Ophthalmology; 1992, module 1.)*

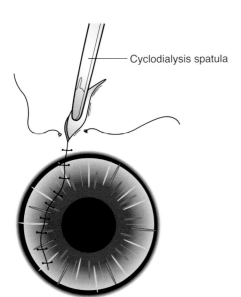

Cyclodialysis spatula

Figure 13-17 Zippering technique of scleral wound closure. Assistant depresses prolapsed uveal tissue while the scleral wound is progressively closed, moving in an anterior to posterior direction. *(Redrawn from Hersh PS, Shingleton BJ, Kenyon KR. Management of corneoscleral lacerations. In: Hersh PS, Shingleton BJ, Kenyon KR, eds. Eye Trauma. St Louis: Mosby-Year Book; 1991.)*

Some posterior wounds are more easily approached with loupes and a headlight, because the open globe should not be rotated too far. If the laceration extends under an extraocular muscle, the muscle may be carefully removed at its insertion and reinserted following repair. Closure of the laceration should continue posteriorly only to the point at which it becomes technically difficult or requires undue pressure on the globe. Very posterior lacerations benefit from effective physiologic tamponade by orbital tissue and are best left alone.

Once the globe is watertight, a decision must be made whether intraocular surgery (if necessary) should be attempted immediately or postponed. Subconjunctival injections of antibiotics to cover both gram-positive and gram-negative organisms are given prophylactically at the conclusion of primary repair. Intravitreal antibiotics such as vancomycin 1 mg and ceftazidime 2.25 mg should be considered for contaminated wounds involving the vitreous.

Essex RW, Yi Q, Charles PG, Allen PJ. Post-traumatic endophthalmitis. *Ophthalmology.* 2004; 111(11):2015–2022.

Secondary repair of intraocular trauma Following primary repair of a corneoscleral laceration, the following secondary measures may be indicated:

- removal of intraocular foreign bodies (eg, using forceps or rare earth magnet)
- iris repair
- cataract extraction
- mechanical vitrectomy
- IOL insertion
- cryotherapy of retinal tears

Deciding whether to pursue such intervention at the time of initial repair is a complex process. The expertise of the surgeon; the quality of the facility, technical equipment, and instruments; the adequacy of the view of the anterior segment structures; and issues of informed consent should be considered. In general, it is recommended that if there are concerns regarding any of these parameters, the surgeon complete the closure of the laceration to maintain globe integrity, and postpone the secondary procedures until a later date. For example, the average anterior segment surgeon should not attempt automated vitrectomy with retina present in the anterior chamber, and even the most expert cataract surgeon might not attempt a lens extraction with limited visualization of the lens. However, intraocular inflammation may worsen, opportunity for placement of an IOL in the capsular bag may be lost, vitreoretinal complications may worsen, and the patient may experience increased pain and expense if these procedures are delayed.

As always, the welfare of the patient should determine the proper course. In general, if a foreign body is visible in the anterior segment and can be grasped, it is reasonable to remove it, either through the wound or through a separate limbal incision. If removal of opacified lens material is attempted, it is helpful to know whether the posterior capsule has been violated and lens–vitreous admixture has occurred. BCSC Section 11, *Lens and Cataract,* also discusses the issues of cataract surgery and IOL placement following trauma to the eye.

Iris repair can be undertaken either primarily or secondarily. Closure of iris lacerations may keep the iris in its proper plane, decreasing the formation of anterior or posterior synechiae. The McCannel technique, using 10-0 polypropylene suture with long needles that may be passed transcamerally, requires only a small additional limbal incision be made (Fig 13-18). Iridodialysis, usually resulting from blunt trauma, may cause monocular diplopia and an eccentric pupil if left untreated. The McCannel technique can also be used to repair an iridodialysis (Fig 13-19). In the event that corneal opacity prevents safe repair of internal ocular injury, repairs can be combined later with penetrating keratoplasty or with placement of a temporary keratoprosthesis, if posterior segment repair is planned.

Postoperative management

After primary repair of penetrating anterior segment trauma, therapy is directed at preventing infection, suppressing inflammation, controlling IOP, and relieving pain. Systemic antibiotics (moxifloxacin 400 mg PO daily) are usually continued for 3–5 days, and topical antibiotics are generally used for about 7 days or until epithelial closure of the ocular surface is complete. Topical corticosteroids and cycloplegics are slowly tapered, depending on the degree of inflammation. A fibrinous response in the anterior chamber may respond well to a short course of systemic prednisone.

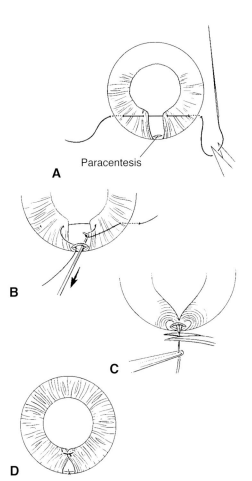

Paracentesis

A

B

C

D

Figure 13-18 The McCannel technique for repairing iris lacerations. With large lacerations, multiple sutures may be used. **A,** A limbal paracentesis is made over the iris discontinuity. Then a long Drews needle with 10-0 polypropylene is passed through the peripheral cornea, the edges of the iris, and the peripheral cornea opposite, and the suture is cut. **B,** A Sinskey hook, introduced through the paracentesis and around the suture peripherally, is drawn back out through the paracentesis. **C,** The suture is securely tied. **D,** After the suture is secure, it is cut, and the iris is allowed to retract. *(Reproduced with permission from Hamill MB. Repair of the traumatized anterior segment. Focal Points: Clinical Modules for Ophthalmologists. San Francisco: American Academy of Ophthalmology; 1992, module 1. Illustrations by Christine Gralapp.)*

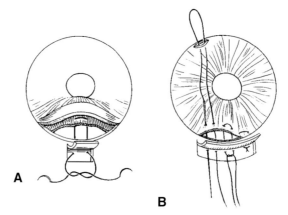

Figure 13-19   Repair of iridodialysis. **A,** A cataract surgery–type incision is made at the site of iridodialysis or iris disinsertion. A double-armed, 10-0 polypropylene suture is passed through the iris root, out through the angle, and tied on the surface of the globe under a partial-thickness scleral flap. The corneoscleral wound is then closed with 10-0 nylon sutures. **B,** In an alternative technique, multiple 10-0 Prolene sutures on double-armed Drews needles are passed through a paracentesis opposite the site of iris disinsertion to avoid the need to create a large corneoscleral entry wound. *(Reproduced with permission from Hamill MB. Repair of the traumatized anterior segment.* Focal Points: Clinical Modules for Ophthalmologists. *San Francisco: American Academy of Ophthalmology; 1992, module 1. Illustrations by Christine Gralapp.)*

Corneal sutures that do not loosen spontaneously are generally left in place for at least 3 months and then removed incrementally over the next few months. Fibrosis and vascularization are indicators that enough healing has occurred to render suture removal safe. Applying fluorescein at each postoperative visit is mandatory to ensure that suture erosion through the epithelium has not occurred, as these eroded sutures can induce infection.

Traumatized eyes are also at increased risk of retinal detachment, so frequent examination of the posterior segment is mandatory. If media opacity precludes an adequate fundus examination, evaluation for an afferent pupillary defect and B-scan ultrasonography are helpful in monitoring retinal status.

Refraction and correction with contact lenses or spectacles can proceed when the ocular surface and media permit. Because of the risk of amblyopia in a child or loss of fusion in an adult, visual correction should not be unnecessarily delayed.

Barr CC. Prognostic factors in corneoscleral lacerations. *Arch Ophthalmol.* 1983;101(6): 919–924.

Brightbill FS, ed. *Corneal Surgery: Theory, Technique, and Tissue.* 4th ed. Philadelphia: Elsevier/ Mosby; 2009.

Spoor TC. *An Atlas of Ophthalmic Trauma.* St Louis: Mosby-Year Book; 1997.

Surgical Trauma

Corneal Epithelial Changes From Intraocular Surgery

The corneal epithelium functions as a barrier to corneal absorption of fluid from tears, including medication instilled topically and pathogens residing on the ocular surface.

Breakdown of the epithelial barrier function, resulting in epithelial edema and stromal swelling, can follow

- inadvertent intraoperative trauma to the epithelium by surgical instruments
- desiccation of the epithelium through inadequate intraoperative hydration
- toxic keratopathy resulting from excessive preoperative instillation of topical ophthalmic preparations (and their preservatives)
- accidental instillation of preoperative periocular facial scrub detergents

Although epithelial damage allows fluid to reach the stroma, it is resisted by the IOP and pumped out by the endothelium. Thus, endothelial damage has a far greater effect on corneal edema than does epithelial damage. Intraoperative damage to the corneal endothelium and/or Descemet's membrane can result in a positive stromal fluid pressure and subsequent epithelial edema. Epithelial edema begins in the basal cell layers of the epithelium and spreads through the epithelium, occasionally resulting in subepithelial bullae.

With epithelial edema, this layer loses its homogeneity, and the corneal surface becomes irregular, leading to symptoms of glare, photophobia, and halos around lights from light scattering. In bright light, edematous epithelium causes enhanced light scattering and can have a marked effect on vision. Surface irregularities caused by epithelial edema are more damaging to vision than stromal edema or scarring. The influence of epithelial surface irregularities on visual acuity is often underestimated, whereas the role of stromal scarring and edema is overestimated.

Descemet's Membrane Changes During Intraocular Surgery

The distensibility of Descemet's membrane allows stretching or distortion, followed by return to its original shape. When the stroma imbibes fluid and thickens, the increased volume is distributed posteriorly, producing bowing and folding of Descemet's membrane (striate keratopathy). Detachment of Descemet's membrane can occur when an instrument or IOL is introduced through the surgical incision or when fluid is inadvertently injected between the membrane and the corneal stroma, resulting in stromal swelling and epithelial bullae localized in the area of detachment (Fig 13-20). Particular care should be taken when clear corneal incisions are enlarged prior to lens implantation during cataract surgery, because Descemet's membrane can be easily stripped off the stroma during reintroduction of the keratome through the incision during this step. The membrane can be reattached with air tamponade. Recurrence may require suturing after repositioning Descemet's membrane in its native position.

Corneal Endothelial Changes From Intraocular Surgery

Normal functioning of the corneal endothelium is highly pertinent to retaining normal stromal and epithelial hydration. Corneal hydration involves the following factors:

- stromal swelling pressure
- barrier function of the epithelium and endothelium
- the endothelial pump
- evaporation from the corneal surface
- IOP

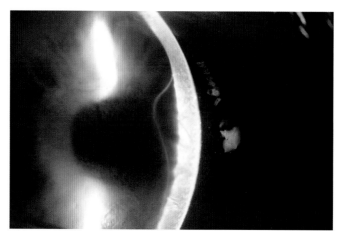

Figure 13-20 Traumatic detachment of Descemet's membrane following cataract extraction accompanied by secondary corneal edema. *(Courtesy of James J. Reidy, MD.)*

Corneal edema following surgical procedures often has many causes; these are related to the health of the patient's endothelium, as well as to iatrogenic factors such as surgical technique, duration of surgery, and intraocular irrigating solutions. Patients with underlying corneal endothelial dysfunction such as Fuchs corneal dystrophy are at risk to develop postoperative corneal edema, even after uncomplicated surgery.

Cataract surgery and IOL implantation

Pseudophakic bullous edema is a leading indication for corneal transplantation, underscoring how surgical trauma can have profound consequences for the health of the endothelium. Manipulation of instruments in the eye through a limbal or clear corneal incision during cataract surgery can impair the functional reserve of an already partially compromised endothelium (as in Fuchs dystrophy), leading to localized edema at the site. During phacoemulsification, heat transferred from the probe to the cornea ("phaco burn") can result in stromal shrinkage, persistent wound leaks, and thinning. A wound that is too tight to allow adequate irrigation fluid flow through the probe or the occlusion of irrigation or aspiration tubing can cause such heat transfer. Closure and repair of phaco burns can be complicated; therefore, every effort should be made to avoid them. The ultrasonic energy of a phaco tip held too close to corneal endothelium during surgery can injure endothelial cells and lead to their loss. Corneal edema in these cases may appear on the first postoperative day or months to years after surgery.

Uncomplicated intracapsular cataract extraction or complicated extracapsular cataract extraction may result in vitreous touch to the corneal endothelium. Persistent corneal edema can occur in the region of vitreocorneal adherence either early or late. Early recognition and treatment with anterior vitrectomy as soon as corneal edema develops can help prevent irreversible corneal edema. More advanced cases with prolonged corneal edema may require endothelial or penetrating keratoplasty combined with vitrectomy.

Current irrigating solutions are superior to those used in the past. They are pH-balanced with bicarbonate buffers, have no epinephrine, and contain glutathione. Endothelial cell loss rates of 8% or less have been reported in multiple series. Preserved solutions either irrigated or inadvertently injected into the anterior chamber can be toxic to the corneal endothelium and cause temporary or permanent corneal edema. Subconjunctival antibiotic injections have been reported to enter the anterior chamber through scleral tunnel incisions or, potentially, by reversing flow through the aqueous outflow tracts.

The presence of iris-fixated or closed-loop flexible anterior chamber IOLs has historically been associated with significant chronic corneal edema and development of pseudophakic bullous keratopathy. Subsequent development of bullous keratopathy often results in reduced visual acuity, chronic foreign-body sensation, photophobia, and epiphora, and predisposes to the development of infectious keratitis.

Laser burns

Endothelial damage occurs following argon laser procedures as a result of the thermal effects of iris photocoagulation. Endothelial burns are usually dense white with sharp margins; they may result in focal endothelial cell loss. Increases in mean endothelial cell size and endothelial cell loss associated with the use of greater laser power have also been reported. In follow-up periods of up to 1 year, endothelial cell loss following laser iridectomy has not been found to be statistically significant, however.

Conjunctival and Corneal Changes From Extraocular Surgery

Conjunctival chemosis with prolapse may result from orbital surgery or trauma. Exposed conjunctiva should generally not be excised but rather reposited and kept in place with patching or, if recurrent, mattress sutures.

Orbital surgery and trauma can cause proptosis of the globe, leading to exposure keratopathy. Therapy includes lubricants, eyelid patching or taping, moist-chamber dressings, and temporary tarsorrhaphy.

CHAPTER 14

Surgery of the Ocular Surface

Introduction

The term *ocular surface* describes the entire epithelial surface of the external eye, encompassing the corneal epithelium as well as the bulbar and palpebral conjunctival epithelium. Moreover, this term stresses the interdependence of the corneal and conjunctival epithelia in maintaining the health of the external eye. Initially, the ocular surface was considered as an anatomical classification based solely on the physical continuity of the stratified nonkeratinizing epithelium of the conjunctiva, limbus, and cornea. More recently, clinical and research insights have offered compelling evidence of important functional relationships within this anatomical entity. This rethinking of the ocular surface as a functional unit has stimulated a complete reorganization of the current approach to the management of ocular surface disease (Table 14-1).

Corneal and Conjunctival Epithelial Wound Healing

Observations of the normal replacement process of corneal epithelium provide valuable insights into the rationale for various ocular surface replacement techniques. Numerous studies have demonstrated that central corneal epithelial mass is maintained by continued

Table 14-1 Indications for Ocular Surface Reconstruction

Conjunctival Autograft	Limbal Autograft or Allograft*	Amniotic† or Mucous Membrane Transplantation
Recurrent pterygium	Chemical injury	Fornix reconstruction
Cicatricial strabismus (bilateral)	Thermal burn	(bilateral)
Fornix reconstruction (unilateral)	Contact lens keratopathy	Chemical injury‡
Postexcision of conjunctival tumor	Persistent epithelial defect (various etiologies)	Immune melts
Symblepharon repair	Post–multiple surgery limbal depletion	Pterygium surgery
	Chronic medication toxicity	Stevens-Johnson syndrome
	Stevens-Johnson syndrome	Ocular cicatricial pemphigiod
	Ocular cicatricial pemphigoid	
	Aniridia	
	Atopy	

*Limbal autograft preferable in unilateral or asymmetric cases; limbal allograft reserved for bilateral cases.
†May be used in conjunction with limbal autograft or allograft.
‡Indicated for fornix reconstruction after cicatrization.

centripetal movement of peripheral corneal epithelium toward the visual axis, as well as by anterior movement from the basal epithelial cells. (The mechanisms of wound healing of the corneal stroma and sclera are covered in BCSC Section 4, *Ophthalmic Pathology and Intraocular Tumors.*)

Role of Stem Cells

Because the corneal epithelium is a highly differentiated cell type that is self-renewing, its stem cells are essential for epithelial replacement and migration. It is believed that the limbal basal layer contains the stem cells of the corneal epithelium that normally repopulate the corneal surface. After severe injuries, this normal process is augmented appreciably in eyes that have a normal reservoir of functioning stem cells. When there is concurrent damage to the limbal stem cells, the conjunctival cells also become involved in repopulating the corneal surface. However, this is a pathologic process often associated with vascularization, surface irregularity, and poor epithelial adhesion.

Conjunctival Epithelium

Healthy conjunctival epithelium has the ability to directly replace damaged corneal epithelium, but, as noted in the preceding section, conjunctival epithelial cells cannot completely restore the function of the corneal epithelium because they do not have the pluripotency of limbal stem cells and cannot differentiate into the corneal phenotype. Following complete traumatic loss of corneal and limbal epithelium, the remaining conjunctival epithelium resurfaces the corneal epithelium by an advancing wave of adjacent conjunctiva. Some of these cells demonstrate morphologic changes, but they do not acquire all the biochemical markers of mature corneal epithelia. It was long believed that conjunctival cells retained the capacity for phenotypic change into corneal epithelium, but we now know this is not the case. The absolute necessity of repopulating the corneal surface epithelium with stem cells forms the rationale for syngeneic or allogeneic limbal stem cell transplantation.

Maintenance of the Ocular Surface and Its Response to Wound Healing

In the mechanically abraded cornea (eg, total epithelial debridement during vitrectomy surgery or following photorefractive keratectomy), reepithelialization and restoration of a relatively normal corneal surface usually occur quickly. In eyes that have suffered severe chemical injury, however, where the insult is to a wide array of cells (corneal, limbal, and conjunctival), the process of cell migration and differentiation may become defective. Consequently, the wave of cells that repopulate the corneal surface often maintains conjunctival characteristics, with variable goblet cells and neovascularization. Based on these observations, autologous conjunctival transplantation has limited value in repopulating the corneal surface unless associated limbal cells are also harvested for grafting. However, conjunctival grafting can be successful in suppressing inflammation and scarring in the traumatized conjunctiva, and thereby providing (indirectly) more support for the proliferating corneal cells. The success of this procedure is contingent on procurement of normal or near-normal donor tissue.

If the goal of surgery is to restore a more functional conjunctival mucosal surface, as in bilateral conjunctival cicatricial disorders or in severe epitheliopathy in keratoconjunctivitis sicca (eg, Sjögren syndrome), then a buccal mucosal graft or amniotic membrane transplant may be employed. Such grafts can restore more normal forniceal architecture and reduce ocular surface inflammation and corneal damage resulting from abnormal eyelid–globe relationships (eg, entropion, trichiasis), chronic exposure (lagophthalmos), and direct corneal trauma (palpebral conjunctival keratinization). In advanced cases of mucosal (conjunctival) disease, complications caused by recurrent corneal epithelial breakdown, secondary infectious keratitis, vascularization, and scarring may lead to corneal blindness.

Mucosal membrane grafting is not, however, by itself effective in repopulating the cornea with normal cells. Rather, its contribution to the health of the corneal surface is indirect: it improves ocular surface wetting by narrowing the palpebral fissure, thereby reducing exposure and evaporation, and it enhances eyelid movement and distribution of the tear film over the cornea and may contribute to mucus formation from the transplanted tissue. Preserved amniotic membrane is another tissue that can be used for ocular surface reconstruction, either by itself, to prevent further stromal degradation, or in conjunction with a limbal autograft or allograft, to repopulate the corneal stem cells.

More recently, stem cell expansion by means of cell culture has proven an effective means of cell surface repopulation. Corneal stem cells have been used for this purpose; however, the long-term survival of these grafts remains uncertain. The use of cultured epithelial stem cells present in the oral mucosa to repopulate the corneal surface has also recently been successful and may hold greater promise for ocular surface reconstruction in a severely damaged eye. At the present time, these approaches are experimental and available in few centers worldwide.

Kinoshita S, Koizumi N, Sotozono C, Yamada J, Nakamura T, Inatomi T. Concept and clinical application of cultivated epithelial transplantation for ocular surface disorders. *Ocul Surf.* 2004;2(1):21–33.

Tseng SCG, Tsubota K. Amniotic membrane transplantation for ocular surface reconstruction. In: Holland EJ, Mannis MJ, eds. *Ocular Surface Disease: Medical and Surgical Management.* New York: Springer-Verlag; 2002:226–231.

Surgical Procedures of the Ocular Surface

This section covers some of the common surgeries performed on the ocular surface, as well as nonsurgical techniques such as the use of bandage contact lenses and cyanoacrylate adhesives. Chapters 15 and 16 of this volume discuss corneal transplantation, and BCSC Section 13, *Refractive Surgery,* covers refractive surgery.

Conjunctival Biopsy

Indications

A conjunctival biopsy can be helpful in evaluating chronic conjunctivitis and unusual ocular surface diseases, including the following:

- squamous lesions of the conjunctiva (eg, conjunctival intraepithelial neoplasia)
- cicatrizing conjunctivitis

- conjunctival lymphoid tumors
- lichen planus
- pemphigus vulgaris
- graft-vs-host disease
- superior limbic keratoconjunctivitis

Surgical technique

After a topical anesthetic agent is administered, a pledget wet with proparacaine or similar agent is applied to the lesion or site for approximately 30 seconds. Subconjunctival anesthesia can also be given but is usually unnecessary. A drop of topical phenylephrine can blanch the conjunctival vessels and reduce bleeding. The surgeon uses forceps and scissors to snip a conjunctival specimen. Lesions are completely excised (excisional biopsy), if possible. For a subepithelial lesion, a wedge or block is excised. Tissue crushing must be minimized by grasping only the edge of the biopsy specimen. Gentle cauterization can be used to facilitate hemostasis; however, it is best to cauterize after excision to minimize burning of the specimen, which severely hinders histologic evaluation.

Tissue processing

The sample is placed in the proper anatomical orientation on a carrier template (eg, filter paper) and inserted into the appropriate fixative, such as formalin (for histology), glutaraldehyde (for electron microscopy), or transport media (Zeus or Michel's) for immunofluorescence microscopy.

Preferred Practice Patterns Committee, Cornea/External Disease Panel. *Conjunctivitis.* San Francisco: American Academy of Ophthalmology; 2008.

Tarsorrhaphy

Tarsorrhaphy is the surgical fusion of the upper and lower eyelid margins. It is one of the safest and most effective procedures for healing difficult-to-treat corneal lesions. Tarsorrhaphy is most commonly performed to protect the cornea from exposure caused by inadequate eyelid coverage, as may occur in Graves disease or facial nerve (CN VII) dysfunctions such as Bell palsy. It can also be used to aid in the healing of indolent corneal ulceration sometimes seen with tear-film deficiency, herpes simplex or zoster, stem cell dysfunction, or CN V dysfunction (neurotrophic lesions). Tarsorrhaphies may be temporary or permanent; in the latter case, raw tarsal edges are created to form a lasting adhesion. They may be total or partial, depending on whether all or only a portion of the palpebral fissure is occluded. Tarsorrhaphies are also classified as lateral, medial, or central, according to the position in the palpebral fissure. BCSC Section 7, *Orbit, Eyelids, and Lacrimal System,* discusses eyelid anatomy and surgical procedures in detail.

Note that the cosmetic effect of a lateral tarsorrhaphy is significant, and patients are often unhappy with the appearance afterward.

Postoperative care

Antibiotic ointment is usually applied to the wound twice a day for the first 5 days. If anterior lamellar sutures are used over a pledget, ointment is applied until the sutures are removed 2 weeks later. Ointment containing corticosteroids should be avoided, because corticosteroids may interfere with rapid healing.

A tarsorrhaphy can be released under local anesthesia. A muscle hook is placed under the tissue, and a blade is used to incise the tarsorrhaphy adhesion parallel to the upper and lower eyelid margins. Iris scissors can also be used to cut along the margin. If the status of the corneal exposure is uncertain, the tarsorrhaphy can be opened in stages, a few millimeters at a time. If the tarsorrhaphy has been performed properly, eyelid margin deformity will be minimal.

Alternatives to tarsorrhaphy

Other therapeutic modalities can help protect the integrity of the ocular surface. Injection of botulinum toxin type A (Botox) into the levator palpebrae muscle, to paralyze the levator muscle, can cause pharmacologic ptosis and provide a temporary protective effect. Applying cyanoacrylate tissue adhesive (discussed later in this chapter) to the eyelid margins may also provide temporary closure of the eyelids for therapeutic purposes. Plastic eyelid splints (Stamler lid splint; Eagle Vision, Memphis, Tennessee) may be placed on the upper eyelid to cause complete closure. If kept dry, these splints may last for a week or more. Tape may also be used for this purpose, but tape rarely lasts for more than 24 hours. As a temporary measure, moisture chambers may be used to protect the ocular surface. These are available commercially or may be constructed with plastic wrap.

Pterygium Excision

A *pterygium* is an abnormal overgrowth of conjunctiva onto the cornea, almost always in the palpebral fissure (see Chapter 12). Indications for pterygium excision include persistent discomfort, vision distortion, significant (>3–4 mm) and progressive growth toward the corneal center/visual axis, and restricted ocular motility.

The aim of microsurgical excision of a pterygium is to achieve a normal, topographically smooth ocular surface. A common surgical technique is to remove the pterygium using a flat blade to dissect a smooth plane toward the limbus. Although it is preferable to dissect down to bare sclera at the limbus, it is not necessary to dissect excessive Tenon tissue medially, as this can sometimes lead to bleeding and later scarring from inadvertent trauma to subjacent muscle tissue and muscle check ligaments. After excision, light cautery is usually applied to the sclera for hemostasis. Options for wound closure include (Fig 14-1)

- *Bare sclera.* No sutures or fine, absorbable sutures are used to appose the conjunctiva to the superficial sclera in front of the rectus tendon insertion, leaving an area of exposed sclera. (Note that this technique has an unacceptably high recurrence rate of 40%–75% and is thus not recommended.)
- *Simple closure.* The free edges of the conjunctiva are secured together (effective only when the conjunctival defect is very small).
- *Sliding flap.* An L-shaped incision is made adjacent to the wound to allow a conjunctival flap to slide into place.

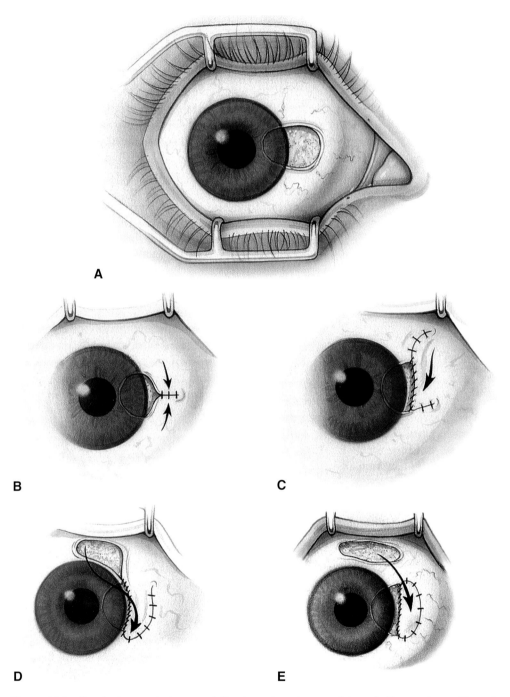

Figure 14-1 Surgical wound closures following pterygium excision. **A,** Bare sclera, although sutures can be placed to tack down conjunctival wound edges. **B,** Simple closure with fine, absorbable sutures. **C,** Sliding flap that is closed with interrupted and/or running suture. **D,** Rotational flap from the superior bulbar conjunctiva. **E,** Conjunctival autograft that is secured with interrupted and/or running suture. *(Reproduced with permission from Gans LA. Surgical treatment of pterygium. Focal Points: Clinical Modules for Ophthalmologists. San Francisco: American Academy of Ophthalmology; 1996, module 12. Illustration by Christine Gralapp.)*

- *Rotational flap.* A U-shaped incision is made adjacent to the wound to form a tongue of conjunctiva that is rotated into place.
- *Conjunctival graft.* A free graft, usually from the superior bulbar conjunctiva, is excised to correspond to the size of the wound and is then moved and either sutured into place or fixated with a tissue adhesive (eg, Tisseel VH; Baxter Healthcare, Deerfield, Illinois). This technique is described in more detail in the next section.
- *Amniotic membrane.* A free amniotic membrane graft has been shown to be a reasonable alternative to conjunctival autograft, particularly when there is a shortage of autologous conjunctiva. Results have generally been reported to be comparable to those of conjunctival autografts. These grafts may be most useful with large pterygia, where a wide excision is needed.

Conjunctival Transplantation

Conjunctival autograft transplantation (see Table 14-1) is appropriate only in cases in which conjunctival inflammation, scarring, or loss is not complicated by extensive damage or destruction of the limbal epithelial stem cells. This technique is essentially a conjunctival free graft designed to

- replace a focal or localized defect in the conjunctiva (eg, after pterygium excision)
- relieve the restriction of extraocular muscle movement caused by scarring of conjunctival and Tenon tissue (after pterygium removal, strabismus surgery, or bulbar tumor excision)
- eliminate problems of conjunctival fornix scarring

Conjunctival transplantation for pterygium

The most common indication for conjunctival transplantation is advanced primary and recurrent pterygium. This technique reduces the risk of pterygium recurrence to approximately 3%–5% and ameliorates the restriction of extraocular muscle function sometimes encountered after pterygium excision. Because the superior bulbar conjunctiva is usually normal and undamaged due to reduced exposure to ultraviolet light and chemical irritants, conjunctival autograft tissue can be obtained from this area in the same eye.

Various techniques of conjunctival transplantation have been used to manage pterygium. The procedure is performed on an outpatient basis, using topical plus peribulbar or retrobulbar anesthetic, especially in recurrent cases complicated by scarring. A traction suture (eg, 6-0 on a spatulated needle) placed at the 12 o'clock position, which can then be clamped down in various positions to the surgical drape, facilitates maximal exposure of the pterygium and the graft site. The pterygium is usually excised with a #57 blade or an angled crescent blade. It is important to remove as much of the fibrovascular scar tissue as possible. If the medial rectus muscle is restricted, it must be isolated, preserved, and carefully freed of all scar tissue. A smooth surface at the site of dissection is a desirable endpoint. With the eye in abduction, the size of the defect is measured with calipers. It is best to allow a little extra tissue for grafting, so the harvested tissue should be approximately 0.5–1.0 mm larger than the size of the defect.

The eye is then turned down to expose the superior bulbar conjunctiva, and the area to be harvested is marked with multiple focal cautery spots or with a surgical pen. The most important aspect of the harvesting is to procure conjunctival tissue with only minimal or no Tenon included. This may be facilitated by injecting a small amount of anesthetic between the conjunctiva and Tenon fascia. Some surgeons make a special point of harvesting limbal stem cells along with the conjunctiva and orienting the donor material in the host bed so that the stem cells are adjacent to the site of corneal lesion excision. The donor site is usually left bare. After the graft is freed, it is transferred to the recipient bed and secured to adjacent conjunctiva (with or without incorporating episclera) with either absorbable (eg, 10-0 Vicryl or 10-0 Biosorb) or nonabsorbable (10-0 nylon) sutures or tissue adhesive. Postoperatively, topical antibiotic-corticosteroid ointment is administered frequently for approximately 4–6 weeks, until inflammation subsides. The surgeon should emphasize to the patient that compliance with this regimen minimizes the chance of recurrence.

If the defect created following dissection of scar tissue is considerably larger than what can be covered with an autologous conjunctival graft, then an amniotic membrane graft may be used in conjunction with a conjunctival graft to cover the entire area of resection. Several authors have noted that this decreases postoperative inflammation and speeds reepithelialization of the surface.

Many authors have described the use of commercially available fibrin tissue adhesive (eg, Tisseel VH) to fixate the conjunctival autograft, thereby eliminating the need for suture fixation. Elimination of sutures decreases postoperative pain and reduces surgical time as well as the recurrence rate, compared with bare sclera techniques. Fibrin tissue adhesive mimics natural fibrin formation, ultimately resulting in the formation of a fibrin clot. Currently, use of this product in pterygium surgery is not FDA approved; its use should be considered off-label. Also, because both pooled human plasma and bovine products are used to obtain some of its components, careful consideration should be given to the potential of the product for disease transmission.

Küçükerdönmez C, Akova YA, Altinörs DD. Comparison of conjunctival autograft with amniotic membrane transplantation for pterygium surgery: surgical and cosmetic outcome. *Cornea.* 2007;26(4):407–413.

Ti SE, Tseng SC. Management of primary and recurrent pterygium using amniotic membrane transplantation. *Curr Opin Ophthalmol.* 2002;13(4):204–212.

Uy HS, Reyes JM, Flores JD, Lim-Bon-Siong R. Comparison of fibrin glue and sutures for attaching conjunctival autografts after pterygium excision. *Ophthalmology.* 2005;112(4):667–671.

Complications   The risk of recurrent pterygium following conjunctival autografting is very low—between 3% and 5%. Self-limited problems include conjunctival graft edema, corneoscleral dellen, and epithelial cysts. Cases of recurrent pterygium after conjunctival autograft transplantation may be substantially improved by either repeated conjunctival autograft, modified limbal autografts, or lamellar keratoplasty. Most studies report that the rate of recurrence with MMC is similar to that with conjunctival grafting. Diplopia resulting from severe scarring rarely occurs but can be most disturbing to the patient. Infections are rare, although *Pseudomonas* sclerokeratitis has been reported, with poor visual outcome.

A large body of literature supports the use of MMC in pterygium surgery to minimize recurrence rates. Although low concentrations of MMC used at the time of surgery (applied to the area of resection with a surgical sponge for up to 2 minutes, followed by irrigation with copious volumes of balanced saline solution) have been shown to be effective in reducing recurrence, it is important to note that any use of topical MMC can be toxic and may cause visually significant complications such as aseptic scleral necrosis and infectious sclerokeratitis. These complications may occur many months, or even years, after the drug's use. If surgery is being performed in a case of recurrent pterygium, and MMC use is contemplated, it is safer to apply it intraoperatively than to give it to the patient for topical postoperative use; in the latter case, overuse may be a problem.

Other indications for conjunctival grafting

In rare cases, an enlarged pinguecula may cause chronic irritation, necessitating removal combined with an autologous conjunctival replacement graft. Conjunctival autografts can also be used for fornix reconstruction when conjunctival fibrosis and cicatrization lead to fornix foreshortening, symblepharon formation, cicatricial entropion, trichiasis, and ocular surface keratinization and vascularization. Occasionally, unilateral fornix foreshortening occurs after localized disease, retinal detachment surgery, or excision of ocular surface tumors or nevi. This foreshortening can be remedied by placing a conjunctival autograft from the opposite eye. Usually, however, conditions associated with fornix obliteration (cicatricial pemphigoid, Stevens-Johnson syndrome) are bilateral, so uninvolved conjunctiva is not available for grafting. Mucous membrane transplantation using buccal mucosa or amniotic membrane has become the preferred ocular surface replacement technique in such instances.

> Koranyi G, Seregard S, Kopp ED. Cut and paste: a no suture, small incision approach to pterygium surgery. *Br J Ophthalmol.* 2004;88(7):911–914.
>
> Tan DTH. Conjunctival autograft. In: Holland EJ, Mannis MJ, eds. *Ocular Surface Disease: Medical and Surgical Management.* New York: Springer-Verlag; 2002:65–89.

Limbal Transplantation

When stem cells are destroyed by disease or injury, the corneal surface becomes covered with conjunctival epithelium, which is less transparent, more irregular, and more prone to erosion and vascularization than normal corneal epithelium (see the discussion of this phenomenon earlier in the chapter). This condition can be diagnosed clinically by the absence of the limbal palisades of Vogt, abnormal epithelium on the cornea, and vascularization, or cytologically with impression cytology or biopsy of the limbal region to show goblet cells. Loss of limbal stem cells is seen most often in chemical injury, but it can also occur as a result of contact lens overwear, multiple surgical procedures, large ocular surface abrasions, repeated infections, or use of topical medications, especially use of toxic chemotherapeutic agents like MMC.

If total loss of limbal stem cells occurs unilaterally, an autograft of limbal epithelium from the fellow eye can repopulate the diseased cornea with normal corneal epithelium (Fig 14-2). In this procedure, corneal epithelium, conjunctiva, and superficial pannus are removed from within 2 mm outside the limbus of the recipient eye, and 2 thin limbal autografts from the fellow eye are then attached to the limbus and allowed to regenerate and proliferate.

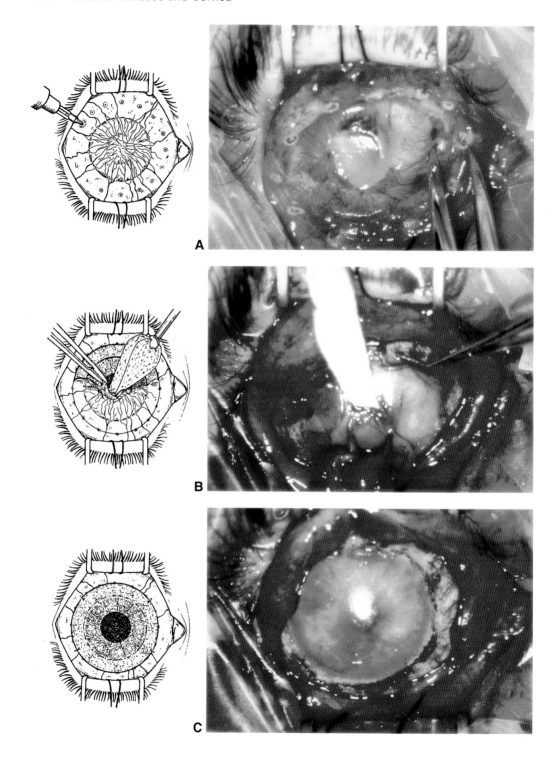

A

B

C

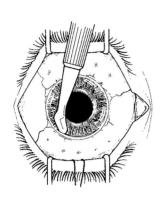

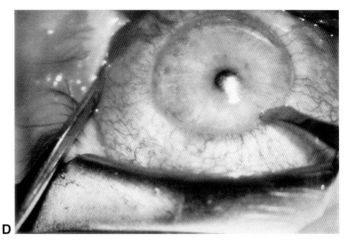

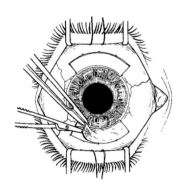

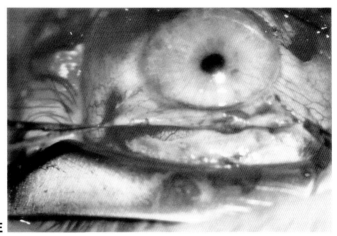

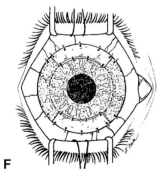

Figure 14-2 Limbal autograft procedure. **A,** With disposable cautery, the area of bulbar conjunctiva to be resected is marked approximately 2 mm posterior to the limbus. **B,** After conjunctival resection, abnormal corneal epithelium and fibrovascular pannus are stripped by blunt dissection using cellulose sponges and tissue forceps. **C,** Additional surface polishing smooths the stromal surface and improves clarity. **D,** Superior and inferior limbal grafts are delineated in the donor eye with focal applications of cautery approximately 2 mm posterior to the limbus. The initial incision is made superficially within clear cornea using a disposable knife. **E,** The bulbar conjunctival portion of the graft is undermined and thinly dissected from its limbal attachment. **F,** The limbal grafts are transferred to their corresponding sites in the recipient eye and are secured with interrupted sutures, 10-0 nylon at the corneal edge and 8-0 Vicryl at the conjunctival margin. *(Reproduced by permission from Kenyon KR, Tseng SC. Limbal autograft transplantation for ocular surface disorders. Ophthalmology. 1989;96(5):709–723.)*

If total loss of limbal stem cells occurs bilaterally, the options for ocular surface transplantation are more limited. The appropriate selection of procedures depends on the relative health of the stem cell population in the prospective donor eye. A limbal stem cell allograft from a living related donor may be considered. A similar procedure, keratolimbal allograft, uses corneolimbal rims from eye bank donor eyes. Although host cells may eventually reject or replace such a tissue, good long-term results have been reported. Technical difficulties, poor epithelial viability, and rejection problems necessitating systemic immunosuppression have limited the usefulness of this modality, but dramatic success has been observed in selected desperate cases. In contrast, the use of cultured limbal epithelium is still not routinely available, even though it is technically feasible and has been used with success. For cases of bilateral stem cell loss, the most promising technique for transferring donor stem cells is limbal allograft transplantation. Use of allogeneic (cultured cell or tissue) grafts requires systemic immune modulation to minimize the chance of rejection of the highly immunogenic limbal tissue.

Ang LP, Tanioka H, Kawasaki S, et al. Cultivated human conjunctival epithelial transplantation for total limbal stem cell deficiency. *Invest Ophthalmol Vis Sci.* 2010;51(2):758–764.

Holland EJ, Schwartz GS. The evolution and classification of ocular surface transplantation. In: Holland EJ, Mannis MJ, eds. *Ocular Surface Disease: Medical and Surgical Management.* New York: Springer-Verlag; 2002:149–157.

Conjunctival Flap

Indications

The conjunctival flap procedure covers an unstable or painful corneal surface with a hinged flap of more durable conjunctiva. Conjunctival flap surgery is performed less frequently now than in the past because of broadened indications for penetrating keratoplasty (PK) (see Chapters 10 and 16), more effective antimicrobial agents, availability of bandage contact lenses, and improved management of corneal inflammatory diseases. Nevertheless, this procedure remains an effective method for managing inflammatory and structural corneal disorders when restoration of vision is not an immediate concern. It should not be used for active microbial keratitis or corneal perforation, because residual infectious organisms may proliferate under a flap if an ulcer is not sterilized first. Any corneal perforation must first be sealed, or it will continue to leak under the flap. The procedure is not meant to provide tectonic support to a very thin cornea. The principal indications for this procedure are

- chronic sterile epithelial and stromal ulcerations (stromal herpes simplex virus keratitis, chemical and thermal burns, keratoconjunctivitis sicca, postinfectious ulcers, neurotrophic keratopathy)
- closed but unstable corneal wounds
- painful bullous keratopathy in a patient who is not a good candidate for PK
- a phthisical eye being prepared for a prosthetic shell

Reduced visualization of the anterior chamber and the creation of a potential barrier against drug penetration are among the disadvantages of conjunctival flap surgery.

However, a successful conjunctival graft, free of buttonholes, will thin out and enable functional vision.

Surgical technique

A complete (Gundersen) flap (Fig 14-3) is highly successful if attention is paid to several fundamental principles:

- complete removal of the corneal epithelium and debridement of necrotic tissue
- reinforcement of thin areas with corneal or scleral tissue
- creation of a mobile, thin conjunctival flap that contains minimal Tenon capsule
- absence of any conjunctival buttonholes
- absence of any traction on the flap at its margins that may lead to flap retraction

Retrobulbar, peribulbar, or general anesthesia may be used. The corneal epithelium and all necrotic tissue are removed, and the eye is retracted inferiorly with an intracorneal traction suture at the superior limbus. Elevation of the flap with subconjunctival injection of lidocaine with epinephrine enhances anesthesia, facilitates dissection, and reduces

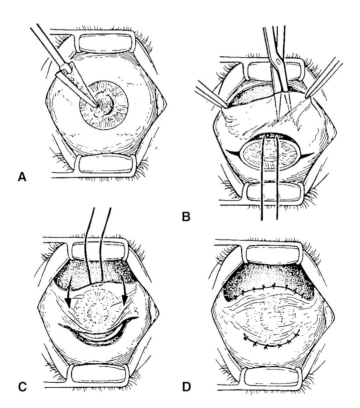

Figure 14-3 Surgical steps for the Gundersen conjunctival flap. **A,** Removal of the corneal epithelium. **B,** A 360° peritomy with relaxing incisions, placement of superior limbal traction suture, superior forniceal incision, and dissection of a thin flap. **C,** Positioning of flap. **D,** Suturing of flap into position with multiple interrupted sutures. *(Reproduced by permission from Mannis MJ. Conjunctival flaps.* Int Ophthalmol Clin. *1988;28(2):165–168.)*

bleeding. The needle for this injection should not pierce the conjunctiva in the area to be used for the flap.

The dissection may start from either the limbus or superior fornix. Dissection of conjunctiva from underlying Tenon fascia must be performed carefully under direct visualization to prevent conjunctival perforation, especially in eyes with previous conjunctival surgery. Once the flap has been dissected, a 360° peritomy is performed, followed by scraping of all remaining limbal and corneal epithelium. Additional undermining of the flap allows it to cover the entire cornea and to rest there without traction. Any residual tension may foster later retraction of the flap. After the flap is positioned over the prepared cornea, it is sutured to the sclera just posterior to the limbus superiorly and inferiorly with absorbable sutures (6-0 to 10-0, depending on surgeon preference).

Partial conjunctival flap A partial, or *bridge,* flap may be used for temporary coverage of a peripheral wound or area of ulceration. Retraction is common despite adequate relaxation of the base. The flap should be well undermined to relieve tension and decrease the chance of retraction. The flaps are fixated to the cornea with nonabsorbable suture (9-0 or 10-0 nylon).

Bipedicle flap This partial, or *bucket handle,* flap can be used for small central or paracentral corneal lesions that do not require complete corneal coverage. It can be useful in a cornea with inferior exposure. The advantage is that the view of the anterior chamber and the remaining uninvolved cornea is not obstructed. The flap is fashioned similar to the Gundersen flap but with only enough dissection required to cover the lesion, plus a small margin (the width of the flap should be 1.3–1.5 times the width of the lesion). Subconjunctival anesthesia is administered, and the epithelium beneath the site of the flap is removed. After marking the bulbar conjunctiva with methylene blue, the surgeon can create the flap and mobilize it into position for suturing with interrupted nylon suture.

Advancement flap Peripheral limbal or paralimbal corneal lesions can be covered with a simple advancement conjunctival flap. A limbal incision is created with relaxing components, and the conjunctiva is simply advanced onto the cornea to cover the defect. Scleral patch grafts and onlay grafts may also be used in conjunction with this technique. The disadvantage of this type of flap is a tendency to retract with time.

Single-pedicle flap Also known as a *racquet flap,* a single-pedicle flap can be used for peripheral corneal lesions that are not large enough to require a total flap. Although a single-pedicle flap is more difficult to dissect than an advancement flap, it is less likely to retract.

Complications

Retraction of the flap is the most common complication, occurring in about 10% of cases. Other complications include hemorrhage beneath the flap and epithelial cysts. In some cases, inclusion cysts enlarge to the point of requiring excision or marsupialization. Ptosis, usually due to levator dehiscence, may also occur postoperatively. Unsatisfactory cosmetic appearance can be improved with a painted contact lens. Progressive corneal disease under the flap is a concern with infective and autoimmune conditions.

Considerations in removal of the flap

If PK is to be performed in an eye with a conjunctival flap, the flap may be removed as a separate procedure or at the time of PK. Simple removal of the flap (without kerato-plasty) is usually unsatisfactory in restoring vision, as the underlying cornea is almost always scarred and/or thinned. Because the conjunctival flap procedure tends to destroy or displace most limbal stem cells, a limbal autograft or allograft after removal of the flap may be necessary to provide a permanent source of normal epithelium before an optical corneal transplant.

Abbott RL, Beebe WE. Corneal edema. In: Abbott RL, ed. *Surgical Intervention in Corneal and External Diseases.* Orlando: Grune & Stratton; 1987:81–84.

Macsai MS, Mannis MJ, Darlington JK. Surface stabilization procedures. In: Holland EJ, Mannis MJ, eds. *Ocular Surface Disease: Medical and Surgical Management.* New York: Springer-Verlag; 2002:137–148.

Mannis MJ. Conjunctival flaps. *Int Ophthalmol Clin.* 1988;28:165–168.

Mucous Membrane Grafting

Indications

The goal of mucuous membrane grafting is to reconstruct a more functional conjunctival mucosal surface so as to ameliorate the fornix obliteration or eyelid margin keratiniza-tion that usually occurs with bilateral cicatricial conjunctival disorders such as Stevens-Johnson syndrome or ocular cicatricial pemphigoid (see Table 14-1). Buccal mucosa or preserved amniotic membrane can be used. Mucous membrane grafting has rarely been used as a treatment for unilateral chemical injury and is performed only in desperate cases of bilateral injury where advancement of the Tenon capsule is not possible and allograft limbal tissue is not available. Nonetheless, this technique has long been a popular method of correcting eyelid position abnormalities caused by cicatrizing conjunctival disorders. Although good results have been reported in inactive cicatricial disorders such as late-stage, nonprogressive Stevens-Johnson syndrome, there is some reluctance to apply this technique to advanced (stage III or IV) ocular cicatricial pemphigoid for fear of exacer-bating this progressive inflammatory disorder. However, advances in immunosuppressive treatment have brought promise that mucous membrane grafting for the eyelid abnormal-ities associated with late-stage ocular cicatricial pemphigoid can achieve some success.

The purpose of grafting mucosal membranes is to achieve better ocular surface wet-ting by improving eyelid movement and distribution of the tear film over the cornea, thereby reducing exposure and evaporation. This procedure also provides favorable ex-tracellular matrix substrate for better epithelial migration and adhesion. However, mu-cous membrane grafting is not effective in replacing normal stem cells. In a small series of patients with advanced ocular cicatricial pemphigoid or Stevens-Johnson syndrome, combinations of allograft limbal transplantation, amniotic membrane transplantation, and tarsorrhaphy, followed by the use of serum-derived tears and systemic immunosup-pression, were shown to reconstruct the ocular surface. These therapeutic modalities ap-pear to provide an alternative to other difficult procedures, such as keratoprosthesis, for treating patients with desperate cicatricial keratoconjunctivitis (see Chapter 16).

There are many surgical techniques for mucosal grafting, and the reader should consult a surgical textbook or video for specifics. Potential complications, regardless of the particular technique, include buttonholing, retraction, trichiasis, surface keratinization of the graft, ptosis, phimosis, depressed eyelid blink, incomplete eyelid closure, submucosal abscess formation, and persistent nonhealing epithelial defects of the cornea.

Fernandes M, Sridhar MS, Sangwan VS, Rao GN. Amniotic membrane transplantation for ocular surface reconstruction. *Cornea.* 2005;24(6):643–653.

Holland EJ. Epithelial transplantation for the management of severe ocular surface disease. *Trans Am Ophthalmol Soc.* 1996;94:677–743.

Tseng SCG, Tsubota K. Amniotic membrane transplantation for ocular surface reconstruction. In: Holland EJ, Mannis MJ, eds. *Ocular Surface Disease: Medical and Surgical Management.* New York: Springer-Verlag; 2002:226–231.

Superficial Keratectomy and Corneal Biopsy

Indications

Superficial keratectomy consists of excision of the superficial layers of cornea (epithelium, Bowman layer, or superficial stroma) without replacement of tissue. The primary indications are

- removal of hyperplastic or necrotic tissue (eg, corneal dermoid, pterygium, Salzmann degeneration, epithelial basement membrane reduplication, degenerative calcification)
- excision of retained foreign material in the cornea
- need for tissue for diagnosis (histopathology or microbiology)
- excision of scarring or superficial corneal dystrophic tissue

If corneal biopsy is performed for histopathology, preservation of tissue integrity and anatomical orientation is crucial. A small specimen can be placed on a filter or thin card to maintain the tissue orientation before fixation or cryosection. For microbiology workup, the biopsied specimens can be minced or homogenized prior to inoculation of the culture media or tissue smearing for histochemical stainings.

Surgical techniques

Mechanical keratectomy   If the corneal lesion is superficial, it may be possible to scrape or peel it away without sharp dissection. When deeper dissection is required, the surgeon can mark the area freehand with an adjustable-depth blade or use a trephine. Care must be taken to maintain the surgical plane and to avoid inadvertent perforation; keeping the dissection plane dry can be very helpful. A lamellar keratectomy can also be performed using a microkeratome, a diamond burr on a surgical drill, or an excimer or femtosecond laser.

Phototherapeutic keratectomy   The excimer laser can remove tissue with much greater precision than is possible with mechanical techniques. One problem with phototherapeutic keratectomy (PTK), however, is that scar tissue may ablate at a different rate than normal tissue, which results in an uneven surface even if the original surface was smooth. Also, if the corneal surface is irregular to begin with and ablates homogeneously, the irregularity will persist. Frequent application of viscous liquid to the corneal surface during ablation fills in the gaps and helps to achieve a smooth surface. Most patients experience a hyperopic shift after PTK from the corneal-flattening effect of the procedure. Nevertheless, PTK may produce marked improvement in vision in selected patients with superficial stromal scarring or dystrophies and obviate the need for corneal transplant surgery. Topical MMC applied to the corneal ablation zone for a brief period following PTK has been shown to decrease postoperative scar formation. Oral vitamin C has been used prophylactically to reduce haze formation in PTK.

Ayres BD, Rapuano CJ. Excimer laser phototherapeutic keratectomy. *Ocul Surf.* 2006;4(4): 196–206.

Kim TI, Pak JH, Lee SY, Tchah H. Mitomycin C–induced reduction of keratocytes and fibroblasts after photorefractive keratectomy. *Invest Ophthalmol Vis Sci.* 2004;45(9):2978–2984.

Management of Descemetocele, Corneal Perforation, and Corneal Edema

Bandage contact lens

Applying a thin, continuous-wear soft contact lens as a therapeutic bandage can protect the loosely adherent remaining or regenerating epithelium from the "windshield wiper" action of the blinking eyelids. Use of bandage contact lenses has significantly improved and simplified the management of recurrent erosions and persistent epithelial defects. Continuous bandaging can reduce stromal leukocyte infiltration and ensure the regeneration of basement membrane and restoration of tight epithelial-stromal adhesion without compromising the patient's vision and comfort.

Frequent lubrication, prophylaxis with antibiotics, and close follow-up are crucial, especially in patients with decreased corneal sensitivity or dry eye. The choice of a soft contact lens for patients with severe dry eye can be difficult. In general, patients with dry eye run a high risk of infection with soft contact lenses. Punctal occlusion can facilitate lens retention and comfort. High-water-content lenses usually are not appropriate because rapid water evaporation further compounds the hypertonicity-induced surface damage in dry eyes. Low-water-content lenses with high oxygen transmissibility (eg, HEMA-silicone polymer) would be the most appropriate choice in this setting. Lenses should be replaced every 2–4 weeks or as deposits accumulate on the lens. The use of an acrylic scleral lens may circumvent the problems encountered with a hydrogel lens.

Even though a hydrogel lens can actually cause corneal hypoxia and increase corneal edema, continuous wear of this type of lens can provide symptomatic relief of painful bullous or filamentary keratopathy. Mild corneal edema can often be managed with hypertonic saline solution and judicious use of topical corticosteroids, if indicated. Chronic use of a bandage contact lens can lead to corneal pannus and compromise the success of future PK for visual rehabilitation. Tarsorrhaphy should be considered for patients who have contact lens complications or a high risk of infection.

Cyanoacrylate adhesive

Tissue adhesives, particularly butylcyanoacrylate, have been used widely as an adjunct in the management of corneal ulceration and perforation. Early application of tissue adhesives in the management of stromal melting has greatly reduced the need for urgent surgical interventions such as therapeutic keratoplasty or conjunctival flap. Although cyanoacrylate tissue adhesives are not approved by the FDA for use on the eye, they have been employed extensively over the past 2 decades to seal perforations or near perforations.

Some perforations are so minimal that they seal spontaneously prior to any ophthalmic examination, with no intraocular damage, prolapse, or adherence. These cases may require only treatment with systemic and/or topical antibiotic therapy, along with close observation. If a corneal wound is leaking but the chamber remains formed, leakage can be reduced or stopped with pharmacologic suppression of aqueous production (topical or systemic), patching, and/or a bandage contact lens. Generally, if these measures fail to seal the wound in 3 days, closure with cyanoacrylate glue or sutures is recommended. Perforations greater than 1–2 mm are usually not amenable to tissue adhesive and require a corneal patch graft.

Cyanoacrylate tissue adhesive applied to thinned or ulcerated corneal tissue may prevent further thinning and support the stroma through the period of vascularization and repair. The adhesive plug is also thought to retard the entry of inflammatory cells and epithelium into the area, thus decreasing the rate of corneal melting. After the lesion has been sealed, new stromal tissue may be laid down, and accompanying corneal vascularization may help to ensure the integrity of the area by providing nutrients and antiproteases.

Surgical technique Tissue adhesive can usually be applied on an outpatient basis using topical anesthetics. However, if adherent or prolapsed uvea in the leakage site or a flat chamber is encountered, the procedure should be performed in the operating room using air or hyaluronate to re-form the anterior chamber. The adhesive is applied under slit-lamp or microscopic observation using a topical anesthetic (eg, 0.5% proparacaine hydrochloride). An eyelid speculum is useful. Before the adhesive is applied, any necrotic tissue and corneal epithelium should be removed from the involved area and a 2-mm surrounding zone. The area is then dried using a cellulose sponge, and a small drop of the fluid adhesive is applied with a 30-gauge needle or a 27-gauge anterior chamber cannula. The glue polymerizes completely within 20–60 seconds and usually adheres well to the deepithelialized surface.

The glue does not polymerize on plastic, so a simple way to handle it is to spread a small amount on a surface such as the inside of the sterile plastic wrapping of any medical product cut to a size slightly larger than the perforation. It should then be applied to the surface of the cornea in as thin a layer as possible using the plastic handle of a cellulose sponge or the wooden stick of a cotton-tipped applicator. The adhesive plug has a rough surface and can be irritating, so a bandage contact lens is used to protect the upper tarsal conjunctiva and to prevent the plug from being dislodged by eyelid blinking.

An alternative to applying cyanoacrylate is to use multiple layers of amniotic membrane that has been cut to the shape of the defect, placing a patch into the defect where the near perforation is located. This patch may be held in place with a larger amniotic membrane patch, nylon sutures, and a bandage contact lens, or by means of fibrin glue. With time, scar tissue will reinforce the deficient area and may mitigate against the need for a corneal transplant.

Chan SM, Boisjoly H. Advances in the use of adhesives in ophthalmology. *Curr Opin Ophthalmol.* 2004;15(4):305–310.

Kim HK, Park HS. Fibrin glue-assisted augmented amniotic membrane transplantation for the treatment of large noninfectious corneal perforations. *Cornea.* 2009;28(2):170–176.

Reconstructive lamellar and patch grafts

See Chapter 16 for discussion and illustration of PK and lamellar keratoplasty.

Corneal Tattoo

Indications and options

Corneal tattooing has been used for centuries to improve the cosmetic appearance of a blind eye with an unsightly leukoma. It has also been used occasionally in seeing eyes to reduce the glare from scars and to eliminate monocular diplopia in patients with large iridectomies, traumatic loss of iris, and congenital iris colobomas.

Different techniques have been used. One involves applying a platinum ion solution to the cornea. When reacted with a second agent, a dark black precipitate is formed in the cornea, producing a dark deposit that can simulate a pupil. A second technique involves using the standard methods used in skin tattooing: applying to the cornea a paste of colored pigment, either india ink or a metal oxide, and then using a hypodermic needle or angled blade to drive the pigment into the corneal stroma in the area that needs coverage. Multiple superficial punctures are made until enough pigment has been applied; multiple pigment colors can be used to give a more natural appearance. However, the method is time-consuming and often needs to be repeated if the pigment uptake is inadequate or the pigment migrates.

Kim JH, Lee D, Hahn TW, Choi SK. New surgical strategy for corneal tattooing using a femtosecond laser. *Cornea.* 2009;28(1):80–84.

Kymionis GD, Ide T, Galor A, Yoo SH. Femtosecond-assisted anterior lamellar corneal staining-tattooing in a blind eye with leukocoria. *Cornea.* 2009;28(2):211–213.

Reed JW. Corneal tattooing to reduce glare in cases of traumatic iris loss. *Cornea.* 1994;13(4):401–405.

Rocher N, Hirst L, Renard G, Doat M, Bourges JL, Mancel E. Corneal tattooing: a series of 14 case studies. *J Fr Ophtalmol.* 2008;31(10):968–974.

CHAPTER 15

Basic Concepts of Corneal Transplantation

Transplantation Immunobiology

Histocompatibility and Other Antigens

Antigens found within the host are known as *endogenous antigens.* The most important group of endogenous antigens is the *homologous antigens,* which are genetically controlled determinants specific to a given species. *Histocompatibility antigens,* homologous antigens found on the surfaces of most cells, are an expression of genetic material on human chromosome 6 in a region referred to as the *major histocompatibility complex (MHC).* In humans, the MHC is known as the *human leukocyte antigen (HLA) system.*

Human leukocyte antigens are found on the surface of all nucleated cells. They are determined by a series of 4 gene loci on chromosome 6 known as HLA-A, HLA-B, HLA-C, and HLA-D. Each zone controls several different antigenic specificities, over 95% of which can be recognized by serologic methods. The histocompatibility antigens are important clinically because they form the basis for graft rejection in organ transplantation and for sensitization to most antigens. It is possible that HLAs are genetic markers rather than actual transplantation antigens and that strong transplantation antigens are closely linked with the HLA markers on the genetic material.

Some grafts are rejected even when donor–recipient pairs are HLA compatible. Although minor histocompatibility antigens such as ABO and Lewis antigens are less potent than major ones, they nonetheless add to the overall antigenicity of a graft. Little is known about the number of minor histocompatibility antigens or their importance in transplantation immunology.

Immune Privilege

The cornea was the first successfully transplanted solid tissue. After other tissues had also been transplanted, it was soon observed that corneas were rejected less frequently than other transplanted tissues. The concept emerged that the cornea was the site of "immunologic privilege" and that corneal grafts were somehow protected from immunologic destruction. Early immunologists attributed ocular immune privilege to "immunologic ignorance" due to the absence of lymphatics draining the anterior segment. It is now evident that corneal grafts are not different from other tissue grafts and that the allogenic cells of the transplant elicit an immune response, but the response is aberrant. There is a profound antigen-specific suppression of cell-mediated immunity, especially T-cell–mediated inflammation, such as delayed hypersensitivity and a concomitant induction of antibody responses.

Tolerance to a corneal graft is now recognized as an active process based on several features:

- absence of blood and lymphatic channels in the graft and its bed
- absence of MHC class II$^+$ antigen-presenting cells (APCs) in the graft
- reduced expression of MHC-encoded alloantigens on graft cells replaced with minor peptides (nonclassical MHC-Ib molecules) to avoid lysis by natural killer cells
- expression of T-cell–deleting CD95 ligand (FasL, or Fas ligand) on endothelium that can induce apoptosis in killer T cells
- immunosuppressive microenvironment of the aqueous humor, including TGF-β_2, α-MSH, vasoactive intestinal peptide, and calcitonin gene–related peptide
- anterior chamber–associated immune deviation (ACAID) involving the development of suppressor T cells. ACAID is a down-regulation of delayed-type cellular immunity. Antigens released into the aqueous humor are, presumably, recognized by dendritic cells of the iris and ciliary body. These APCs can then enter the venous circulation and induce regulatory T cells in the spleen, bypassing the lymphatic system.

For an immune response to occur, an antigenic substance is introduced and "recognized" (afferent limb), producing the synthesis of specific antibody molecules and the appearance of effector lymphocytes that react specifically with the immunizing antigen (efferent limb). Although antibodies to foreign tissues are formed during graft rejection, they are not believed to be important in the usual type of allograft rejection. Rather, extensive evidence indicates that allograft rejection is associated with cellular immune mechanisms. The term *delayed hypersensitivity,* or *type IV,* reaction is used to describe such T-lymphocyte–mediated responses. Other mechanisms are also probably involved. For the endothelial cells to be rejected, they must express MHC class II antigens. Streilein suggests that in the presence of inflammatory stress (including mediators TNF-α and IFN-γ), the endothelial cells' endogenous minor H antigens, which are recognized by the CD4$^+$ T cells, lead to delayed hypersensitivity and graft rejection.

See also the discussion of immune-mediated disorders in Chapters 6 and 7 of this volume. BCSC Section 9, *Intraocular Inflammation and Uveitis,* discusses and illustrates the principles of immunology in greater detail.

Niederkorn JY. Ocular immune privilege: Nature's strategy for preserving vision. *Science and Medicine.* 2003;9(Pt 6):320–331.

Streilein JW. New thoughts on the immunology of corneal transplantation. *Eye.* 2003;17(8): 943–948.

Eye Banking and Donor Selection

Before reliable storage or preservation methods were available, it was imperative that corneas be transplanted immediately from donor to recipient. The McCarey-Kaufman tissue transport medium developed in the early 1970s significantly reduced endothelial cell attrition, allowing corneal buttons to be safely transplanted after being stored for up to 4 days at 4°C. Improvements in storage media over the past 2 decades have extended the viable storage period to as long as 2 weeks, not only increasing the availability of donor corneas but also allowing penetrating keratoplasty to be performed on a less exigent basis. The most commonly used preservation medium in the United States today is Optisol-GS (Bausch & Lomb, Irvine, CA), which includes such components as 2.5% chondroitin sulfate, 1% dextran, ascorbic acid, vitamin B_{12}, adenosine triphosphate precursors, and the antibiotics gentamicin and streptomycin. Currently under investigation is the addition of insulin, epidermal growth factor, broader-spectrum antibiotics, and other components to storage media. These changes may further improve endothelial cell viability and function and enhance sterility in the future.

Organ culture storage techniques are commonly practiced in Europe and have the potential to provide improved donor quality in the future. Organ culture offers a relatively long storage time, which allows optimal use of available donor corneas in areas where there is a relative shortage. An added benefit of organ culture is the delivery of a donor cornea with sterility control of the medium prior to transplantation. Its disadvantages include increased complexity and cost as well as a thick, opaque cornea at the time of surgical transplantation.

Some eye banks in the United States are now offering precut tissue for *Descemet stripping automated endothelial keratoplasty (DSAEK),* otherwise known as *endothelial keratoplasty,* and Intralase (Abbott Laboratories, Abbott Park, IL)-enabled keratoplasty (IEK). This means that donors arriving at an eye bank are screened and then cut with a microkeratome to produce a thin posterior lamella suitable for DSAEK or are cut in a preselected wound shape for IEK. Such shaped wounds include top hat, mushroom, and zigzag donor configurations. These open the door to more precise wound apposition with better wound-healing strength. The long-term effect on transplant outcome and astigmatism still must be determined.

In the United States, not all eye banks are members of the Eye Bank Association of America (EBAA), but all eye banks must comply with US Food and Drug Administration regulatory requirements (Good Tissue Practices) implemented in 2005 to ensure the safety of human cells, tissue, and cellular- and tissue-based products.

Criteria Contraindicating Donor Cornea Use

The EBAA has developed extensive criteria for screening donor corneas prior to distribution to avoid transmissible infections and other conditions. Contraindications include

- death of unknown cause
- unknown CNS disease or certain infectious diseases of the central nervous system (eg, Creutzfeldt-Jakob disease, subacute sclerosing panencephalitis, progressive multifocal leukoencephalopathy, congenital rubella, Reye syndrome, rabies, active viral encephalitis, encephalitis of unknown origin, or progressive encephalopathy)
- active septicemia (bacteremia, fungemia, viremia)
- social, clinical, or laboratory evidence suggestive of HIV infection, syphilis, or active viral hepatitis

- leukemias or active disseminated lymphomas
- active bacterial or fungal endocarditis
- active ocular or intraocular inflammation such as iritis, scleritis, conjunctivitis, vitritis, retinitis, choroiditis
- intrinsic malignancies such as malignant anterior segment tumors, adenocarcinoma in the eye of primary or metastatic origin, and retinoblastoma (eyes with posterior choroidal melanoma may be considered acceptable, but most medical eye bank directors decline their use)
- congenital or acquired eye disorders that would preclude successful surgical outcome: any central donor corneal scar or pterygia involving the central 8-mm clear zone (optical area of the donor button), keratoconus, keratoglobus, or Fuchs dystrophy
- prior refractive corneal surgery such as radial keratotomy (RK), photorefractive keratectomy (PRK), LASIK, and lamellar inserts, although for use in endothelial keratoplasty such as DSAEK, refractive laser surgery may not disqualify a donor
- hepatitis B surface antigen-positive donors, hepatitis C seropositive donors, HIV seropositive donors, HIV or high-risk-for-HIV patients meeting any of the EBAA's behavioral or history exclusionary criteria (eg, inmates, drug users, homosexuals, or guidelines as prescribed by the CDC)

Corneas from patients with prior intraocular surgery (cataract, IOL implants, glaucoma filtration) may be accepted if endothelial adequacy is documented by specular microscopy and meets the local eye bank's prescribed standards; those from patients with prior laser surgical procedures such as automated lamellar keratoplasty (ALT) and retinal photocoagulation may be used if cleared by the eye bank's medical director. Diseases known or suspected to be transmitted by corneal transplantation are listed in Table 15-1.

Table 15-1 Disease Transmission From Donor Corneas

Proven transmission by corneal transplantation
  Rabies
  Hepatitis B
  Creutzfeldt-Jakob disease (previously diagnosed)
  Retinoblastoma
  Bacterial or fungal keratitis
  Bacterial or fungal endophthalmitis
Possible transmission by corneal transplantation
  Human immunodeficiency virus (HIV)
  Herpes simplex virus (HSV)
  Prion diseases
Other diseases that exclude corneal donors
  Hepatitis C, HTLV-I or -II infection, ocular adenocarcinoma, malignant tumors of the anterior segment, Reye syndrome, subacute sclerosing panencephalitis, progressive multifocal leukoencephalopathy, leukemias, active disseminated lymphomas, active infectious endocarditis, active septicemias, variant CJD (vCJD), dementia of unknown cause, recipient of nonsynthetic dura mater graft

---

Even with these standards, the ultimate responsibility for accepting donor tissue rests with the surgeon. Other factors to be considered include the following:

- slit-lamp appearance of donor tissue
- specular microscopic data (generally, endothelial cell counts <2000 cells/mm² are not used)
- death-to-preservation time (optimal range <12–18 hours)
- tissue storage time prior to keratoplasty
- donor age

Most surgeons do not use corneas from donors younger than 24 months, as these corneas are extremely flaccid and can result in high corneal astigmatism and myopia postoperatively. Most eye banks establish a lower age limit of 24 months and an upper age limit of 70 years, as older corneas tend to have lower endothelial cell counts. The acceptable age of donors who provide tissue for transplantation is up to the individual surgeon.

For various reasons, including the potential decline in suitable donor tissue because of widespread refractive surgery, the EBAA and National Eye Institute sponsored the Cornea Donor Study (CDS) in 1999. The study completed enrollment in 2002 and has been extended from 5-year to 10-year follow-up. The 1100 patients, 40–80 years old, who had endothelial dysfunction as indication for the first graft in the study eye, were randomized to receive tissue from donors aged 10–64 or 65–75 years. The primary endpoint is graft failure for all causes. A secondary endpoint is the analysis of ABO mismatches in the rate of rejection and failures. The Specular Microscopy Ancillary Study (SMAS) is analyzing the loss of endothelial cells in a subset of the study population. The study showed no difference in transplant outcome at 5 years' follow-up between the groups.

Cornea Donor Study Investigator Group; Gal RL, Dontchev M, Beck RW, et al. The effect of donor age on corneal transplantation outcome results of the cornea donor study. *Ophthalmology.* 2008;115(4):620–626.e6.

Cornea Donor Study Investigator Group; Lass JH, Gal RL, Dontchev M, et al. Donor age and corneal endothelial cell loss 5 years after successful corneal transplantation. Specular microscopy ancillary study results. *Ophthalmology.* 2008;115(4):627–632.e8.

CHAPTER 16

Clinical Approach to Corneal Transplantation

Corneal Transplantation

Corneal transplantation refers to surgical replacement of a full-thickness or lamellar portion of the host cornea with that of a donor eye. If the donor is another person, the procedure is called an *allograft;* use of donor tissue from the same or fellow eye is called an *autograft* (see Corneal Autograft Procedures later in this chapter). In 2007, there were 34,806 *penetrating keratoplasties (PKs),* accounting for approximately 68% of all corneal grafts. *Descemet stripping automated endothelial keratoplasty (DSAEK)* accounted for 28% of transplants, or 14,159 procedures in 2007, an increase of over 135% from the previous year. In addition, as surgeons strive for selective removal of pathologic tissue while preserving the healthy cornea, the indications and use of *superficial anterior lamellar keratoplasty (SALK)* and *deep anterior lamellar keratoplasty (DALK)* have expanded. See Tables 16-1 and 16-2.

Surgical Approach to Corneal Disease

There are many options for surgical intervention to treat the large spectrum of corneal disease. If the pathology is limited to the superficial 50–75 µm of the cornea, *photothera-peutic keratectomy (PTK)* may be the best choice (see also Chapter 15). For corneal scarring or disease confined to the anterior third of the cornea, SALK is an excellent option. In patients with more extensive stromal disease and a healthy endothelium, such as with keratoconus, postinfectious keratitis, and corneal dystrophy or scarring, DALK is increasingly popular. In cases of primary endothelial dysfunction such as Fuchs corneal dystrophy, pseudophakic bullous keratopathy (PBK), or a failed corneal graft, EK has become the procedure of choice. However, full-thickness PK is a viable alternative for any type of corneal pathology and is particularly useful in patients with combined epithelial, stromal, and endothelial disease or with a failed graft with high astigmatism; or in cases where the surgical plan requires extensive anterior segment reconstruction and corneal surgery simultaneously. In the subset of patients with severe ocular surface disease or multiple graft failures, a keratoprosthesis may be the best prognosis for visual rehabilitation.

The discussion of corneal transplantation in this chapter is intended to provide a basic understanding of surgical techniques involved with the procedures and is not meant to be comprehensive. Many excellent resources available for this purpose are listed in the

Table 16-1 Indications for Penetrating and Lamellar Keratoplasty by Frequency

Indications	Frequency (percent)
Penetrating keratoplasty	
Keratoconus	19.6
Repeat graft	15.7
Post–cataract surgery edema	15.7
Corneal dystrophies and degenerations	12.6
Fuchs dystrophy	9.2
Mechanical or chemical trauma	2.9
Microbial/postmicrobial keratitis	2.8
Congenital opacity	1.7
Postrefractive surgery	0.2
Other causes of corneal opacification or distortion	19.3
Lamellar keratoplasty	
Unspecified anterior stromal scarring	32.7
Keratoconus	27.6
Ulcerative keratitis or perforations	16.2
Corneal degenerations	14.3
Pterygium	4.3
Trauma	3.2
Postkeratectomy	1.4
Reis-Bücklers dystrophy	0.3

From Eye Bank Association of America. *2007 Eye Banking Statistics Report.* www.restoresight.org.

references. Although most ophthalmologists do not perform corneal transplantation, all should be familiar with the preoperative evaluation for appropriate referral of patients and postoperative managment if problems should arise.

Eye Bank Association of America [www.restoresight.org]. *Statistical Report on Eye Banking Activity for 2008.*

Preoperative Evaluation and Preparation

A complete eye examination is necessary prior to corneal transplantation, including a detailed social history to help determine whether the patient will be compliant with the postoperative regimen and report quickly if problems arise. Simple clinical tests, such as those for color recognition or an afferent pupillary defect, can be very important in evaluating patients with media opacity. Ocular surface problems such as dry eye, trichiasis, exposure, blepharitis, and rosacea must be recognized and treated prior to transplantation. In older patients, the increased risk of problems with anesthesia and the rare complication of expulsive hemorrhage must also be considered. In addition, the postoperative course may be more problematic due to the increased incidence of chronic epithelial defects, poor blink rate, infections, and wound dehiscence or slippage associated with slower wound healing.

The preoperative evaluation should also address any neurologic or intraocular factors that could compromise the final visual result, such as other media opacity, uncontrolled glaucoma, amblyopia, macular abnormalities, retinal disease, or optic nerve damage.

Table 16-2 Comparison of Procedures for Penetrating and Selective Keratoplasty

Procedure	Penetrating Keratoplasty	Descemet Stripping Automated Endothelial Keratoplasty (DSAEK)	Superficial Anterior Lamellar Keratoplasty (SALK)	Deep Anterior Lamellar Keratoplasty (DALK)
Indications	Any stromal or endothelial corneal pathology	Endothelial dystrophy Pseudophakic bullous keratopathy ICE syndrome Failed corneal grafts	Superficial stromal dystrophies and degenerations Salzmann nodular degeneration Scars/trauma/dermoids Infections	Keratoconus Infections Corneal stromal dystrophies not involving endothelium Corneal thinning Corneal ectasia secondary to LASIK
Intraoperative complications	Hemorrhage Damage to lens/iris Irregular trephination Poor graft centration Iris or vitreous incarceration in the wound Damage to donor endothelium	Poor microkeratome dissection of donor tissue Inability to strip Descemet's tissue Loss of orientation of tissue Poor centration of trephination, leading to a thick edge and possible epithelial ingrowth Intraocular hemorrhage leading to heme in the interface Excessive manipulation of tissue, leading to cell loss	Poor microkeratome dissection Corneal perforation	Corneal perforation requiring transition to PK Descemet's membrane splitting
Postoperative complications	Wound leak Flat chamber Glaucoma Endopthalmitis Persistent epithelial defect Recurrent primary disease Primary graft failure Eroded infected sutures Graft rejection Corneal astigmatism	Pupillary block Dislocation of lenticule Difficulty following intraocular pressure Primary graft failure Epithelial ingrowth	Loss of donor lenticule	Opacification and vascularization of interface Allograft rejection Inflammatory necrosis of the graft

(Continued)

Table 16-2 *(continued)*

Procedure	Penetrating Keratoplasty	Descemet Stripping Automated Endothelial Keratoplasty (DSAEK)	Superficial Anterior Lamellar Keratoplasty (SALK)	Deep Anterior Lamellar Keratoplasty (DALK)
Advantages	Full-thickness tissue eliminates interface-related visual problems	Rapid visual rehabilitation Independent of ocular surface wound healing Stable corneal curvature for triple procedures Tectonically strong Eliminates suture-related problems	Selective removal of pathologic tissue More rapid visual rehabilitation Less need for sutures Minimal requirements for donor tissue Reduced risk for graft rejection Reduced risk of penetration into the anterior chamber Less risk for poorly compliant patient, eye rubber	Tectonically stronger wound than in PK Early removal of sutures Less dependence on topical corticosteroids Minimal requirements for donor tissue
Disadvantages	Difficult to determine anterior corneal curvature, leading to significant refractive error Postoperative astigmatism Ocular surface disease or neurotrophic cornea leads to prolonged healing or persistent epithelial defect	Significant stromal haze, subepithelial fibrosis, or epithelial irregularity may require second procedure Possible higher rate of endothelial cell loss	Irregular interface Irregular surface if lenticule shifts Interface vascularizaton	Irregular interface

Preexisting glaucoma or ocular inflammation should be controlled before transplantation is considered. Active keratitis or uveitis is treated medically if possible, and the eye should ideally remain quiet for several months prior to surgery. An inflamed eye at the time of surgery is associated with a higher incidence of postoperative complications, such as graft rejection and failure, glaucoma, and cystoid macular edema. For example, corneal perforations in an acutely inflamed eye should, if possible, be closed either with cyanoacrylate tissue adhesive for a small perforation or by means of a lamellar corneal graft in order to restore the integrity of the globe and allow the eye to become quiet. A vision-restoring transplant may then be undertaken at a later date. A lamellar graft should at least be considered in any case with normal endothelium.

Fluorescein angiography or optical coherence tomograpy (OCT) can be helpful in detecting retinal problems such as cystoid macular edema and age-related macular degeneration. If the media are completely opaque, standard B-scan for evaluating the posterior segment or ultrasound biomicroscopy (UBM) for evaluating the anterior segment may reveal problems that could affect the visual prognosis after transplant. The potential visual acuity meter, laser interferometer, blue-field entoptic phenomenon testing, visual fields, color discrimination, 2 points of light separation, and visually evoked cortical potentials may also help in preoperative assessment of the afferent system.

In general, deep corneal vascularization, ocular surface disease, active anterior segment inflammation, peripheral corneal thinning, previous graft failures, poor compliance, and increased IOP worsen the prognosis for transplantation and thus influence the appropriateness of this procedure for the affected patient.

Surgical Technique for Penetrating Keratoplasty

Preparation of donor cornea

Donor tissue is most commonly prepared by trephination of the tissue—that is, centering the previously excised corneoscleral donor tissue, endothelial side up, in the concave well of a cutting block apparatus that approximates the cornea's shape. Sharp disposable blades are vertically advanced along a guiding shaft to punch the button in a precise, crisp, guillotine fashion. The main goal is to obtain a central donor button with smooth vertical side cuts. Currently, femtosecond laser technology allows for the creation of mushroom-shaped or inverted mushroom–shaped side incisions, top-hat configurations, and zigzag shapes. These wound configurations can also be fashioned with a manual lamellar dissection using an artificial anterior chamber for the donor tissue and a suction trephine for the host. The new side configurations are reported to produce more rapid wound healing, allow early suture removal, create a stronger and more stable graft-vs-host interface, and induce less astigmatism. At this point, however, there are no studies demonstrating the clinical superiority of the shaped incisions. Each of these techniques has advantages and disadvantages relative to experience, cost, convenience, availability, and clinical scenario.

Most surgeons size the donor button 0.25–0.50 mm larger than the diameter of the host corneal opening (eg, an 8.0-mm-diameter corneal button for a 7.5-mm wound). This size disparity may reduce postoperative glaucoma, enhance watertight wound closure, prevent peripheral anterior synechiae formation and excessive postoperative corneal flattening, and provide the recipient eye with more endothelial cells. In keratoconus, especially in eyes with high axial length, sizing the donor tissue to match the exact size of the wound may flatten the corneal contour and thereby reduce postoperative myopia.

Preparation of recipient eye

For safety purposes, it is recommended that all donor preparations be completed before trephination of the recipient eye. For preparation of the host bed, use of the traditional handheld trephine is still one of the most common methods because it offers convenience and low cost, requires only sharp disposable blades, and has design simplicity. However, hand fixation and rotation may lead to tilting and irregularity of cut as well as to unanticipated anterior chamber entry. Corneal vacuum trephines offer improved accuracy and consistency of cut, depth control, disposability, suture placement marking points, and relatively low cost. Disadvantages include outward beveling of the posterior corneal edges in deep trephination, slightly reduced observation, and more complexity than with a traditional trephine. The Hanna Trephine System (I-Med Pharma, Quebec, Canada) offers the advantages of less recipient edge undercutting and precision of cut depth. Its disadvantages include cost, complexity, and the surgeon's reduced visualization of the cornea when applying the device. Femtosecond laser technology can also be used to prepare the host bed so it matches the shaped side incisions in the donor tissue. Difficulties encountered with the use of the femtosecond laser include limited accessibility, increased costs, and the possibility that the treatment must be performed at a different location or time from the rest of the procedure.

After completion of the trephination and excision of the diseased cornea, the donor corneal button is placed onto the recipient's eye, endothelial side down. Use of viscoelastic material helps protect the donor endothelium during surgical manipulation, keeps the anterior chamber formed, and shields the iris while the donor button is being sutured into the wound.

Suture techniques

The donor button is secured with at least 4 interrupted cardinal sutures. The second cardinal suture is the most important because a mistake at this stage in anchoring the button 180° away from the first suture has the greatest mathematical potential, in principle, for misalignment error and subsequent astigmatism. Complete wound closure is achieved with interrupted sutures, 1 or 2 continuous sutures, or a combination.

The suture knots may be positioned in either donor or host tissue and are buried in the corneal stroma, not left in the wound interface. Most corneal surgeons prefer deep partial-thickness corneal suture bites over full-thickness bites. Incorporating 95% of the donor's and host's relative corneal thickness avoids posterior wound gape. Full-thickness bites may be associated with a higher chance of leakage along suture tracks and serve as a portal of entry for microorganisms or epithelial ingrowth. The advantages of deep suture placement with either technique are decreased posterior wound gape and enhanced wound stabilization and healing.

A variety of techniques are used to complete the suturing, depending on the clinical situation and preference of the surgeon. Vascularized, inflamed, or thinned corneas tend to heal unevenly and unpredictably. *Interrupted sutures,* usually 16–24 in number, are the technique of choice in such corneas, as well as in pediatric keratoplasties, where wound

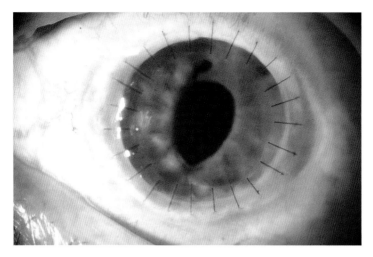

Figure 16-1 PK for syphilitic interstitial keratopathy, with 24 interrupted 10-0 nylon sutures in place.

healing is rapid (Fig 16-1). The tension of each interrupted suture acts as an independent vector, generating central steepening and local flattening. Sutures may be removed selectively in the presence of sufficient donor–recipient interface healing if they attract blood vessels or if they loosen because of wound contraction. Astigmatism may be reduced postoperatively by selective removal of sutures in the steep corneal meridian, although premature removal risks wound dehiscence or slippage.

In the absence of vascularization, focal inflammation, or thinning, single or double *continuous sutures* or *combined interrupted and continuous sutures* can be used to secure the PK (Figs 16-2, 16-3). If properly placed, continuous sutures may allow more even distribution of tension and healing around the wound. Suture passes may be placed radially to the donor–recipient wound or be placed torque-free. The advantages of running sutures include their ease of removal postoperatively. Disadvantages include sectoral loosening, or cheese wiring, which may compromise the entire closure.

The combined interrupted and continuous suture technique offers several of the advantages of both methods. The interrupted sutures may be removed earlier after PK in order to reduce corneal astigmatism, whereas the continuous suture remains to protect against wound dehiscence. There is no consensus as to whether the combined technique or the running techniques produce less astigmatism. Many variables contribute to astigmatism, but the key suturing principle is uniform placement to minimize uneven suture tension, tissue torque, and distortion, thereby achieving secure closure without override or posterior wound gape.

Combined Procedures

Penetrating keratoplasy may be combined with other procedures such as cataract extraction, primary or secondary IOL implantation, IOL removal or exchange, glaucoma surgery, vitrectomy, and retinal procedures. Synechiolysis can be performed with caution—excessive

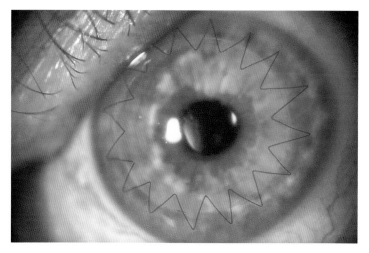

Figure 16-2 PK for pseudophakic corneal edema, with single continuous 10-0 nylon suture in place.

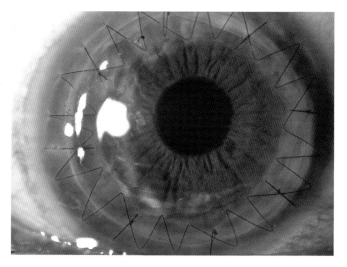

Figure 16-3 Combined suturing technique employs both interrupted and continuous 10-0 nylon sutures. *(Courtesy of Robert W. Weisenthal, MD.)*

bleeding, tearing, or tissue and inflammatory exudation must be avoided. Iris defects may be repaired with 10-0 Prolene sutures to achieve pupil constriction, eliminate monocular diplopia, improve spectacle acuity, reduce glare, and minimize chances of iridocorneal adhesion. Iris segments and combined iris and IOL prostheses (eg, devices by Morcher and Ophtec) may be available under a Humanitarian Device Exemption application (see BCSC Section 13, *Refractive Surgery*). In eyes at risk for postoperative uveitis (eg, those with herpes simplex or interstitial keratitis), a peripheral iridectomy may reduce the chance of postoperative pupillary-block glaucoma.

Intraoperative Complications

Complications that can occur during PK include the following:

- damage to the lens and/or iris from the trephine, scissors, or other instruments
- irregular trephination
- inadequate vitrectomy resulting in vitreous contact with graft endothelium
- poor graft centration on the host bed
- excessive bleeding from the iris and wound edge (in vascularized host corneas)
- choroidal hemorrhage and effusion
- iris incarceration in the wound
- damage to the donor endothelium during trephination and handling

In severely edematous corneas, recipient Descemet's membrane may be inadvertently left behind after corneal excision, as it is easily stripped completely from the stroma. Thus, the recipient eye must be carefully examined for retained Descemet's membrane; donor endothelium resting against host Descemet's membrane may severely compromise the graft.

Postoperative Care and Complications

The postoperative care of a corneal transplant is far more complex than that following cataract surgery. The long-term success of a PK depends on the quality of the postoperative care as much as on the performance of the operative technique. Routine postsurgical care—use of topical antibiotics, tapering topical corticosteroids, and frequent office visits—is directed at prevention and early recognition of the myriad complications that can occur after PK, as well as optimizing postoperative wound healing and facilitating rapid visual rehabilitation. This section covers some of the more common postsurgical complications. Astigmatism and graft rejection are discussed separately.

Wound leak

The wound is always checked carefully for leakage at the end of surgery. Small wound leaks that do not cause anterior chamber shallowing frequently close spontaneously. Patching, therapeutic contact lenses, and use of aqueous production inhibitors may hasten wound closure. Resuturing is advised for leaks lasting longer than 3 days.

Flat chamber/iris incarceration in the wound

Both flat chamber and iris incarceration in the wound imply either poor wound integrity or excessive posterior pressure, and early surgical intervention is advised.

Glaucoma

High IOP may occur at any time after PK. Often, the first clinical sign is the loss of folds in Descemet's membrane, usually seen in the early postoperative period. Glaucoma should be treated aggressively with medical, laser, or surgical intervention as indicated. Unusual causes include epithelial downgrowth or fibrous ingrowth. (See BCSC Section 10, *Glaucoma*.)

Endophthalmitis

After PK, endophthalmitis may arise from intraoperative contamination, donor button contamination, or postoperative invasion by organisms. Aggressive intervention can save the eye and vision in some cases. (See BCSC Section 9, *Intraocular Inflammation and Uveitis.*)

Primary endothelial failure

When a graft is edematous from the first postoperative day and remains so without inflammatory signs, a deficiency of donor endothelium is presumed (Fig 16-4). Most surgeons allow at least 4 weeks and up to 2 months for spontaneous resolution of edema and only then consider a regraft.

Persistent epithelial defect

Large epithelial defects are common after PK, but they should heal within 14 days. After this time, irreversible scarring and ulceration may occur. Ocular surface disease (such as dry eye, exposure, rosacea, blepharitis, or trichiasis) should be ruled out or treated. Lubrication, patching, therapeutic contact lenses, punctal occlusion with plugs or cautery, and tarsorrhaphy may be helpful in difficult cases. If these are not successful, herpetic keratitis should be considered in the differential diagnosis, even in cases where this was not the underlying reason for the graft (Fig 16-5). Oral antivirals may be used as a therapeutic trial. Otherwise, management is similar to that used in treating neurotrophic keratitis.

Recurrence of primary disease

Bacterial, fungal, viral, and amebic keratitis can recur in a graft. Medical treatment directed at the causative agent in recurrent infections is the initial form of therapy. In patients with superficial recurrent corneal stromal dystrophies such as granular or lattice dystrophy, PTK can be used to remove visually significant lesions (Fig 16-6).

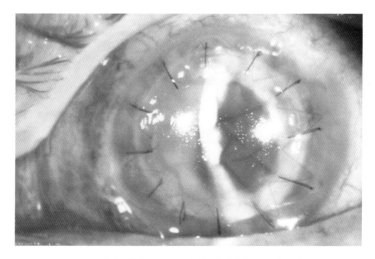

Figure 16-4   Primary endothelial failure after PK.

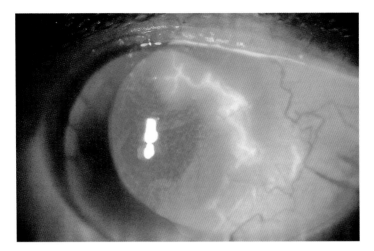

Figure 16-5 Herpes simplex virus keratitis recurring in a graft.

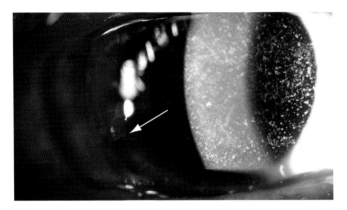

Figure 16-6 Recurrence of granular corneal dystrophy after corneal transplantation. *Arrow* high-lights deposition of new granular material within suture tract. *(Courtesy of Robert W. Weisenthal, MD.)*

Suture-related problems

Postoperative problems related to sutures include the following:

- excessive tightness
- loosening (usually as a result of wound contraction, resolution of graft–host junction edema, suture breakage, or suture cheese wiring) (Fig 16-7)
- breakage of running suture
- infectious abscesses (usually localized around loose, broken, or exposed sutures; Fig 16-8)
- noninfectious (toxic) suture infiltrates (Fig 16-9)
- giant papillary conjunctivitis from exposed knots
- vascularization along suture tracks

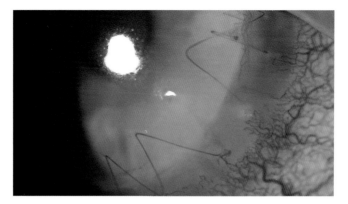

Figure 16-7 Broken running suture after PK. It should be removed to avoid further vascularization, infection, and graft rejection. *(Courtesy of Robert W. Weisenthal, MD.)*

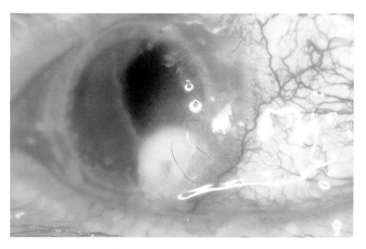

Figure 16-8 Suture abscess caused by *Streptococcus pneumoniae,* 2 years after PK.

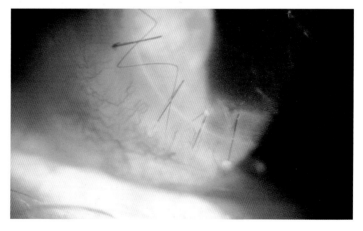

Figure 16-9 Deep, noninfectious toxic suture infiltrates after PK.

Loose and broken sutures do not contribute to wound stability and, therefore, should be removed as soon as possible. Totally buried interrupted suture fragments may be left. Vascularization along the suture indicates that the wound is adequately healed in the vicinity and that sutures may be removed safely. Vascularized sutures are also prone to loosening and may increase the chance of graft rejection. If only a small segment of the running suture is eroded, it is possible to remove this portion while leaving the remainder intact, especially if no significant corneal astigmatism is present. Patients should be warned to return if a foreign-body sensation is noted, as contiguous portions of a running suture may loosen and erode at a later date. After the sutures are removed, there may be a dramatic shift in refractive error or astigmatism, so the patient should be seen for follow-up to ensure wound stability and to recheck refraction.

Microbial keratitis

The use of topical corticosteroids, the presence of epithelial defects or edema, and exposed sutures predispose the PK patient to infectious keratitis, sometimes with unusual organisms. Decreased corneal sensation and topical corticosteroid use may also delay presentation. Lesions must be scraped immediately for diagnosis, and broad-spectrum antibiotic therapy initiated, in order to preserve the graft. A peculiar form of keratitis, *infectious crystalline keratopathy,* is seen in grafts and other immunocompromised corneas (Fig 16-10). Branching colonies of organisms proliferate in the deep corneal stroma with no visible inflammatory response. Many organisms have been implicated, but *Streptococcus viridans* is seen most frequently.

Late nonimmune endothelial failure

When a graft becomes edematous after months to years without inflammatory signs, 2 causes are possible. First, the tissue might have originally possessed a marginal number of endothelial cells, and the normal spreading of these cells has resulted in inability to maintain graft clarity. Alternatively, significant loss of endothelial cells might have

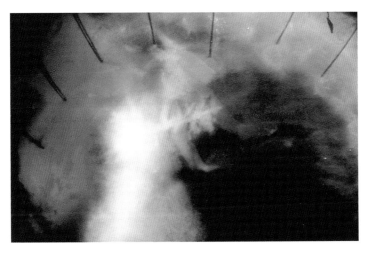

Figure 16-10 Infectious crystalline keratopathy after PK.

occurred later in the postoperative period; possible causes of such a loss include success-fully treated rejection episodes, retention of an intraocular lens that caused endothelial damage, or persistent loss due to peripheral anterior synechiae.

Control of Postoperative Corneal Astigmatism and Refractive Error

A corneal transplant was once considered successful merely if the graft remained clear. Only later in the refinement of surgical procedures was the vexing and relatively common problem of high corneal astigmatism after surgery seriously addressed. Severe astigma-tism may be associated with decreased visual acuity, anisometropia, aniseikonia, image distortion, and monocular diplopia, thus rendering an otherwise successful operation in-effective. Astigmatism is the most frequent complication of PK. It may result in anisome-tropic asthenopic symptoms or in the inability to wear contact lenses. Many methods have been used to reduce the occurrence, including

- varying suture techniques
- making intraoperative adjustments
- improving trephines and use of new technology, such as the femtosecond laser, to better match donor and host
- selective suture removal or adjustment of the running suture using computerized videokeratography and wavefront analysis for postoperative management

The primary method to minimize astigmatism in the corneal graft postoperatively is to readjust or remove the sutures. If a single running suture technique has been used, the surgeon may redistribute the suture tension at 1 month postoperatively using corneal to-pography as a guide. Alternatively, if there is a combination of running and interrupted sutures, the interrupted sutures can be removed starting at 1 month. If the patient has only interrupted sutures, then suture removal should begin at a later stage to avoid wound slippage or dehiscence. Clinicians must be especially careful with older patients placed on long-term topical corticosteroid therapy, as the wound healing may be even slower.

Managing astigmatism is similar with any type of suturing technique. The most criti-cal step is to identify the steep axis using corneal topography, handheld keratoscopy, pho-tokeratoscopy, or manual keratometry. For example, in Figure 16-11 the SIM K readings show the steep axis of 49.93 at 11 and the flat axis of 44.06 at 101. The photokeratoscopy shows clear rings that are ovalized, with the shorter axis horizontally corresponding to the steep axis. The presence of distinct rings demonstrates the smooth surface indicative of regular astigmatism. Rings that are very irregular or indistinct indicate irregular astigma-tism. In the latter case, caution or delayed suture removal or adjustment is required.

A manifest refraction is helpful to confirm the steep axis (positive cylinder). The au-torefraction in Figure 16-11 is –9.00 + 6.75 at 4°. The manifest refraction is –7.00 + 5.00 at 4°, providing 20/25 acuity; the good visual acuity confirms the presence of regular astig-matism. Removing the interrupted sutures at the 4° meridian or adjusting the running suture will compensate for the induced astigmatism. After manipulation or removal of the sutures, the patient is placed on a topical antibiotic for 4 days, and a return visit scheduled for 1 month for repeat corneal topography and manifest refraction.

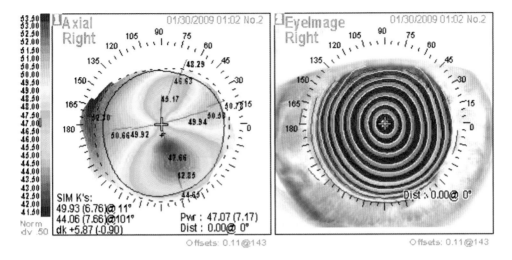

tam	SPH	CYL	AXIS	SimK1	SimK2	dK	e(Q)	SA@4.0	Pupil
R	-9.00	6.75	4 E	49.93(6.76)@ 11	44.06(7.66)@101	+5.87(-0.90)	-0.58(0.33)	O+0.184 C+0.135	6.33 6.

Figure 16-11 Corneal topography with a Nidek OPD showing the astigmatism after corneal transplantation. *(Courtesy of Robert W. Weisenthal, MD.)*

Relaxing incisions are used to reduce astigmatism if a large amount of residual astigmatism is present after all sutures have been removed. Incisions are placed either in the donor cornea anterior to the graft–host junction or in the graft–host interface at the steep (plus cylinder) meridian in an arcuate manner for maximum effect (astigmatic keratotomy [AK]). The effect can be augmented by suture placement at the flat meridian. LASIK, photorefractive astigmatic keratectomy, and femtosecond laser–assisted astigmatic keratoplasty have also been used to manage astigmatism (see BCSC Section 13, *Refractive Surgery*).

All of these procedures are associated with the potential for micro- or macroperforation, infection, rejection, under- and overcorrections, chronic epithelial defects, and worsening of irregular astigmatism.

Bahar I, Levinger E, Kaiserman I, Sansanayudh W, Rootman DS. Intralase enabled astigmatic keratotomy for postkeratoplasty astigmatism. *Am J Ophthalmol.* 2008;146(6):897–904.

Speaker MG, Haq F, Latkany R, Reing CS. Postkeratoplasty astigmatism. In: Krachmer JH, Mannis MJ, Holland EJ, eds. *Cornea.* 2nd ed. Vol 2. Philadelphia: Elsevier/Mosby; 2005:1527–1539.

Diagnosis and Management of Graft Rejection

Corneal allograft rejection rarely occurs within 2 weeks, and it may occur as late as 20 years after PK. Fortunately, most episodes of graft rejection do not cause irreversible graft failure if recognized early and treated aggressively with corticosteroids. Early recognition is the key to survival of an affected corneal graft. Corneal transplant rejection takes

4 clinical forms, described in the following sections, which may occur either singly or in combination.

Epithelial rejection

The immune response may be directed entirely at the donor epithelium (Fig 16-12). Lymphocytes cause an elevated, linear epithelial ridge that advances centripetally. Because host cells replace lost donor epithelium, this form of rejection is problematic only in that it may herald the onset of endothelial rejection. Epithelial rejection has been reported at a rate of 10% of those patients experiencing rejection, and it is usually seen early in the postoperative period (1–13 months).

Subepithelial rejection

Corneal transplant rejection may also take the form of subepithelial infiltrates (Fig 16-13). When seen alone, they may cause no symptoms. It is not known whether these lymphocytic

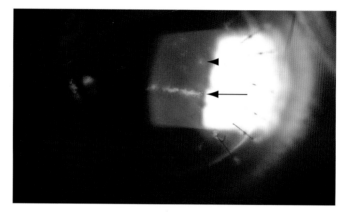

Figure 16-12   An epithelial rejection line *(arrow)* with subepithelial infiltrates *(arrowhead)* after PK. *(Courtesy of Robert W. Weisenthal, MD.)*

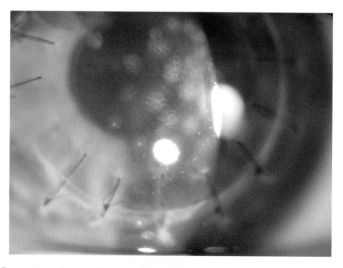

Figure 16-13   Corneal graft rejection manifested by subepithelial infiltrates. *(Courtesy of Charles S. Bouchard, MD.)*

cells are directed at donor keratocytes or at donor epithelial cells. A cellular anterior chamber reaction may also accompany this form of rejection. Easily missed on cursory examination, subepithelial infiltrates can best be seen with broad, tangential light. They resemble infiltrates of adenoviral keratitis. Subepithelial graft rejection leaves no sequelae if treated, but it may presage the more severe endothelial graft rejection.

Stromal rejection

Isolated stromal rejection is not common but can be seen as stromal infiltrates, neovascularization, or typically noninfiltrative keratolysis within the graft–host interface not extending into the peripheral recipient stroma. In very aggressive severe or prolonged bouts of graft rejection, the stroma can become necrotic.

Endothelial rejection

The most common form of graft rejection is endothelial rejection, with reported rates of 8%–37%. It is also the most serious form of corneal transplant rejection, because endothelial cells destroyed by the host response can be replaced only by a regraft. Inflammatory precipitates are seen on the endothelial surface in fine precipitates, in random clumps, or in linear form under an area of corneal edema (Khodadoust line; Fig 16-14). Inflammatory cells are usually seen in the anterior chamber as well. As endothelial function is lost, the corneal stroma thickens and the epithelium becomes edematous. Patients have symptoms related to inflammation and corneal edema, such as photophobia, redness, irritation, halos around lights, and fogginess of vision.

Treatment

Frequent administration of corticosteroid eyedrops is the mainstay of therapy for corneal allograft rejection. Either dexamethasone 0.1% or prednisolone 1.0% eyedrops are used as often as every 15 minutes to 2 hours, depending on the severity of the episode. Although topical corticosteroid ointments may be used on occasion, their bioavailability is not as beneficial as that of frequently applied eyedrops.

Corticosteroids may be given by periocular injection (triamcinolone acetonide 40 mg) for severe rejection episodes or noncompliant patients. In particularly fulminant cases,

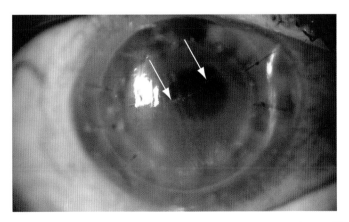

Figure 16-14   Endothelial graft rejection with stromal and epithelial edema. Note the Khodadoust line *(arrows). (Courtesy of Robert W. Weisenthal, MD.)*

systemic corticosteroids may be administered either orally (40–60 mg per day tapered as the graft rejection responds) or intravenously (125–500 mg methylprednisolone as a 1-time dose).

Prevention

A number of practices will minimize or reduce rejection. Attention to surgical techniques to avoid the peripheral cornea and ensure proper graft–host junction alignment will minimize rejection, for example, as will early attention to loosening sutures and infections. Chronic topical corticosteroids or immunosuppressing agents such as cyclosporine may reduce episodes of rejection as well. In high-risk cases, the use of various immunosuppressing agents, including oral cyclosporine, tacrolimus, and CellCept, have been reported, but these require very careful follow-up because of the narrow therapeutic index of these medications. Topical tacrolimus has also been advocated in high-risk patients.

Bahar I, Kaiserman I, Srinivasan S, Ya-Ping J, Slomovic AR, Rootman DS. Comparison of three different techniques of corneal transplantation for keratoconus. *Am J Ophthal.* 2008;146(6):905–912.

Dhaliwal JS, Mason BF, Kaufman SC. Long-term use of topical tacrolimus (FK506) in high-risk penetrating keratoplasty. *Cornea.* 2008;27(4):488–493.

Krachmer JH, Mannis MJ, Holland EJ, eds. *Cornea.* 2nd ed. Vol 2. Part IX: Penetrating Keratoplasty. Philadelphia: Elsevier/Mosby; 2005:1413–1666.

Pediatric Corneal Transplantation

Corneal transplantation in infants and children presents special challenges. The issues involved in preoperative evaluation and anesthesia concerns are summarized by Maxwell. Improvements in pediatric anesthesia and the recognition that development of amblyopia is a major impediment to useful vision have led to PK being performed in neonates as early as 2 weeks after birth. Increased understanding of the special problems associated with pediatric grafts and advances in surgical methods have improved the outlook for corneal transplants in this group. However, the prognosis in pediatric transplantation is still guarded and, in many cases, dependent on the extent of coexisting ocular abnormalities. For example, the most common indication for pediatric keratoplasty is Peters anomaly. In type 1 disease, with a central corneal opacity and a normal anterior segment, the survival rate for a clear graft ranges from 48% to 67%. In type 2 disease, characterized by adhesions among the cornea, iris, and lens; corneal neovascularization; glaucoma; cataract; and corneal staphyloma, more extensive surgery is required. Unsurprisingly, the survival rate of the transplant decreases to 0%–22%. The probability of a repeat graft surviving for 3 years is less than 10%.

In addition, the success of the procedure is very dependent on the dedication of the family to follow a rigorous postoperative regimen, including repeat examinations under anesthesia and compliance with medications. Postoperative glaucoma, strabismus, self-induced trauma, and immune rejection are extremely common. Prior to surgery, the physician must reserve time to discuss with the family the many difficult issues associated with surgery, including significant risks, guarded prognosis, high costs, loss of time from

Table 16-3 Guidelines for Suture Removal in Pediatric Corneal Transplants

Age of Child	Timing of Suture Removal
6–9 months	Approximately 5 weeks postoperatively
12–24 months	6–8 weeks postoperatively
2–3 years	8–12 weeks postoperatively
4–6 years	4 months postoperatively
10 years until teens	6 months postoperatively
Teenage	Approximately 9 months postoperatively

work (with associated loss of income), the extensive ongoing care required by the child, disruption of home life, and less time to attend to other dependents.

Corneal grafting in children under the age of 2 is associated with rapid neovascularization, especially along the sutures. As the wound heals, erosions may occur along the sutures, leading to eye rubbing, epithelial defects, vascularization, and mucus accumulation. Suture erosion has been reported to occur as early as 2 weeks postoperatively in infants, which necessitates suture removal.

In general, suture removal is best performed in the operating room for pediatric cases. Table 16-3 lists guidelines for the timing of suture removal. Also, it must be stressed that until all sutures are removed in infants or young children, frequent examinations are required.

Early fitting with a contact lens (as early as the time of PK) and ocular occlusive therapy are necessary to stem development of amblyopia in children with monocular aphakia.

As lamellar surgery has become more popular in the adult population, DALK may be an option for certain pediatric patients with stromal scarring without any other corneal pathology. If the disease is primarily endothelial, then EK may be a good alternative in the appropriate patient. Some surgeons favor the use of a keratoprosthesis in pediatric patients with previous graft failures, multiple surgeries, or inflamed eyes.

Botelho PJ, Congdon NG, Handa JT, Apek EK. Keratoprosthesis in high-risk pediatric corneal transplantation: first 2 cases. *Arch Ophthalmol.* 2006;124(9):1356–1357.

Dana MR, Schaumberg DA, Moyes AL, Gomes JA. Corneal transplantation in children with Peters anomaly and mesenchymal dysgenesis. Multicenter Pediatric Keratoplasty Study. *Ophthalmology.* 1997;104(10):1580–1586.

Maxwell, G. Age-associated issues in preoperative evaluation, testing, and planning: pediatrics. *Anesthesiol Clin North America.* 2004;22:27–43.

Yang LL, Lambert SR, Lynn MJ, Stulting RD. Long-term results of corneal graft survival in infants and children with Peters anomaly. *Ophthalmology.* 1999;106(4):833–848.

Corneal Autograft Procedures

The greatest advantage of a corneal autograft is the elimination of allograft rejection. Although cases with clinical circumstances appropriate for autograft are uncommon, an astute ophthalmologist who recognizes the possibility of a successful autograft can spare a patient the risk of long-term topical corticosteroid use and the necessity of lifelong vigilance against rejection.

Rotational Autograft

A rotational autograft can be used to reposition a localized corneal scar that involves the pupillary axis. By making an eccentric trephination and rotating the host button prior to resuturing, the surgeon can place a paracentral zone of clear cornea in the pupillary axis. The procedure is particularly useful in children, who have a poorer prognosis for PK, and in areas with tissue scarcity. Graft edema can still be a problem, because both the preexisting disease or scar and the rotational procedure usually cause endothelial cell loss. Residual postoperative astigmatism is also a problem because of the eccentric location of the graft. Wound leaks occur frequently.

Bourne WM, Brubaker RF. A method for ipsilateral rotational autokeratoplasty. *Ophthalmology*. 1978;85(12):1312–1316.

Murthy S, Bansal AK, Sridhar MS, Rao GN. Ipsilateral rotational autokeratoplasty: an alternative to penetrating keratoplasty in nonprogressive central corneal scars. *Cornea*. 2001;20(5): 455–457.

Contralateral Autograft

A contralateral autograft is reserved for patients who have in 1 eye a corneal opacity with a favorable prognosis for visual recovery and in the other eye both a clear cornea and severe dysfunction of the afferent system (eg, retinal detachment, severe amblyopia). The clear cornea is transplanted to the first eye, and the cornea from the second eye is replaced either with the diseased cornea from the first eye or with an allograft, or the eye is eviscerated or enucleated. Such bilateral grafting carries the risk of bilateral endophthalmitis.

Keratoprosthesis

Some patients have an extremely guarded prognosis for corneal transplantation due to a history of multiple graft failures or associated ocular surface disease, as seen with chronic bilateral inflammation from Stevens-Johnson syndrome or pemphigoid. These patients may be good candidates for a synthetic keratoprosthesis. Claes Dohlman, a pioneer in the development of the keratoprosthesis, divides these high-risk patients into 2 groups: those with a good blink and wet eye and those with significant conjunctival scarring, dry eye, and exposure. In the first group of patients, the Boston Keratoprosthesis (KPro) Type I (Massachusetts Eye and Ear Infirmary, Boston), made of medical-grade polymethylmethacrylate, works well (Fig 16-15). Another option is the AlphaCor keratoprosthesis (Addition Technology, Sunnyvale, CA).

The prognosis with a keratoprosthesis has improved dramatically due to innovations in the design of keratoprostheses and a better understanding of the postoperative management of these patients. The use of a soft contact lens and long-term prophylactic antibiotics have reduced the incidence of infection and breakdown of tissue around the keratoprosthesis. For patients with end-stage dry eye, the Boston Type II KPro is an excellent alternative. Other types of keratoprostheses are available for these high-risk patients, such as the TKPro, which uses tibia bone tissue, and the osteo-odonto-keratoprosthesis (OOKP), which uses dentine and alveolar bone tissue.

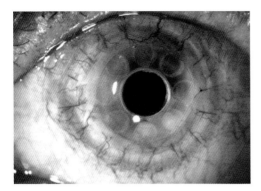

Figure 16-15 Boston keratoprosthesis. *(Courtesy of James J. Reidy, MD.)*

The most common complications associated with keratoprosthesis implantation include necrosis of tissue around the synthetic device, postoperative inflammation producing retroprosthesis membranes, vitreous opacities, retinal detachment, and macular edema. There is also the risk of significant glaucoma and infection. However, in general, the success rate with keratoprostheses has improved significantly due to the evolution in design of the synthetic devices and better patient care postoperatively.

Dohlman CH, Barnes S, Ma J. Keratoprosthesis. In: Krachmer JH, Mannis MJ, Holland EJ, eds. *Cornea.* 2nd ed. Vol 2. Philadelphia: Elsevier/Mosby; 2005:1719–1728.

Hille K, Hille A, Ruprecht KW. Medium term results in keratoprostheses with biocompatible and biological haptic. *Graefes Arch Clin Exp Ophthalmol.* 2006;244(6):696–704.

Nouri M, Terada H, Alfonso EC, Foster CS, Durand ML, Dohlman CH. Endophthalmitis after keratoprosthesis: incidence, bacterial causes, and risk factors. *Arch Ophthalmol.* 2001;119(4):484–489.

Lamellar Keratoplasty

With advances in instrumentation and techniques, the selective removal of corneal tissue with *lamellar keratoplasty (LK)* has become a much more popular procedure. The general ophthalmologist should be familiar with the special indications and limitations of the major techniques of LK, including SALK, DALK, and EK.

Anterior Lamellar Transplantation

Lamellar corneal grafting may be indicated in patients who present with opacities or loss of tissue that, for the most part, does not involve the full thickness of the cornea (Fig 16-16). These conditions include

- superficial stromal dystrophies and degenerations (eg, Reis-Bücklers dystrophy, Salzmann nodular degeneration, band keratopathy)
- superficial corneal scars
- multiple recurrent pterygium
- corneal thinning (eg, Terrien marginal degeneration, descemetocele formation, pellucid marginal degeneration)

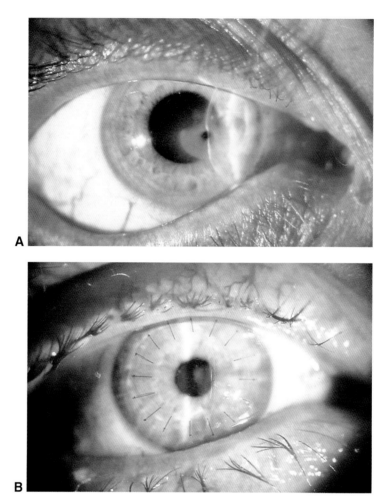

Figure 16-16 **A,** Descemetocele in a patient with rheumatoid arthritis. **B,** Same patient after lamellar keratoplasty.

- superficial corneal tumors
- congenital lesions (eg, dermoid)
- corneal perforations that are not amenable to resuturing or that occur in patients with ocular surface disease (eg, keratoconjunctivitis sicca)
- keratoconus
- selective infections, including acanthamoeba

Advantages

LK has the following advantages over PK:

- minimal requirements for donor material (as preservation of endothelium is not mandatory)

- reduced risk of entry into the anterior chamber (avoids risks of glaucoma, cataract, retinal detachment, cystoid macular edema, expulsive hemorrhage, and endophthalmitis)
- shorter wound healing time and convalescence
- reduced incidence of allograft rejection and, consequently, decreased need for topical corticosteroids

LK is less risky than PK in patients who have ocular surface disease, show poor compliance with medical instructions, or experience difficulty in obtaining frequent follow-up.

Disadvantages

Anterior LK does not replace damaged endothelium, which severely restricts its indications. The procedure is technically more difficult than PK and more time-demanding, and it may cause opacification and vascularization of the interface, which may limit visual function.

Surgical Technique

Superficial anterior lamellar keratoplasty

SALK is most commonly performed in 2 stages. In the initial procedure, a lamellar flap that encompasses the corneal pathology is created using a microkeratome. The flap is lifted to ensure that the underlying stroma is clear and then replaced. After a 4–6-week interval that allows the flap to stabilize and partially adhere, the second stage is performed. A trephine is centered over the pupil and used to incise the previously made flap to a depth slightly below the initial lamellar dissection, ideally leaving a 1-mm flap rim. A blunt spatula is gently introduced at the plane of the lamellar flap, and the abnormal tissue is separated and lifted off. The donor tissue is then prepared using an artificial anterior chamber and a microkeratome with the same thickness head as in the initial procedure. The superficial donor disk remains on the microkeratome and is transferred to a cutting block. A trephine of the same or slightly oversized (0.25 mm) diameter is used to excise the tissue. The donor disk is then transferred to the host bed and, if there is a good match, the donor tissue may adhere spontaneously without sutures, although several 10-0 nylon cardinal anchoring sutures can be used to ensure proper alignment. To avoid the creation of striae and irregular astigmatism, care must be taken not to suture too tightly. A bandage lens can also be placed to facilitate adherence. Using a 2-stage approach, the diameter of the host bed can be matched precisely with the diameter of the donor tissue with nice vertical incisions from trephination.

The femtosecond laser may also be used to perform the lamellar dissections of both the host and donor tissue, which may allow better matching of the thickness and diameter of the resection, in a 1-stage procedure.

Deep anterior lamellar keratoplasty

In DALK, the objective is to remove the abnormal stromal tissue without inducing scarring or interface haze. The Anwar big-bubble technique is the most popular method for consistently exposing Descemet's membrane to provide the best interface over the pupillary zone.

Initially, a disposable or suction trephine is used to make an approximate 300-μm-depth incision. The anterior stromal tissue is excised, debulking the corneal scarring and allowing better exposure for the remainder of the procedure. The trephine incision is then slightly deepened with a sharp blade. A 27-gauge needle on a 5-cc syringe is bent at a 60° angle, approximately 3 mm from the tip, bevel facing down. The needle is inserted deep into the groove and advanced for 2–3 mm parallel to the surface of the cornea to avoid perforation of Descemet's membrane. The air is then forcefully injected, producing a white and opaque stroma. The air enters the pre-Descemet's plane, causing the sudden appearance of a big air bubble outlined by a circular white band.

A limbal paracentesis is made to drain aqueous from the eye in order to reduce the pressure and help prevent perforation of the cornea while exposing Descemet's membrane. The anterior wall of the bubble is then entered with a sharp 15° blade to create a 1-mm opening. Once incised, the bubble collapses; some surgeons then inject viscoelastic into the collapsed bubble to help with the meticulous dissection. A spatula is used to enter the pre-Descemet's plane and advanced to the 6 o'clock position. When the spatula is lifted anteriorly, the stroma on the top of the spatula is incised using a sharp blade. As the stroma is severed, Descemet's membrane is exposed. To improve visualization, air may be injected into the anterior chamber, highlighting Descemet's membrane. A similar maneuver is performed in the opposite direction. A 0.12 forceps and blunt-pointed Vannas scissors are used to fashion 2 long perpendicular incisions, creating 4 quadrants of residual stroma; then each quadrant is excised, baring Descemet's membrane.

Only after recipient bed preparation is completed is the donor tissue prepared because inadvertent entry into the anterior chamber necessitates conversion to a full-thickness PK. In the early learning curve stages, such inadvertent entry is not infrequent.

The donor tissue is prepared by punching an appropriate-sized button with a trephine. Descemet's membrane is teased off the donor graft with a 0.12 forceps or Weck-Cel sponge and then sutured into position using 10-0 nylon in a running or interrupted fashion.

Postoperative Care and Complications

Opacification and vascularization of the interface

Meticulous irrigation and cleaning of the lamellar bed at the time of surgery may reduce opacification and vascularization, which can occur despite corticosteroid therapy. Postoperatively, best-corrected visual acuity is usually limited to 20/40 or worse.

Allograft rejection

Because the endothelium is not transplanted, endothelial rejection cannot take place. Epithelial rejection, subepithelial infiltrates, and stromal rejection occasionally occur, but they respond to corticosteroid therapy. If graft edema occurs, another cause must be sought for endothelial dysfunction.

Inflammatory necrosis of the graft

Although inflammatory necrosis of the graft has previously been described as an allograft reaction, no immunohistopathologic evidence has confirmed this, and recent series have not demonstrated this phenomenon. The mechanism probably relates to the preexisting corneal disease. Prognosis for retention of a clear graft is poor despite corticosteroid therapy.

Anwar M, Teichmann KD. Big-bubble technique to bare Descemet's membrane in anterior lamellar keratoplasty. *J Cataract Refract Surg.* 2002;28(3):398–403.

Anwar M, Teichmann KD. Deep lamellar keratoplasty: surgical techniques for anterior lamellar keratoplasty with and without baring of Descemet's membrane. *Cornea.* 2002;21(4): 374–383.

Gorovoy MS. Advances in lamellar corneal surgery. *Focal Points: Clinical Modules for Ophthalmologists.* San Francisco: American Academy of Ophthalmology; 2008, module 4.

John T. *Surgical Techniques in Anterior and Posterior Lamellar Keratoplasty.* New Delhi, India: Jaypee Brothers Medical Publishers; 2006:L1–L687.

Descemet Stripping Automated Endothelial Keratoplasty

Gerrit Melles in Holland introduced the technique of posterior endothelial lamellar keratoplasty in 1998. Since then, significant modifications in surgical technique have led to a new procedure called *Descemet stripping automated endothelial keratoplasty (DSAEK)* that has reduced the learning curve for surgeons and improved the outcome for patients. In this procedure, Descemet's membrane and endothelium are stripped in the host eye (descemetorhexis), producing a smooth posterior stromal bed in the host. Then an automated microkeratome is used to prepare the donor tissue, producing a smoother stromal bed and potentially less irregularity in the graft–host interface.

DSAEK is now the procedure of choice for endothelial dysfunction, including Fuchs corneal dystrophy, pseudophakic bullous keratopathy (PBK), and repeat corneal grafts due to endothelial cell failure. It has also been advocated for the treatment of iridocorneal endothelial syndrome (ICE) and posterior polymorphous dystrophy (PPMD) in the absence of visually significant corneal scarring.

Gorovoy MS. Descemet-stripping automated endothelial keratoplasty. *Cornea.* 2006;25(8): 886–889.

Melles GR, Eggink FA, Lander F, et al. A surgical technique for posterior lamellar keratoplasty. *Cornea.* 1998;17(6):618–626.

Melles GR, Wijdh RH, Nieuwendaal CP. A technique to excise the Descemet membrane from a recipient cornea (descemetorhexis). *Cornea.* 2004;23(3):286–288.

Price FW Jr, Price MO. Descemet's stripping with endothelial keratoplasty in 200 eyes: early challenges and techniques to enhance donor adherence. *J Cataract Refract Surg.* 2006;32(3): 411–418.

Advantages

DSAEK has the following advantages over PK:

- better globe integrity and stability with a scleral or clear corneal incision, as compared to a full-thickness central corneal incision
- elimination of corneal suture–related problems
- increased accuracy in IOL power calculations when combined with cataract extraction, although the shape of the lenticule in DSAEK may produce hyperopic shift

- less induced postoperative corneal astigmatism
- more rapid visual rehabilitation with less concern for ocular surface disorders

Disadvantages

In DSAEK, the best spectacle-corrected visual acuity may not be 20/20, often ranging between 20/25 and 20/40. This may be from optical degradation associated with the graft–host lamellar interface or persistent stromal haze. Evaluation of patients with Fuchs corneal dystrophy who underwent DSAEK revealed that corneal light scatter was still increased as compared to the norm 6 months after the procedure and correlated with the age of the recipient at the time of surgery. Also, anterior lamellar keratoplasty or corneal epithelial debridement may be required for full visual rehabilitation in the presence of anterior basement membrane dystrophy or subepithelial fibrosis. Long- term graft survival is unknown.

Patel SV, Baratz KH, Hodge DO, Maguire LJ, McLaren JW. The effect of corneal light scatter on vision after Descemet stripping with endothelial keratoplasty. *Arch Ophthalmol.* 2009; 127(2):153–160.

DSAEK Surgical Technique

Preparation of donor tissue

Corneal surgeons have the option of obtaining precut tissue from an eye bank or preparing the tissue in the operating room using an automated microkeratome and artificial anterior chamber. Recent studies have shown that there is no clinical difference in outcomes between tissue obtained from the eye banks and tissue prepared in the operating room.

To prepare the donor tissue using an automated microkeratome for the lamellar dissection, the tissue is placed on an artificial anterior chamber. The epithelium may be removed prior to the lamellar dissection with a Weck-Cel sponge. The corneal thickness can be measured using a pachometer to select the appropriate size microkeratome head, 250 μm to 350 μm, with a goal of leaving approximately 100–150 μm of posterior stroma with Descemet's membrane and endothelium. The donor corneoscleral rim is then pressurized with balanced salt solution (BSS), optisol storage medium, or viscoelastic to ensure a deep and smooth dissection. After the lamellar dissection is performed, the corneal stroma may be marked with an outline of the area of the trephine cut to allow proper centration of the tissue. Gentian violet has been shown to produce endothelial toxicity, so the surgeon must be careful to limit the amount of ink used.

The donor tissue, with or without the anterior stromal free cap, is then placed in a concave well. A trephine is used to create a disk-shaped lamella of donor tissue from 8 to 9 mm in diameter.

Chen ES, Terry MA, Shamie N, Hoar KL, Friend DJ. Precut tissue in Descemet's stripping automated endothelial keratoplasty: donor characteristics and early postoperative complications. *Ophthalmology.* 2008;115(3):497–502.

Price MO, Baig KM, Brubaker JW, Price FW Jr. Randomized prospective comparison of precut vs. surgeon-dissected grafts for Descemet stripping automated endothelial keratoplasty. *Am J Ophthalmol.* 2008;146(1):36–41.

Terry MA, Shamie N, Chen ES, Phillips PM, Hoar KL, Friend DJ. Precut tissue for Descemet's stripping automated endothelial keratoplasty: vision, astigmatism, and endothelial survival. *Ophthalmology.* 2009;116(2):248–256.

Surgical technique for recipient eye

Some surgeons perform DSAEK under topical anesthesia; however, many prefer a retrobulbar block. The surgeon decides whether the incision will be limbal, clear corneal, or scleral. The length of the incision varies from 3 to 6 mm. Several studies using vital dye staining of the endothelium after insertion of the donor corneal tissue have shown that placing tissue through a 3-mm incision causes 2–4 times more acute damage to the endothelium than does using a 5-mm incision, regardless of the technique used to place the tissue. However, new methods of tissue insertion may eliminate the trauma associated with the use of a smaller incision size.

If the surgeon prefers, Descemet's membrane can be stripped (Fig 16-17A) using a variety of instruments, including a Sinskey hook (BD Visitec, Franklin Lakes, NJ), a specially designed Descemet stripper, or an irrigation–aspiration handpiece. The stripping can be performed under viscoelastic, air, or irrigation with BSS. Some surgeons feel that it is necessary to strip Descemet's membrane only in Fuchs dystrophy and not to do so in patients with failed PK or pseudophakic bullous keratopathy. Whether the retention of Descemet's membrane in these cases may predispose to dislocation of the graft is controversial.

Initially, the primary method for graft insertion was to fold the donor tissue into a 60/40 "taco" shape that required gently unfolding within the anterior chamber. However, laboratory studies using vital dye staining, specular microscopy, and scanning electron microscopy have demonstrated a 30%–40% endothelial loss with this technique. As a result, some excellent newer methods have been developed that are less traumatic to the endothelium. These include the Busin glide; Tan EndoGlide; modified lens cartridges, using an IOL sheet glide to push or pull the tissue into place; Neusidl injector; and a suture pull-through technique (Fig 16-17B). The object is to insert the tissue in a single plane, stromal side up, without having the endothelial cells touch each other, while also maintaining proper orientation of the tissue and reducing the need for intraocular manipulation to unfold it.

After tissue placement in the anterior chamber, air is injected to appose the donor graft against the host stromal bed (Fig 16-17C). It is not clear what factors are responsible for tissue adherence, but it is probably a combination of physical and physiologic factors. Intraoperative maneuvers to facilitate adhesion include scraping the peripheral recipient bed, draining fluid from the interface through vertical midperipheral vent incisions, sweeping the surface of the cornea with a roller, and presoaking the donor tissue in BSS. The required duration and pressure of the air fill to ensure adherence of the tissue is controversial. Techniques vary from a full air fill in the operating room for 10 minutes followed by release and replacement with a partial air fill; a full air fill for up to 1 hour, with subsequent partial release at a slit lamp; and a complete air fill overnight, combined with an inferior iridectomy or use of acetazolamide (Diamox).

If the air is removed at the slit lamp within the first hour, it must be released slowly to prevent sudden and dramatic loss of pressure in the eye. Patients are then advised to

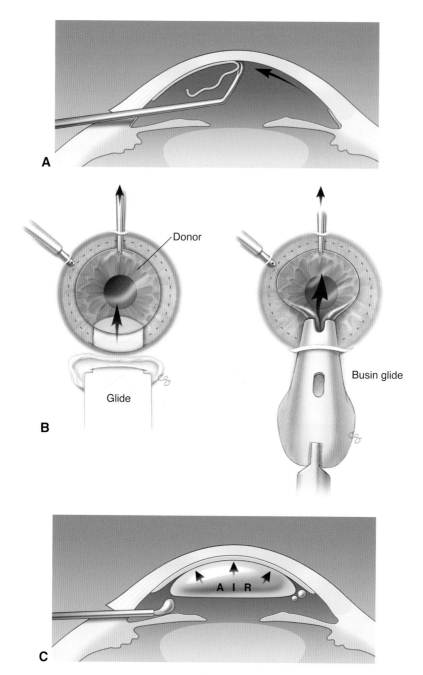

Figure 16-17 A, Stripping Descemet's membrane. **B,** Glide insertion of donor tissue *(left);* Busin glide insertion of donor tissue *(right).* **C,** Air is tamponaded to appose the donor graft to the host stromal bed. *(Illustration by Christine Gralapp.)*

lie on their back for the first 24 hours to tamponade the donor graft against the posterior stroma with the retained air bubble, although some surgeons have relaxed the positioning requirements. Placement of an inferior anchoring suture may prevent graft dislocation while minimizing the need for the patient to remain supine.

Busin M, Bhatt PR, Scorcia V. A modified technique for Descemet membrane stripping automated endothelial keratoplasty to minimize endothelial cell loss. *Arch Ophthalmol.* 2008; 126(8):1133–1137.

Mehta JS, Por YM, Beuerman RW, Tan DT. Glide insertion technique for donor cornea lenticule during Descemet's stripping automated endothelial keratoplasty. *J Cataract Refract Surg.* 2007;33(11):1846–1850.

Mehta JS, Por YM, Poh R, Beuerman RW, Tan D. Comparison of donor insertion techniques for Descemet stripping automated endothelial keratoplasty. *Arch Ophthalmol.* 2008;126(10): 1383–1388.

Terry MA, Saad HA, Shamie N, et al. Endothelial keratoplasty: the influence of insertion techniques and incision size on donor endothelial survival. *Cornea.* 2009;28(1):24–31.

Intraoperative complications

Complications that can occur during DSAEK include the following:

- poor microkeratome dissection, precluding use of the donor tissue
- incomplete removal of Descemet's tissue
- poor centration of the donor tissue during trephination, leading to a thick edge and possibly retained epithelial cells that could be implanted into the anterior chamber
- intraocular hyphema and blood in the interface (Fig 16-18)
- excessive manipulation of the donor tissue, risking endothelial cell loss
- posterior dislocation of the donor tissue
- disorientation during placement of the donor tissue, leading to placement of the endothelium against the host stromal cornea

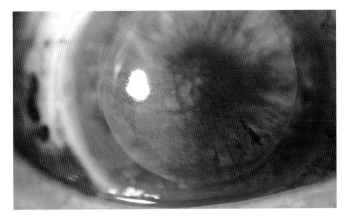

Figure 16-18 Hemorrhage in the interface after DSAEK. *(Courtesy of Robert W. Weisenthal, MD.)*

Postoperative care and complications

During this discussion the emphasis will be on issues specific to DSAEK. Problems common to PK and DSAEK, such as graft rejection, were covered earlier in the chapter.

In a typical postoperative follow-up, the patient is seen on postoperative day 1 to ensure that the lenticule is in good position and that no fluid is in the interface. Typically, there is about a 40% air bubble (Fig 16-19). Over a 4-day period, the air bubble absorbs and the cornea begins to clear. After 6 months, it is difficult to visualize the interface centrally (Fig 16-20A, B).

The postoperative medication regimen is similar to that of PK, although some surgeons recommend maintaining the patient on topical corticosteroids for a longer period of time.

Chen ES, Terry MA, Shamie N, Hoar KL, Friend DJ. Descemet-stripping automated endothelial keratoplasty: six-month results in a prospective study of 100 eyes. *Cornea.* 2008;27(5): 514–520.

Suh LH, Yoo SH, Deobhakta A, et al. Complications of Descemet's stripping with automated endothelial keratoplasty: survey of 118 eyes at one institute. *Ophthalmology.* 2008;115(9): 1517–1524.

Pupillary block Inadequate release of the intraoperative air fill may lead to pupillary block from migration of the air behind the iris, thus closing the angle. The acute rise in pressure produces pain and can potentially exacerbate underlying glaucoma. Pupillary dilation beyond the retained air bubble for the first 24 hours may reduce the incidence of this complication. An inferior iridectomy may also prevent pupillary block.

Dislocation of the donor graft See Figure 16-21. The rate of dislocation of the donor graft varies greatly in reported case series, from 4% with experienced surgeons up to 35%–40% with novice surgeons (those who have had fewer than 10 cases). Dislocation of the donor graft occurs primarily within the first 24 hours, although occasionally inadvertent trauma from eye rubbing or a sudden blow to the eye has caused the donor disk to be displaced at a later time.

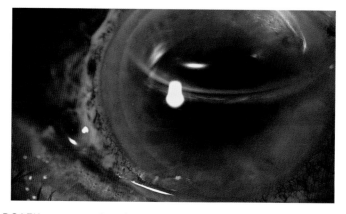

Figure 16-19 DSAEK postoperative day 1 showing a residual air bubble. *(Courtesy of Robert W. Weisenthal, MD.)*

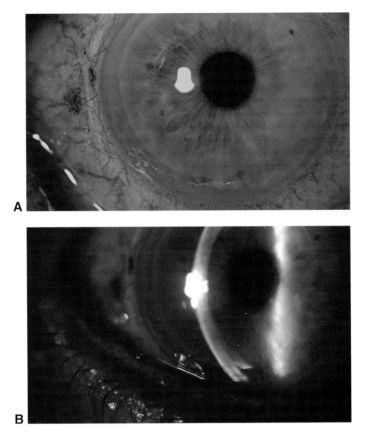

Figure 16-20 **A,** Slit-lamp picture of healed DSAEK. **B,** Side illumination. *(Courtesy of Robert W. Weisenthal, MD.)*

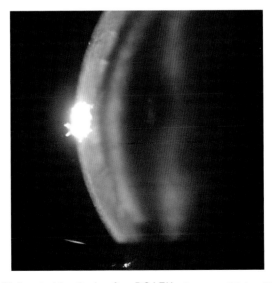

Figure 16-21 Dislocated lenticule after DSAEK. *(Courtesy of Robert W. Weisenthal, MD.)*

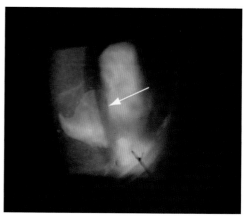

Figure 16-22 Epithelial ingrowth in the interface after DSAEK *(arrow)*. *(Courtesy of Robert W. Weisenthal, MD.)*

Epithelial ingrowth   Epithelial ingrowth may first be seen as a white deposit within the interface that can be relatively stable and asymptomatic (Fig 16-22). In rare cases, epithelial ingrowth may lead to graft failure that is missed on clinical examination but recognized on histologic examination of the tissue after a second procedure. The source of the ingrowth may be host surface epithelial cells implanted within the eye during placement of the donor tissue or donor epithelial cells inadvertently left in place and implanted following eccentric trephination beyond the microkeratome dissection. In early reports, the prognosis with epithelial ingrowth appears to be similar to that seen with epithelial seeding under the lamellar LASIK flap—that is, often limited and asymptomatic—as compared with the progressive and devastating course that is seen with the intraocular epithelial downgrowth associated with intracapsular cataract extraction or corneal transplantation. In reported cases of graft failure where epithelial ingrowth was noted only after histopathologic examination of the removed lenticule, the second procedures have done well, without recurrence of the ingrowth.

Koenig SB, Covert DJ. Epithelial ingrowth after Descemet-stripping automated endothelial keratoplasty. *Cornea.* 2008;27(6):727–729.

Primary graft failure   The primary failure rate seen in published reports varies between 3% and 12%, with higher numbers associated with surgeons in the early stages of the learning curve and lower numbers associated with more experienced surgeons. The improved results probably reflect better surgical technique leading to less endothelial trauma as a consequence of less tissue manipulation and a lower rate of dislocations.

Endothelial cell loss   Additional manipulation of tissue risks endothelial cell loss from microkeratome dissection, placement and orientation of the tissue within the anterior chamber, air tamponade, and additional exposure of the donor graft to air in rebubbling. In 2 different studies, mean endothelial cell loss at 6 months was 34%. However, in a 6-month to 3-year follow-up by Price and colleagues, further cell loss was only 8%, which compared favorably to the CDS PK study that showed 42% cell loss between 6 months and 3 years. Price attributed these results to the increased diameter of the DSAEK grafts (8.75 to 9 mm), which provided more surface area and thus more transplanted endothelial cells than the traditional PK; to removal of a smaller area of endothelium on the recipient, which allowed for overlap of the donor tissue onto host endothelium; and to use of corticosteroids for a longer duration postoperatively. Long-term follow-up is necessary to confirm these results.

Additional complications associated with DSAEK are similar to those seen in PK, including suprachoroidal hemorrhage, retinal detachment, cystoid macular edema, and graft rejection. The rate of graft rejection may be lower in DSAEK than in PK due to the absence of sutures, which reduces vascularization and reduces the incidence of both late suture erosion inciting inflammation and fewer donor epithelial cells stimulating an immune reaction. Long-term follow-up is necessary to confirm this observation.

Cornea Donor Study Investigator Group; Lass JH, Gal RL, Dontchev M, et al. Donor age and corneal endothelial cell loss 5 years after successful corneal transplantation. Specular microscopy ancillary study results. *Ophthalmology.* 2008;115(4):627–632.

Price FW Jr, Price MO. Does endothelial cell survival differ between DSEK and standard PK? *Ophthalmology.* 2009;116(3):367–368.

Price MO, Jordan CS, Moore G, Price FW Jr. Graft rejection episodes after Descemet stripping with endothelial keratoplasty: part two: the statistical analysis of probability and risk factors. *Br J Ophthalmol.* 2009;93(3):391–395.

Terry MA, Chen ES, Shamie N, Hoar KL, Friend DJ. Endothelial cell loss after Descemet's stripping endothelial keratoplasty in a large prospective series. *Ophthalmology.* 2008;115(3): 488–496.

Descemet's Membrane Endothelial Keratoplasty

Another modification in EK, recently suggested by Melles, is to transplant only donor Descemet's membrane and endothelial cells and not to include stromal tissue, as in DSAEK. This promising procedure has been named *Descemet's membrane endothelial keratoplasty (DMEK).* At the time of this publication, there are only early reports on DMEK and its possible advantages and disadvantages.

Ham L, van der Wees J, Melles GR. Causes of primary donor failure in Descemet membrane endothelial keratoplasty. *Am J Ophthalmol.* 2008:145(4):639–644.

Melles GR, Ong TS, Ververs B, van der Wees J. Preliminary clinical results of Descemet membrane endothelial keratoplasty. *Am J Ophthalmol.* 2008;145(2):222–227.

Basic Texts

External Disease and Cornea

Albert DM, Miller J, Azar D, Blodi B, eds. *Albert & Jakobiec's Principles and Practice of Ophthalmology.* 3rd ed. 4 vols. Philadelphia: Elsevier/Saunders; 2008.

Arffa RC, Grayson M, eds. *Grayson's Diseases of the Cornea.* 4th ed. St Louis: Mosby; 1997.

Brightbill FS, McDonnell PJ, McGhee CN, Farjo AA, Serdarevic O. *Corneal Surgery: Theory, Technique, and Tissue.* 4th ed. Philadelphia: Elsevier/Mosby; 2009.

Catania LJ. *Primary Care of the Anterior Segment.* 2nd ed. Norwalk, CT: Appleton & Lange; 1996.

Corbett M, Rosen ES, O'Brart DP. *Corneal Topography: Principles and Applications.* London: BMJ Books; 1999.

Coster DJ. *Cornea.* Fundamentals of Clinical Ophthalmology series. London: BMJ Books; 2002.

Foster CS, Azar DT, Dohlman CH, eds. *Smolin and Thoft's The Cornea: Scientific Foundations and Clinical Practice.* 4th ed. Philadelphia: Lippincott Williams & Wilkins; 2004.

Kaufman HE, Barron BA, McDonald M, eds. *The Cornea.* 2nd ed. Boston: Butterworth-Heinemann; 1998.

Krachmer JH, Mannis MJ, Holland EJ, eds. *Cornea.* 2nd ed. 2 vols. Philadelphia: Elsevier/Mosby; 2005.

Krachmer JH, Palay DA. *Cornea Color Atlas.* St Louis: Mosby; 1999.

Leibowitz HM, Waring GO III, eds. *Corneal Disorders: Clinical Diagnosis and Management.* 2nd ed. Philadelphia: Saunders; 1998.

Murray PR, Baron EJ, Jorgensen JH, et al, eds. *Manual of Clinical Microbiology.* 9th ed. 2 vols. Washington, DC: ASM Press; 2007.

Ostler HB, Ostler MW. *Diseases of the External Eye and Adnexa: A Text and Atlas.* Baltimore: Urban and Schwarzenberg; 1993.

Pepose JS, Holland GN, Wilhelmus KR, eds. *Ocular Infection and Immunity.* St Louis: Mosby; 1996.

Rapuano CJ, Luchs JI, Kim T. *Anterior Segment: The Requisites.* Requisites in Ophthalmology series. St Louis: Mosby; 2000.

Seal DV, Pleyer U, eds. *Ocular Infection: Investigation and Treatment in Practice.* 2nd ed. New York: Informa Healthcare; 2007.

Related Academy Materials

Focal Points: Clinical Modules for Ophthalmologists

Colby KA. Chemical injuries of the eye (Module 1, 2010).

Dunn SP. Iris repair: putting the pieces back together (Module 11, 2002).

Garcia-Ferrer FJ, Schwab IR. New laboratory diagnostic techniques for corneal and external diseases (Module 9, 2002).

Goins KM, Wagoner MD. Imaging the anterior segment (Module 11, 2009).

Gorovoy MS. Advances in lamellar corneal surgery (Module 4, 2008).

Heidemann, DG. Atopic and vernal keratoconjunctivitis (Module 1, 2001).

Hirst LW. Pterygium surgery (Module 3, 2009).

Koreishi AF, Karp CL. Ocular surface neoplasia (Module 1, 2007).

Mamalis N. Toxic anterior segment syndrome (TASS) (Module 10, 2009).

Mets MB, Noffke AS. Ocular infections of the external eye and cornea in children (Module 2, 2002).

Nordlund ML, Brilakis HS, Holland EJ. Surgical techniques for ocular surface reconstruction (Module 12, 2006).

Pflugfelder SC. Dry eye (Module 5, 2006).

Schultze RL, Singh GD. Neurotrophic keratitis (Module 2, 2003).

Tuli SS. Herpetic corneal infections (Module 8, 2008).

Zloty P. Diagnosis and management of fungal keratitis (Module 6, 2002).

Print Publications

Arnold AC, ed. *Basic Principles of Ophthalmic Surgery*. (2006).

Dunn JP, Langer PD, eds. *Basic Techniques of Ophthalmic Surgery*. (2009).

Parke DW II, ed. *The Profession of Ophthalmology: Practice Management, Ethics, and Advocacy*. (2005).

Rockwood EJ, ed. *ProVision: Preferred Responses in Ophthalmology*. Series 4. Self-Assessment Program, 2-vol set (2007).

Wang MX. *Corneal Dystrophies and Degenerations: A Molecular Genetics Approach* (Ophthalmology Monograph 16, 2003).

Wilson FM II, Blomquist PH, eds. *Practical Ophthalmology: A Manual for Beginning Residents*. 6th ed. (2009).

Preferred Practice Patterns

Preferred Practice Patterns are available at http://one.aao.org/CE/PracticeGuidelines/PPP.aspx.

Preferred Practice Patterns Committee, Cornea/External Disease Panel. *Bacterial Keratitis* (2008).
Preferred Practice Patterns Committee, Cornea/External Disease Panel. *Blepharitis* (2008).
Preferred Practice Patterns Committee, Cornea/External Disease Panel. *Conjunctivitis* (2008).
Preferred Practice Patterns Committee, Cornea/External Disease Panel. *Dry Eye Syndrome* (2008).

Ophthalmic Technology Assessments

Ophthalmic Technology Assessments are available at http://one.aao.org/CE/PracticeGuidelines/Ophthalmic.aspx and are published in the Academy's journal, *Ophthalmology*. Individual reprints may be ordered at http://www.aao.org/store.

Ophthalmic Technology Assessment Committee, Cornea Panel. *Confocal Microscopy* (2004; reviewed for currency 2009).
Ophthalmic Technology Assessment Committee, Cornea Panel. *Corneal Endothelial Photography* (1997; reviewed for currency 2008).
Ophthalmic Technology Assessment Committee, Cornea Panel. *Corneal Topography* (1999; reviewed for currency 2008).
Ophthalmic Technology Assessment Committee, Cornea and Anterior Segment Disorders Panel. *Descemet's Stripping Endothelial Keratoplasty: Safety and Outcomes* (2009).
Ophthalmic Technology Assessment Committee, Cornea and Anterior Segment Disorders Panel. *Safety of Overnight Orthokeratology for Myopia* (2008).

CDs /DVDs

Basic and Clinical Science Course (Sections 1–13) (DVD-ROM, 2010).
Johns KL, ed. *Eye Care Skills: Presentations for Physicians and Other Health Care Professionals*, version 3.0 (CD-ROM, 2009).

Online Materials

For Preferred Practice Patterns and Ophthalmic Technology Assessments, go to http://one.aao.org/CE/PracticeGuidelines/default.aspx.

Basic and Clinical Science Course (Sections 1–13); http://one.aao.org/CE/EducationalProducts/BCSC.aspx

Clinical Education Cases; http://one.aao.org/CE/EducationalContent/Cases.aspx

Clinical Education and Ethics Courses; http://one.aao.org/CE/EducationalContent/Courses.aspx

Focal Points modules; http://one.aao.org/CE/EducationalProducts/FocalPoints.aspx

Maintenance of Certification Exam Study Kit, MOC version 2.0 (2007); http://one.aao.org/CE/MOC/default.aspx

Maintenance of Certification Exam Study Kit, Compass version 2.0 (2008); http://one.aao.org/CE/EducationalContent/CompassExam.aspx

Price FW, Baig K, Price MO. Descemet's Stripping with Endothelial Keratoplasty (December 2008); http://one.aao.org/CE/Educational Content/Courses.aspx

Rockwood EJ. ProVision: Preferred Responses in Ophthalmology. Series 4. Self-Assessment Program, 2-vol set (2007); http://one.aao.org/CE/EducationalProducts/Provision.aspx

Wilhelmus KR, Huang AJ, Hwang DG, Parrish CM, Sutphin JE. Ocular Surface Disease (April 2006); http://one.aao.org/CE/Educational Content/Courses.aspx

---

To order any of these materials, please order online at www.aao.org/store or call the Academy's Customer Service toll-free number 866-561-8558 in the U.S. If outside the U.S., call 415-561-8540 between 8:00 AM and 5:00 PM PST.

Credit Reporting Form

Basic and Clinical Science Course, 2011–2012
Section 8

The American Academy of Ophthalmology is accredited by the Accreditation Council for Continuing Medical Education to provide continuing medical education for physicians.

The American Academy of Ophthalmology designates this enduring material for a maximum of 15 *AMA PRA Category 1 Credits™*. Physicians should claim only credit commensurate with the extent of their participation in the activity.

If you wish to claim continuing medical education credit for your study of this Section, you may claim your credit online or fill in the required forms and mail or fax them to the Academy.

To use the forms:

1. Complete the study questions and mark your answers on the Section Completion Form.
2. Complete the Section Evaluation.
3. Fill in and sign the statement below.
4. Return this page and the required forms by mail or fax to the CME Registrar (see below).

To claim credit online:

1. Log on to the Academy website (www.aao.org/cme).
2. Select Review/Claim CME.
3. Follow the instructions.

Important: These completed forms or the online claim must be received at the Academy by June 2013.

I hereby certify that I have spent _____ (up to 15) hours of study on the curriculum of this Section and that I have completed the study questions.

Signature: _____
                                                                                                    Date

Name: _____

Address: _____

City and State: _____ Zip: _____

Telephone: (_____) _____ Academy Member ID# _____
                     area code

Please return completed forms to: **Or you may fax them to:** 415-561-8575
American Academy of Ophthalmology
P.O. Box 7424
San Francisco, CA 94120-7424
Attn: CME Registrar, Customer Service

2011–2012
Section Completion Form

Basic and Clinical Science Course

Answer Sheet for Section 8

Question	Answer	Question	Answer	Question	Answer
1	a b c d	18	a b c d	35	a b c d
2	a b c d	19	a b c d	36	a b c d
3	a b c d	20	a b c d	37	a b c d
4	a b c d	21	a b c d	38	a b c d
5	a b c d	22	a b c d	39	a b c d
6	a b c d	23	a b c d	40	a b c d
7	a b c d	24	a b c d	41	a b c d
8	a b c d	25	a b c d	42	a b c d
9	a b c d	26	a b c d	43	a b c d
10	a b c d	27	a b c d	44	a b c d
11	a b c d	28	a b c d	45	a b c d
12	a b c d	29	a b c d	46	a b c d
13	a b c d	30	a b c d	47	a b c d
14	a b c d	31	a b c d	48	a b c d
15	a b c d	32	a b c d	49	a b c d
16	a b c d	33	a b c d	50	a b c d
17	a b c d	34	a b c d		

Section Evaluation

Please complete this CME questionnaire.

1. To what degree will you use knowledge from BCSC Section 8 in your practice?

   ☐ Regularly

   ☐ Sometimes

   ☐ Rarely

2. Please review the stated objectives for BCSC Section 8. How effective was the material at meeting those objectives?

   ☐ All objectives were met.

   ☐ Most objectives were met.

   ☐ Some objectives were met.

   ☐ Few or no objectives were met.

3. To what degree is BCSC Section 8 likely to have a positive impact on health outcomes of your patients?

   ☐ Extremely likely

   ☐ Highly likely

   ☐ Somewhat likely

   ☐ Not at all likely

4. After you review the stated objectives for BCSC Section 8, please let us know of any additional knowledge, skills, or information useful to your practice that were acquired but were not included in the objectives.

5. Was BCSC Section 8 free of commercial bias?

   ☐ Yes

   ☐ No

6. If you selected "No" in the previous question, please comment.

7. Please tell us what might improve the applicability of BCSC to your practice.

Study Questions

Although a concerted effort has been made to avoid ambiguity and redundancy in these questions, the authors recognize that differences of opinion may occur regarding the "best" answer. The discussions are provided to demonstrate the rationale used to derive the answer. They may also be helpful in confirming that your approach to the problem was correct or, if necessary, in fixing the principle in your memory. The Section 8 faculty would like to thank the Self-Assessment Committee for working with them to provide these study questions and discussions.

1. Phlyctenular keratoconjunctivitis is an example of which type of hypersensitivity response?
   a. type I
   b. type II
   c. type III
   d. type IV

2. Immune privilege in the cornea results in part from expression of which of the following:
   a. interleukin-8 (IL-8)
   b. multifocal choroiditis and panuveitis syndrome-1(MCP-1)
   c. Fas ligand
   d. major histocompatibility complex (MHC) class II

3. A soluble mediator of ocular inflammation in the tear film that promotes angiogenesis and vascular permeability is
   a. intercellular adhesion molecule 1 (ICAM-1)
   b. vascular endothelial growth factor (VEGF)
   c. substance P
   d. interleukin-1 (IL-1)

4. The normal conjunctiva typically contains which of the following cell types:
   a. plasma cells
   b. basophils
   c. eosinophils
   d. killer lymphocytes

5. The immunoglobulin involved in atopic keratoconjunctivitis is
   a. IgE
   b. IgA
   c. IgG
   d. IgM

6. Ligneous conjunctivitis is treated with

    a. systemic antibiotics

    b. topical antibiotics

    c. topical plasminogen

    d. topical interferon-α

7. Peripheral ulcerative keratitis (PUK), which is associated with systemic immune-mediated disease is typically caused by which of the following?

    a. type IV hypersensitivity reactions

    b. vasculitis and immune-complex deposition

    c. contact lenses

    d. staphylococcal blepharitis

8. In Mooren ulcer, which type of cells are present in increased concentration in the conjunctiva adjacent to the ulcerated area?

    a. suppressor T cells

    b. plasma cells

    c. dendritic cells

    d. mast cells

9. Which of the following ocular structures produces mucin, which contributes to the stabilization of the tear film?

    a. conjunctival epithelium

    b. tarsus

    c. meibomian glands

    d. glands of Moll

10. Which of the following layers of the cornea continues to thicken from birth to adulthood?

    a. epithelium

    b. stroma

    c. Descemet's membrane

    d. endothelium

11. The major refractive power of the eye comes from the

    a. cornea

    b. lens

    c. vitreous

    d. aqueous

12. Which of the following metabolic disorders that affect the cornea is X-linked recessive?

   a. Sanfilippo syndrome

   b. Hurler syndrome

   c. Scheie syndrome

   d. Hunter syndrome

13. Which of the following drugs is associated with corneal verticillata?

   a. metoprolol

   b. amiodarone

   c. erythromycin

   d. tetracycline

14. Prominent corneal nerves may be seen in which condition?

   a. multiple endocrine neoplasia (MEN)

   b. pulmonary adenocarcinoma

   c. lattice corneal dystrophy type I

   d. macular corneal dystrophy

15. A slit-lamp finding of corneal protrusion superior to a band of thinning in the inferior cornea describes which of the following conditions?

   a. keratoglobus

   b. keratoconus

   c. polymorphic amyloid degeneration

   d. pellucid marginal degeneration

16. In which of the following corneal disorders are recurrent corneal erosions most likely to occur?

   a. pellucid marginal degeneration

   b. macular dystrophy

   c. lattice dystrophy

   d. keratoglobus

17. Slit-lamp findings of fingerprint lines, maplike lines, and dots at the level of the corneal epithelial basement membrane are all associated with which of the following conditions?

   a. corneal thinning and protrusion

   b. polymorphic amyloid degeneration

   c. recurrent corneal erosion

   d. autosomal recessive disorder

18. Which of the following conjunctival reactions is most commonly seen with a herpes simplex virus (HSV) infection?

    a. follicular response

    b. papillary response

    c. pseudomembrane formation

    d. pyogenic granuloma formation

19. Papillary conjunctivitis is associated with which of the following conditions?

    a. herpes simplex (HSV) conjunctivitis

    b. atopic keratoconjunctivitis

    c. adult inclusion conjunctivitis

    d. molluscum conjunctivitis

20. Which examination technique uses the Placido disk?

    a. specular microscopy

    b. retinoscopy

    c. keratoscopy

    d. wavefront analysis

21. Central corneal opacity present at birth, iridocorneal adhesions, cataract, elevated IOP, and cardiac abnormalities may be associated with which of the following disorders?

    a. congenital hereditary endothelial dystrophy (CHED)

    b. congenital glaucoma

    c. Peters plus

    d. Peters anomaly

22. Corneal changes due to birth trauma typically manifest as which of the following:

    a. ruptures of Descemet's membrane

    b. breaks in Bowman layer

    c. epithelial reduplication

    d. stromal thinning

23. Which of the following is a typical corneal finding in congenital glaucoma?

    a. small corneal diameter

    b. Haab striae

    c. Vogt striae

    d. guttae

24. Which of the following would render a donor cornea unsuitable for penetrating keratoplasty?

    a. cell count of 2500 cells/mm^2

    b. negative serology for hepatitis B

    c. positive serology for cytomegalovirus (CMV)

    d. previous LASIK eye surgery

25. Corneal transplant rejection is believed to be uncommon because
    a. the cornea has immune privilege
    b. the cornea has immune processing cells in the stroma only
    c. the human body has developed tolerance to corneal tissue
    d. there are no histocompatibility antigens in the cornea

26. Which of the following characteristics of a progressive corneal infiltrate is a contraindication for corneal biopsy?
    a. located deep in the cornea
    b. unresponsive to appropriate antimicrobial therapy
    c. culture-negative on superficial scrapings
    d. atypical clinical course

27. Which technique should be avoided in pterygium excision surgery?
    a. excision with conjunctival autograft
    b. excision with sliding conjunctival flap
    c. simple excision with bare sclera
    d. excision with amniotic membrane graft

28. Which of the following is the best technique for achieving a permanent fusing of the eyelids?
    a. taping the eyelid margins
    b. injecting botulinum toxin into the eyelid
    c. suturing the eyelid margins
    d. applying cyanoacrylate adhesive to eyelid margins

29. Which of the following is an appropriate way to alleviate chronic pain associated with a postinflammatory corneal opacity in an eye with poor vision potential?
    a. performing a corneal tattooing procedure
    b. performing a conjunctival flap
    c. prescribing tinted glasses
    d. prescribing a topical anesthetic agent

30. Immediate surgical treatment is indicated for which complication following penetrating keratoplasty?
    a. choroidal detachment
    b. suture abscess
    c. primary graft failure
    d. wound leak with flat anterior chamber

31. An 83-year-old woman with prominent corneal edema and central corneal scarring in both eyes has episodic foreign-body pain OD. Her best-corrected visual acuity is finger counts at 5 feet OD and 20/100 OS. There is a slight cataract in the left eye only, and IOP is normal. Which is the best management option to restore visual function to the right eye?

    a. anterior stromal puncture

    b. epithelial debridement

    c. lamellar keratoplasty

    d. penetrating keratoplasty

32. Band keratopathy can be caused by the deposition of which of the following materials?

    a. calcium hydroxyapatite

    b. hyaline

    c. amyloid

    d. calcium hydroxide

33. Which of the following is an indication for surgery on a pterygium?

    a. induced myopia

    b. tear deficiency

    c. induced astigmatism

    d. macular degeneration

34. Which of the following is the best initial management for irregular astigmatism post-keratoplasty?

    a. lamellar keratoplasty

    b. excimer laser

    c. astigmatic keratotomies

    d. rigid gas-permeable contact lens fitting

35. Which of the following is the most serious complication associated with silicone punctal occlusion?

    a. dacryocystitis

    b. migration into the canaliculus

    c. loss of the silicone plug

    d. epiphora

36. Aqueous tear deficiency may be treated with which of the following?

    a. 0.2% brimonidine tartrate

    b. 0.15% hyaluronic acid

    c. 0.005% latanoprost

    d. 1% trifluridine

37. Common clinical findings in aqueous tear deficiency include which of the following?
    a. rapid tear-film breakup time
    b. increased tear meniscus
    c. lack of debris in the tear film
    d. increased Schirmer test

38. In order to establish a diagnosis of Sjögren syndrome, which of the following laboratory tests should be ordered?
    a. anti-Ro/Sjögren syndrome-A (SS-A) antigen
    b. p-antineutrophil cytoplasmic antibody (p-ANCA)
    c. c-antineutrophil cytoplasmic antibody (c-ANCA)
    d. erythrocyte sedimentation rate (ESR)

39. What is the most common presentation of meibomian gland dysfunction?
    a. anterior uveitis
    b. central corneal ulceration
    c. posterior eyelid margin disease
    d. anterior eyelid margin disease

40. What is the most common presentation of ocular rosacea?
    a. scleritis
    b. central corneal ulceration
    c. recurrent erosions
    d. chronic eyelid margin injection

41. A persistent epithelial defect is most commonly associated with which of the following conditions:
    a. pellucid marginal degeneration
    b. herpes zoster keratitis
    c. posterior polymorphous corneal dystrophy (PPCD)
    d. superficial punctate keratitis (SPK) of Thygeson

42. Which of the following dermatologic disorders is included in the differential diagnosis for persistent corneal epithelial defect?
    a. sebaceous cell carcinoma
    b. acne rosacea
    c. melanoma
    d. basal cell carcinoma

43. Dysfunction of the ophthalmic branch of the trigeminal ganglion may result from
    a. aneurysm
    b. pituitary adenoma
    c. myasthenia gravis (MG)
    d. prostaglandin analogue

44. Corneal limbal stem cells reside
    a. within the superficial epithelial layer of the corneal limbus
    b. over the entire surface of the bulbar conjunctiva
    c. in the central and paracentral cornea
    d. within the basal epithelial layer of the corneal limbus

45. Which of the following conditions may be associated with epiphora?
    a. megalocornea
    b. sclerocornea
    c. conjunctivochalasis
    d. pingueculum

46. A major risk factor for the development of bacterial keratitis is
    a. age
    b. contact lens wear
    c. frequent use of nonpreserved tears
    d. systemic bacterial infection

47. Parinaud oculoglandular syndrome is most commonly caused by which of the following organisms:
    a. *Rhinosporidium seeberi*
    b. *Treponema pallidum*
    c. *Bartonella henselae*
    d. *Mycobacteria* spp

48. Corneal signs typically associated with acanthamoeba keratitis include
    a. subepithelial infiltrates
    b. ring infiltrate
    c. corneal neovascularization
    d. crystalline midstromal infiltrate

49. Which of the following is a type of intraepithelial neoplasia of the conjunctiva?

    a. vascular

    b. actiniform

    c. ulcerative

    d. leukoplakic

50. An elevated, vascular, darkly pigmented lesion at the interpalpebral limbus may represent which entity?

    a. malignant melanoma

    b. conjunctival intraepithelial neoplasia

    c. conjunctival papilloma

    d. limbal dermoid

Answers

1. **d.** Phlyctenular keratoconjunctivitis is a type IV delayed hypersensitivity response. Type IV delayed hypersensitivity reactions are mediated by T cells (CD4+ Th1 lymphocytes) that release lymphokines in order to attract macrophages.

2. **c.** The cornea's relative immune privilege is due to many factors, including expression of Fas ligand (CD95 ligand) by corneal cells, which is thought to play a critical role in inducing apoptosis (programmed cell death) of activated lymphocytes.

3. **b.** VEGF may be found in the tear film of inflamed eyes. It acts by promoting the growth of new blood vessels and by increasing vascular permeability.

4. **a.** Plasma cells are the only cells present in normal conjunctiva. The other cells may be present in diseased conjunctiva.

5. **a.** IgE is the immunoglobulin that mediates allergic reactions, including allergic conjunctivitis and atopic keratoconjunctivitis.

6. **c.** Ligneous conjunctivitis is thought to result from a deficiency of type I plasminogen. Topical application of plasminogen may be an effective therapy.

7. **b.** Conjunctival biopsies from patients with PUK have shown vaso-occlusive disease, which supports this process as the etiology for peripheral corneal ulceration. Type IV hypersensitivity reactions are associated with phlyctenular disease. Staphylococcal marginal infiltrates are not associated with systemic vasculitic disease.

8. **b.** Mooren ulcer is an example of immune-mediated corneal inflammation, in which corneal autoantigens may be generated as a response to injury or infection. An autoantibody response may then be generated, presumably by plasma cells.

9. **a.** Goblet cells, which account for up to 10% of the basal cells of the conjunctival epithelium, produce mucin. Corneal epithelial cells also produce some mucin.

10. **c.** Descemet's membrane is the basement membrane of the corneal endothelium (which comes from neural crest cells). It increases in thickness from 3 μm at birth to 10–12 μm in adults.

11. **a.** The curvature of the central cornea contributes about 74% or 43.25 diopters of the total 58.6 dioptric power of a normal human eye.

12. **d.** Most of the metabolic disorders that affect the cornea are autosomal recessive. Two exceptions are Hunter syndrome and Fabry disease, which are both X-linked recessive.

13. **b.** Amiodarone, an antiarrhythmic agent, produces lysosomal deposits in the basal corneal epithelial layer, creating a whorl-like pattern. This pattern may also be seen in Fabry disease and has been associated with long-term treatment with chloroquine, chlorpromazine, and indomethacin.

14. **a.** MEN type 2B has been associated with prominent corneal nerves. It is an autosomal dominant disease characterized by medullary carcinoma of the thyroid, pheochromocytoma, and mucosal neuromas. (Some patients with MEN type 2A also have enlarged corneal nerves.)

15. **d.** Pellucid marginal degeneration is characterized by a band of inferior thinning and protrusion of the cornea above it. Keratoconus shows protrusion at the point of maximal

thinning. Polymorphic amyloid degeneration is characterized by stromal amyloid deposits. Keratoglobus is characterized by a globular deformation of the entire cornea.

16. **c.** Lattice is often accompanied by recurrent erosions. Erosions are less common in macular dystrophy and not characteristic of either pellucid marginal degeneration or keratoglobus.

17. **c.** Maps, dots, and fingerprints are typical for corneal epithelial basement membrane dystrophy (EBMD). Approximately 10% of patients with EBMD have recurrent erosions, and 50% of patients with recurrent erosions have evidence of this dystrophy.

18. **a.** Epithelial infections with HSV are associated with follicular reactions of the conjunctiva. They do not result in a papillary reaction, membrane or pseudomembrane formation, or a pyogenic granuloma.

19. **b.** Atopic keratoconjunctivitis results in a typical papillary reaction of the tarsal conjunctiva. HSV, adult inclusion conjunctivitis, and molluscum all cause a follicular conjunctivitis.

20. **c.** In 1880, Antonio Placido developed a disk composed of a series of concentric circles that, when held in front of the cornea, are reflected off the tear film. The corneal surface affects the shape of the circles. Analysis of the corneal shape using this type of device is known as *keratoscopy*.

21. **d.** The appropriate answer is Peters anomaly. Peters plus refers to the same finding associated with limb dwarfism. CHED does not have elevated IOP. Corneal opacity and iridocorneal adhesions are not consistent with congenital glaucoma alone.

22. **a.** Progressive corneal edema developing during the first few postnatal days, accompanied by vertical or oblique posterior striae, may be caused by birth trauma. Ruptures occur in Descemet's membrane. Healing usually takes place, often leaving a hypertrophic ridge(s) of Descemet's membrane.

23. **b.** Haab striae is correct. Vogt striae occur in keratoconus. A large corneal diameter would be expected, but guttae are not typically present.

24. **d.** Only a cell count of less than 2000 would disqualify this donor. Negative serology for hepatitis B is a requirement. Serology that is positive for CMV will not disqualify the donor. Previous LASIK surgery will disqualify the donor for full penetrating keratoplasty, as curvature of the cornea and bonding of the 2 layers cannot be ensured.

25. **a.** The cornea has a way of causing tolerance in the body that can be called "immune privilege."

26. **a.** A corneal biopsy would not be done in a posterior lesion, as this would require a full-thickness removal of tissue that would leave a perforation requiring a corneal transplant. A biopsy is a good option when a keratitis has not responded to antimicrobial therapy, is culture-negative on usual scrapings, or is following an atypical course. Fungal infections, acanthamoeba, and mycobacterial infections may elude routine scrapings.

27. **c.** In pterygium surgery, the recurrence rate with simple bare excision is quite common, often quoted at up to 75%. It is therefore not recommended and not justified unless no other means is available. The other methods of excision with covering of the bare sclera generally lead to an acceptable cosmetic and functional result with a small risk of recurrence.

28. **c.** For permanent closure of the eye fissure, suturing the eyelid margins, with removal of a small amount of the margin, will result in a permanent closure of the eyelids. The other choices are good options when a temporary closure of the eyelids is required.

29. **b.** In an eye with chronic ocular surface pain and poor visual potential, a Gunderson conjunctival flap that covers the cornea is the best option. One would never prescribe a topical anesthetic agent, as it can be toxic and lead to ulceration and perforation. Tinted glasses will not remedy the pain, and corneal tattooing is useful only in improving the cosmetic appearance of a scar and will not improve the pain associated with chronic corneal pain.

30. **d.** Small wound leaks with a deep anterior chamber can be managed conservatively with a bandage lens and topical aqueous suppressants; however, a flat anterior chamber with a large wound leak should be managed acutely. Choroidal detachments may resolve without intervention, a suture abscess can be treated with topical antibiotics, and primary graft failure can be handled electively.

31. **d.** The combination of stromal scarring and corneal edema from endothelial dysfunction requires penetrating keratoplasty in order to address the pathology in both the stroma and endothelial layers.

32. **a.** Band keratopathy is caused by the deposition of calcium hydroxyapatite in the superficial cornea. Amyloid deposition is seen with lattice dystrophy; hyaline deposition is associated with granular dystrophy; and calcium hydroxide is seen in lime, which is very harmful to the cornea.

33. **c.** The major indication for pterygium excision is induced or irregular astigmatism that reduces a patient's vision. Pterygia do not cause myopia or macular degeneration. Tear deficiency may exacerbate the symptoms of the pterygium but is not related to its pathogenesis.

34. **d.** Regular astigmatism after corneal transplantation can be treated with astigmatic keratotomy or the excimer laser. However, irregular astigmatism should be primarily managed with a rigid gas-permeable contact lens. Ultimately, the best treatment is prevention, with meticulous surgical technique and suturing.

35. **a.** Dacrocystitis is the most serious complication because it can require dacrocystorhinostomy, a major surgical procedure to remove the plug—effectively a foreign body—from the lacrimal drainage system. If severe enough, secondary infection could result in orbital cellulitis.

36. **b.** The addition of hyaluronic acid to topical tear replacement formulations has been found to be helpful in the treatment of moderate to severe aqueous deficiency states. Trifluridine is a topical antiviral agent that has secondary epithelial toxic effects that will worsen the effect of aqueous deficiency. Brimonidine and latanoprost are antiglaucoma preparations and are not indicated for the treatment of dry-eye syndrome.

37. **a.** Rapid tear-film breakup time is arguably the most sensitive test of tear-film deficiency. It is easily carried out and readily available.

38. **a.** The presence of Sjögren syndrome autoantibodies (SS-A and SS-B) has been correlated with the severity of symptoms and ocular surface disease in patients with Sjögren syndrome. An elevated ESR is a nonspecific finding in many inflammatory disorders. Elevated ANCA autoantibodies are found in both Wegener granulomatosis and polyarteritis nodosa, not Sjögren syndrome.

39. **c.** Posterior eyelid margin disease is consistent with the location of the meibomian glands and their orifices.

40. **d.** The association of rosacea with ocular surface disease is often missed, in part because of the variability of the severity of rosacea and the fact that it is not always obvious in dimly lit ophthalmologic offices. Hyperemia of the eyelid margin is a common early clinical finding. Corneal ulceration may occur as a late finding in severe ocular rosacea. Scleritis may occur in association with rosacea, but it is uncommon. Recurrent erosion of the cornea is not a common feature of rosacea.

41. **b.** Herpes zoster keratitis is perhaps the most common cause of neurotrophic keratopathy leading to corneal ulceration. Pellucid marginal degeneration and PPCD do not lead to neurotrophic keratopathy. SPK of Thygeson does not result in loss of corneal sensitivity.

42. **b.** Rosacea has a number of ophthalmic manifestations, and this association is important.

43. **a.** Although perhaps not the most common cause, a cerebral aneurysm within the cavernous sinus is potentially life-threatening and therefore important in the differential. Pituitary adenoma, MG, and systemic prostaglandin analogues do not cause selective dysfunction of the ophthalmic branch of the trigeminal ganglion.

44. **d.** Corneal stem cells reside within the basal epithelial layer of the corneoscleral limbus. They are not present in the central cornea. Conjunctival stem cells are found throughout the bulbar conjunctiva but do not transform into the cornea phenotype.

45. **c.** Conjunctivochalasis is associated with epiphora when redundant nasal bulbar conjunctiva occludes the puncta. Megalocornea and sclerocornea are not typically associated with epiphora. Uninflamed pingueculae are usually asymptomatic.

46. **b.** Contact lens wear is the most common risk factor for the development of bacterial keratitis because of presumed microtrauma to the corneal epithelium combined with bacterial adherence factors.

47. **c.** Rhinosporidiosis is a rare cause of conjunctival granuloma but has not been reported to cause Parinaud oculoglandular syndrome. *Bartonella henselae* is the most common causative agent.

48. **b.** A ring infiltrate is often associated with acanthamoeba keratitis. Radial keratoneuritis, pseudodendrite(s), and pain out of proportion with clinical findings are also typical findings. Subepithelial infiltrates, crystalline infiltrates, and corneal neovascularization are not characteristic of acanthamoebal keratitis.

49. **d.** The 3 types of conjunctival intraepithelial neoplasia are papilliform, leukoplakic, and gelatinous.

50. **a.** Malignant melanoma of the conjunctiva is usually darkly pigmented, elevated, and often vascular. Limbal dermoids are usually located inferotemporally and are not pigmented. Conjunctival papilloma and intraepithelial neoplasia are not pigmented.

Index

(*f* = figure; *t* = table)